2014 EDITION

PROVIDER'S GUIDE

Value-Based Medicare Reimbursement

FOR HOSPITALS & PHYSICIANS

Ray Tew 6/6/14

[signature]

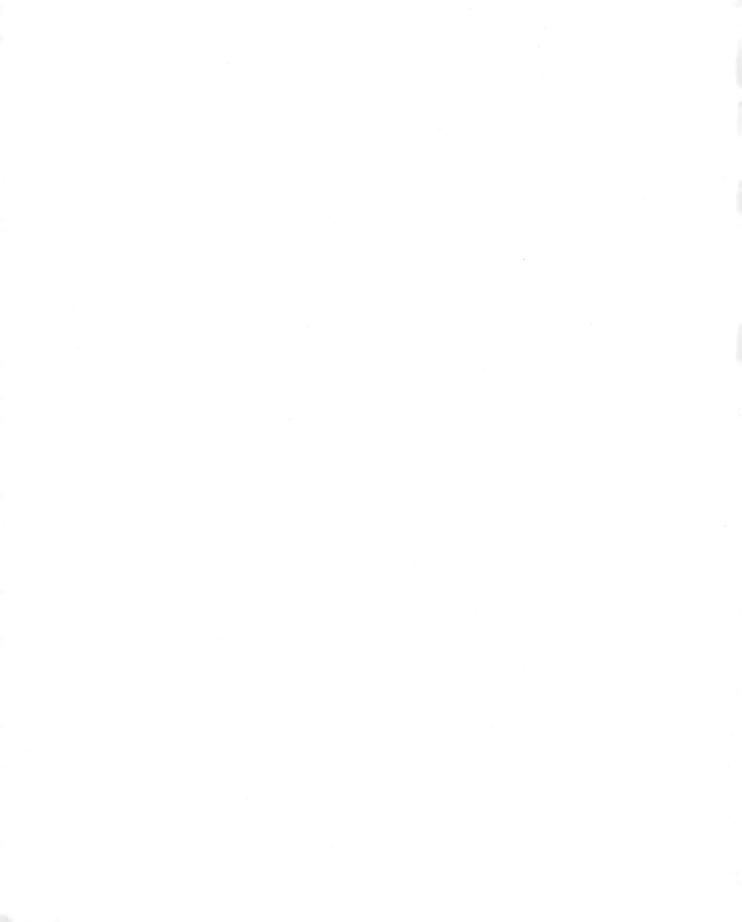

2014 EDITION
PROVIDER'S GUIDE

Value-Based Medicare Reimbursement

FOR HOSPITALS & PHYSICIANS

By J. Duncan Moore Jr., Raymond Paul Tew & Steven L. Owen

Editor: Alison Szot | Designer: Nicole Lombardo Ganz

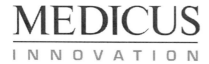

Content Outline

Preface

Our interest in Medicare's value-based reimbursement programs began with a client engagement in the summer of 2012. We were tasked by this progressive organization to assist them in understanding the emerging transformation of Medicare from its traditional role as a "passive payer of services" to that of an "active purchaser of quality." Further, we were asked to help them assess the potential impact on customers, patients, and their organization to determine how best to align strategic objectives and internal resources to most effectively meet customer challenges presented by a rapidly changing health care environment.

As a starting point, we reached out to physicians and hospital executives for perspective. What we discovered was that while many of these key members of the health care team had a general awareness about Medicare's value-based reimbursement programs and initiatives, very few had the effective working knowledge needed to act proactively. We found that the most significant barrier to provider engagement wasn't a lack of interest, but was the result of a complex mix of changing program regulations, time constraints, and an internal focus on the professional silo. Health care professionals have not been able to understand program design well enough to take proactive steps to maximize incentive payments, minimize potential penalties, or develop effective marketing strategies. We identified four key groups that struggle to adapt to this new reimbursement paradigm, due primarily to a lack of actionable information.

Physicians:

One of your largest payers informs you that 6 percent of your reimbursement would potentially be cut, based on quality and cost of care benchmarks, over the next twenty-four months and the amount at risk could increase to 9.0 percent in the years ahead. However, there is also a chance to avoid payment cuts and actually increase your reimbursements based on these same benchmarks. Should you invest the time to learn the details of the programs?

Hospital Management:

Your largest payer is placing 5.75 percent of your inpatient reimbursement at risk by holding you responsible for meeting quality and cost benchmarks on the inpatient care you provide. There is also a chance to increase your reimbursements based on these same benchmarks. How important is it for the physicians who are providing inpatient care in your hospital to understand the quality and cost benchmarks that determine how much you are reimbursed?

Health Care Lawyers and Consultants:

Your clients are in the midst of a transformational change regarding how they are compensated for their services. These payment reforms involve quality and cost benchmarks against which your customers will be measured and determine how much they are paid for their services. Can you continue to be a trusted advisor if you don't know the details about these programs and provide clients with current updates as they occur? Equally important, is spending weeks and months of your professional time finding and digesting literally thousands of pages of regulations the highest and best use of your time?

Health Care Industry Professionals:

If your company sells products or services to the health care industry, is it critical that you understand the underlying challenges that these new clinical quality, safety, and cost benchmarks create for your customers? Can you understand your customers and develop effective market strategies if those in your organization don't know these new quality and cost measures and benchmarks?

Clearly, the answers to these questions have significant implications for all health care providers and professionals.

For each of these groups, an overall lack of understanding about value-based reimbursement can be attributed to a variety of factors. The most significant factor is the absence of an easy-to-use, sole source reference guide that explains these Medicare reimbursement programs and provides companion narrative from key opinion leaders covering the rationale and current impact of these regulations on the health care environment.

To solve this challenge, our Medicus Innovation team undertook an eighteen-month journey, meticulously navigating through thousands of pages of regulations and conducting numerous interviews with health care key opinion leaders. The result is the first-of-its-kind resource: the *Provider's Guide to Value-Based Medicare Reimbursement for Hospitals and Physicians*.

Seen through another lens, health care providers are in the midst of the largest change management initiative in the history of the United States. If a similarly large US corporation undertook such a massive structural realignment, change management strategies would have been launched prior to the implementation of changes taking effect in order to support colleague education and gain buy-in concerning these complex changes that affect Medicare reimbursement.

The time has come for health care providers and industry professionals to develop an effective working knowledge about these new Medicare value-based reimbursement programs. Your leadership and collaboration across silos will be necessary, but not sufficient for success. Utilizing a common "sourcebook" as these discussions occur across health care silos will be critical. Our role is to support this process by providing you with an important resource to begin that dialogue. It is our hope that the *Provider's Guide to Value-Based Medicare Reimbursement* becomes only one of many tools that will be available to support this national dialogue in the years ahead. Good luck, and we look forward to hearing from you.

How to Use
the *Provider's Guide*

During our research we received a wealth of feedback about how to create the *Provider's Guide*. Through that process three primary hurdles were identified: a) how to present these topics in an interesting and engaging manner, b) how to keep the data updated, and c) how to format it to satisfy the needs of an intensely time-constrained audience while making it easy to navigate large volumes of information.

To address these challenges the book is organized and updated in the following way:

Chapter Organization:

Each chapter is organized into three distinct sections. Each chapter section essentially approaches the same topic from a different perspective.

- **Section 1: The Flash Read – Read Time: 5 minutes**

  - The Flash Read provides a concise overview, presented in two to three page bulleted summaries, to include program description and design, potential fiscal impact, and information critical to effective implementation. The Flash Read contains the "must know" information for readers who "only have five minutes" and need to know the basics.

- **Section 2: Provider Perspectives – Read Time: 15 minutes**

  - Through interviews with nationally recognized key opinion leaders, the Provider Perspectives provide a window into why the programs were developed and how specific value-based programs and initiatives are impacting the medical community. Examples of effective program implementation are presented along with challenges to provide a balanced real-world view.

- **Section 3: Technical Appendix – Comprehensive Content**

  Read Time: As needed

  - This section provides the information necessary for effective implementation and execution of a specific value-based Medicare reimbursement program or initiative.

  - Information is presented in a straightforward, bullet-pointed, easily understood manner. It is not a recitation of all of the Federal Regulations; however, the information is highly referenced and hyperlinked to source documents for accuracy confirmation.

  - Complete coverage of the value-based program or initiative is provided to include the legislative and regulatory history; current program design, metrics, process, incentives, and penalties; links to related information, reports, and quality measures.

  - Graphs, tables, and additional topics are included as appropriate to support easy understanding of the program details.

  - Each Appendix contains an Acronym Guide for the related chapter.

  - Where available, the Appendix will contain the most current program requirements for future program years.

Ease of Use:

The *Provider's Guide* is available as both a soft-cover book and in a digital format. Each contains an extensive table of contents to allow for quick and efficient location of needed information.

The digital version is organized in a "click and go" format to make it easy to navigate through the book and meet the informational needs of a diverse cross section of health care providers and professionals.

- Readers simply click on a topic in the table of contents and are taken directly to that specific section of the book.

- A "key word" search function also enables readers to go directly to specific topics of interest quickly, without having to search piecemeal via the Internet or through multiple files of data.

- As an electronically delivered digital resource, the *Provider's Guide* contains links throughout to assist with topic selection and to access additional reference sources.

- The table of contents is accessible from each page of the *Provider's Guide* and is fully linked to key topic headings to facilitate seamless transitions.

- Reference sources are footnoted at the bottom of the respective page and, where possible, are active links to source documents.

Updates:

- To preserve the integrity of the *Provider's Guide* as a trusted source of information, customers will receive timely and accurate updated information as it becomes available. With the purchase of the *Provider's Guide*, you will be able to sign up for a twelve-month update service at no additional cost. You will receive message alerts with links to download the latest information relating to Medicare value-based reimbursement regulations.

Table of Contents

Introduction

In 2010, the US Congress passed the Patient Protection and Affordable Care Act (ACA). This law represents one of the biggest transformations to the US health care system since the rapid expansion of employer-based health care in the 1950s and the launch of Medicare in 1965. The ACA was drafted and passed by the Democratic majority in Congress with the support of President Barack Obama and has survived numerous attempts to invalidate it, including constitutional challenges that the Supreme Court heard in 2012.

It may be helpful to conceive of the health reform law as an attempt to accomplish two separate yet interdependent goals:

1. Extend insurance coverage to a large swath of the population, both through an expansion of public programs such as Medicaid as well as numerous restrictions on insurance companies that guarantee access for segments of the population previously shut out of private policies. Despite these protections, the law was designed to preserve a competitive, private sector, market-based insurance industry (much to the dismay of advocates for a single-payer, or Medicare-for-all, system).

2. Reform the delivery and reimbursement system to enhance value by improving quality while simultaneously reducing costs, again using primarily free-market levers. Instead of instituting price controls or utilization clampdowns, the ACA focuses providers' attention on those aspects of the system that have underserved the true needs of patients and payers, including: too many unwarranted procedures and tests; insufficient attention to the cumulative costs of care; lack of follow-up after care transitions; and an underfunded primary care infrastructure.

Most interest and media attention has been devoted to the first goal. In fact, the preponderance of the ACA media stories and controversy in the years since its passage—opposition to the individual mandate to buy coverage, the Supreme Court case, the states' various responses to Medicaid expansion, the troubled rollout of the online exchanges—concern reforms to the insurance industry. At first glance, these reforms affect consumers most directly, both in their pocketbooks and in their access to the providers they choose. They are, in effect, the front yard of health reform—the items that everybody sees immediately from the street.

The *Provider's Guide to Value-Based Medicare Reimbursement* is about the backyard of the ACA: all the activities that happen out of sight of most of the public in the health care system. While the insurance reforms are updating how health care is paid for in America, the value-based reimbursement policies and programs hold the potential to forever alter the fundamental structure of how hospitals and physicians are reimbursed for patient care.

The law assigned to Medicare the role of change agent, and charged it with leading the way for transformational changes that lawmakers intended to ripple through to the entire system. The ACA gave the Centers for Medicare & Medicaid Services (CMS) new tools with which to experiment, and even created a new organization to oversee these transformative efforts: the Center for Medicare & Medicaid Innovation (CMMI). The CMMI has a portfolio of experiments that tests various payment and delivery models intended to improve care for patients and the health of communities, as well as save the government money along the way.

"Medicare administrators have largely forborne from using coverage policy or financial incentives to discourage ineffective or needlessly costly methods of care," Brookings Institution Analyst Henry J. Aaron noted. Members of Congress have not been so restrained, he added. "They have pressured those same administrators on coverage policies and passed laws to impose them."[1] The case could be made that Medicare's vast expenditures—combined with its reluctance to take an activist stance on payment reform, quality improvement, or value enhancement—have been the major enablers of excessive cost growth throughout the medical industrial complex.

Therefore, the changes in the ACA cast the giant agency in an unfamiliar role: that of innovator and disciplinarian. Now, the federal government intends to use its extraordinary purchasing power to influence the shape of the health care industry, in the same way that the Pentagon reconfigured the defense contracting industry a decade ago. Small, independent physicians' practices are being rolled up into larger units that can afford the investments in

---

[1] *Henry J. Aaron, "The Independent Payment Advisory Board—Congress's 'Good Deed'", New England Journal of Medicine, 364:25. June 23, 2011.*

information technology and coordinated care that the standard of medical care now demands. Standalone hospitals are finding merger partners to help them cover the capital requirements and skill development needed to compete in a coming era of scarcity.

Rewarding Quality, Not Quantity

The reforms move US health care away from the classic fee-for-service model—which has notoriously given providers a financial incentive to focus on quantity—to one that holds providers accountable for rigorous quality and cost targets set by the CMS. The shift creates extraordinary challenges for health care providers, as hospitals and physicians scramble to identify and implement strategies they hope will improve quality, lower costs, and maximize their reimbursements. These CMS-ordained changes are also designed to alter the relationships among health care providers, taking them out of their silos and compelling them to work together to reduce waste and improve collaboration, and thereby, outcomes.

These value-based reimbursement reforms are poised to have an even more profound effect on the evolution of US health care in the long run than the ACA's insurance reforms and coverage expansions. Certainly, these value-based reimbursement reforms are harder to understand and don't produce the same shocks and thrills in the public media. Yet, critically, they hold the prospect of changing the value equation for the better.

The most immediate challenge is for health care providers to understand these new regulations. The patient care strategies necessary to effectively and successfully meet the new requirements can only be created by those who are affected the most: hospital managers and physicians. That can only happen if providers have a clear understanding of the new regulations: It's hard to meet a reimbursement quality or cost "benchmark" if you don't know what it is.

Michael E. Porter of the Harvard Business School stated in economic terms the basic problem that the ACA is trying to address: The current delivery system is not organized around value for patients. "Our system rewards those who shift costs, bargain away, or capture someone else's revenues, and bill for more services, not those who deliver the most value. The focus is on minimizing the cost of each intervention and limiting services rather than on maximizing value over the entire care cycle."[2] Incremental reforms have not lived up to expectations. A more comprehensive approach is needed.

Perhaps because the proponents of reform needed to gather such a head of steam to move it to actuality, the law as it was drafted included virtually every innovation, pet health care project, and "innovative" concept that had been conceived of during the previous twenty years. Some were free-market approaches, and some were informed by concepts of social equity favored by Democrats and progressives.

Thus, the bill that resulted was loaded with many complicated and heterogeneous provisions, especially the regulations on the thousands of changes relating to value-based provider reimbursement. Indeed, the complexity of the law is a major contributing factor to its continued political fragility, even four years after it was passed. It's so hard to explain that the ACA's sponsors have been unable to build the basis of comprehension and support that they undoubtedly counted on to ease its way through implementation and toward success, with concomitant political rewards for themselves.[3]

As of this writing, any rewards have proved highly theoretical, while the ACA's downsides and risks are tangible, and probably growing. Certainly the law's massive size and miscellanea have made the ACA an easy target for its opponents, both from the right and the left. The intricacy resembles a game of three-dimensional chess—each move affects every other chess piece on the board, often in unexpected and contradictory ways. For instance, it's not possible to loosen the requirement on individuals to buy insurance without turning upside down the actuarial assumptions behind the enlarged risk pool. It's also hard to mandate that citizens buy something they might not want or be able to afford unless provisions are included to rein in cost inflation in the underlying services.

The need for higher value in health care is urgent, virtually all observers agree. "The goal of high-value health care is to produce the best health outcomes at the lowest cost," wrote Gregory D. Curfman, MD, Stephen Morrissey, and Jeffrey M. Drazen, MD "Health care professionals are increasingly given incentives to deliver high-value care by virtue of such payment-reform measures as pay-for-

---

[2] *Michael E. Porter, "A Strategy for Health Care Reform—Toward a Value-Based System," New England Journal of Medicine, 361:2. July 9, 2009.*

[3] *Paul Starr, Remedy and Reaction: The Peculiar American Struggle over Health Care Reform, Yale, 2011.*

performance policies, bundled-payment strategies, global budgets, and financial risk sharing within accountable care organizations."[4]

These incentives are being invented across the spectrum of payers, and private payers have been using many of these methods for decades, but our focus in this book will be on Medicare reimbursement and the core value-oriented programs and policies included in Section 3000 of the ACA, plus related legislation enacted in the several years before and since. For hospitals, our focus in the first edition of the *Provider's Guide* is the Inpatient Quality Reporting System (IQR), the Hospital Value-Based Purchasing Program (HVBP), the Hospital Readmission Reduction Program (HRRP), and the Hospital Acquired Condition Reduction Program (HAC). For physicians, we focus on the Physician Quality Reporting System (PQRS), the Electronic Health Records (EHR) Incentive Program, the Value-Based Payment Modifier (VBM) Program, and two care models endorsed in the ACA: Accountable Care Organizations and the Patient Centered Medical Home. These models seek to link improved quality and lower cost of services to increased provider reimbursement for services.

The CMS has traditionally been the most conservative of agencies, resistant to change, subject to political agendas, and beholden to interest groups in the health care industry. The federal program has been lacking in utilization controls, notoriously accommodating of bad actors and fraudsters on the provider/supplier side, and generous to beneficiaries, on whom it has placed few restrictions. In fact, many providers lament the fact that there is insufficient patient "skin in the game" for some of the new value-based reimbursement measures to be truly effective. Medicare, the country's largest single buyer of health care, has employed largely blunt methods as a payer, using its leverage mostly to effect price changes but not often using it to effect reforms or steer spending toward higher-value services.

Slowing Health Care Costs

Arguments exist on both sides of the debate about whether the recent reforms may already be having an effect on cost inflation. For forty years, from 1970 to 2010, health care costs grew faster than the economy as a whole, outstripping economic growth by about 2.4 percent on average per year, the Kaiser Family

---

[4] *Gregory D. Curfman, MD, Stephen Morrissey, and Jeffrey M. Drazen, MD, "High-Value Health Care—A Sustainable Proposition," New England Journal of Medicine, 2013; 369:1163–64, September 19, 2013.*

Foundation reported.[5] Yet recently, health care cost growth has slowed, finally moving along more in sync with the rest of the US economy.

The Office of the Actuary at CMS is projecting that overall health spending in the United States will grow at an average annual rate of 5.8 percent from 2012 to 2022, or 1.0 percent faster than the average annual economic growth predicted for that period. By contrast, from 1990 to 2006, health spending grew at 7.4 percent per year. Medicare spending growth in 2012 was 4.6 percent, down from 6.2 percent in 2011, the actuaries estimated.[6]

A number of factors may have contributed to the cost-growth slowdown, including general weakness in the economy, higher cost-sharing for patients, cutbacks in Medicaid spending, and tighter Medicare payment policies. Some economists and actuaries believe cost growth may resume once the economy picks up again and after the newly insured come on board via the ACA. In addition, the health care industry has historically responded to the threat (now the reality) of health reform by restraining its cost growth, as happened during the Clinton reform era.

Still, some have argued that the law has accelerated changes already taking place in the health care marketplace. "Most providers anticipate that, in the future, they will be paid based less on how much they do than on how well they do it. And that anticipation is leading to significant change today," said Peter Orszag, President Obama's former director of the Office of Management and Budget. "The biggest government expense of all may be improving faster than policy makers yet appreciate."[7]

Nevertheless, a chorus of contrarians has risen up to knock down the notion that the law could have had so much impact so fast. "These assertions border on nonsense," wrote Thomas Miller and Abby McCloskey, of the American Enterprise Institute, a free-market think tank, in *The Wall Street Journal*. Annual health spending growth rates started declining after 2002, they pointed out. That year, health spending growth hit almost 10 percent, and it had calmed down to 3.9 percent by 2009, a year before the health reform law was enacted.

---

[5] *Health Care Costs: A Primer. Key Information on Health Care Costs and Their Impact. Henry J. Kaiser Family Foundation, May 2012.*

[6] *Gigi A. Cuckler, et al., "National Health Expenditure Projections, 2012–22: Slow Growth Until Coverage Expands And Economy Improves," Health Affairs, October 2013.*

[7] *Peter Orszag, "Are Hospitals Already Saving Money for Medicare?" Bloomberg, August 26, 2013.*

Changes in health-spending growth rates normally lag two years behind overall economic growth rates anyway. "The persistently weak economic recovery" is the main explanation for the slowdown in health spending, they argued.[8]

Robert Laszewski, an influential blogger, wrote that claiming the ACA is "even partly responsible" for the slowdown is "silly." The law does have some limited cost-containment features, "but these are either pilot projects or are years from being fully implemented," he said.[9]

The Need to Adapt

In conclusion, this *Provider's Guide* represents the first sole-source, easy-to-use guide to value-based reimbursement regulations that affect the revenue for physicians and hospitals. We want to emphasize that we won't be rehashing political points of view on the insurance reforms in the ACA. Our intention is to write a guidebook for providers that avoids the ideological litmus tests, skirmishes, and turf wars that have accompanied the law's passage and implementation. We suspect that physicians who participate in organized medicine and hospital executives who have to lead their complicated organizations into uncharted territory have had quite enough of those conversations.

Instead, we simply accept the reform law as a given, and help health care providers understand and navigate through these technical requirements. Information on this topic has been neither quick to access nor easy to understand. The experimentation process to improve quality and reduce costs is taking root throughout the health-delivery system, both in the private and public sectors. But while hundreds of transitional programs are being created to address the challenges inherent in value-based reimbursement regulations, the definitive solutions have yet to be created. Only when our country's best and brightest—our health care professionals—fully understand the details of these regulations will we be able to harness their intellect and creativity to design solutions to the challenges these new policies and programs present.

---

[8] Thomas Miller and Abby McCloskey, "The Next Obamacare Mirage," *The Wall Street Journal*, November 25, 2013.

[9] Robert Laszewski, "Is Obamacare Responsible For the Recent Slowdown in Health Care Costs?" *Health Care Policy and Marketplace Review* blog, December 5, 2013.

Charles Darwin is often misquoted as saying "only the strongest survive." What he actually said was, "It's NOT the strongest of the species who survive, nor even the most intelligent, but the ones most responsive to change." This quote is especially relevant to health care providers during these times of transformational change. Health care providers who commit the time and energy to learn and adapt will thrive in a value-based reimbursement environment. This guide is but one of many new tools that will be needed as we navigate through the new reimbursement landscape. As a health care provider, you are among the most important and trusted members of our society. Your success is everyone's success. Everyone will have to work closely to adapt to these changes and ensure success for all of us today and for generations to come. Good luck.

PART 1

Value-Based Medicare
Reimbursement Programs
Affecting Hospitals

PART 1

Value-Based Medicare
Reimbursement Programs
Affecting Hospitals

CHAPTER 1

Inpatient Quality Reporting (IQR)

Section 1.1: Flash Read!

The hospital IQR program was developed to encourage hospitals and clinicians to improve the quality of inpatient care they provide as well as to provide consumers with the information they need to make more informed health care decisions. The hospital IQR program requires most hospitals to submit data for specific quality measures for their Medicare patients, and imposes financial penalties on those that don't. Quality information gathered through IQR is available to consumers on the Hospital Compare website. The hospital IQR program is the foundation for the Affordable Care Act's (ACA) Hospital Value-Based Purchasing Program (HVBP), the Hospital Readmissions Reduction Program (HRRP), and the Hospital-Acquired Conditions (HAC) Program.

- The hospital IQR program uses a combination of hospital-reported chart-abstracted measures and CMS claims-extracted data for a given program year to determine annual payment adjustments for hospitals' Medicare reimbursement.

- Data collected through the hospital IQR program are also used to calculate the performance metrics of all CMS hospital value-based reimbursement programs.

- IQR data collection occurs during a specific calendar year and IQR penalties are imposed for a specific fiscal year:

- o Data collection for the hospital IQR program occurs during the calendar year preceding the beginning of the fiscal program year. For example, data collected from January 1, 2013–December 31, 2013, will be used to determine IQR penalties for FY2015 (October 1, 2014–September 30, 2015).

- Hospitals that did not successfully participate in CY2013 reporting will receive a -2.0 percent adjustment to their FY2015 Annual Payment Update (APU).

- Hospitals that do not successfully participate in CY2014 IQR reporting will receive a negative adjustment in FY2016 equal to 25 percent of their total APU.

- Of 3,296 IQR-applicable hospitals for the FY2014 program:
  - o 40 hospitals received a -2.0 percent adjustment to their APU for unsuccessful IQR participation
  - o 36 hospitals elected nonparticipation and received a -2.0 percent adjustment

- For CY2014, the hospital IQR program contains 63 individual measures, including:
  - o 40 chart-abstracted measures requiring hospital reporting
  - o 6 measures reportable by hospitals via a web-based tool
  - o 17 measures that are CMS-extracted from claims and do not require hospital reporting

- For CY2014 reporting, 16 clinical measures are available for reporting through an electronic health record (EHR). Measure sets include: stroke (STK), venous thromboembolism (VTE), emergency department (ED), and perinatal care (PC). CMS estimates that using the EHR option will save an individual hospital some $47,000 in labor-related costs for CY2014 IQR reporting.

- CY2014 EHR reporting incentives include:

  - reduction in labor hours, estimated at 800 hours per individual hospital

  - the requirement to report only one-quarter (instead of four-quarters) of measures

  - non-inclusion of EHR-reported measures in the Hospital Compare website

- To achieve successful participation and avoid negative payment adjustments, data must be submitted no later than 11:59 p.m. PT on submission deadlines with the exception of validation medical records, which must be received by the Clinical Data Abstraction Center (CDAC) no later than 4:30 p.m. ET.

- Newly added CMS claims-extracted measures reportable for the FY2016 program year include:

MEASURES:	EXTRACTED FROM CLAIMS:
30-day Mortality for STK and Chronic Obstructive Pulmonary Disease (COPD)	July 1, 2012–June 30, 2015
30-day Readmissions for STK and COPD	July 1, 2012–June 30, 2015
AMI Payment Per Episode of Care	July 1, 2012–June 30, 2015

Section 1.2:
Provider Perspectives

Medicare's Inpatient Quality Reporting (IQR) program was one of the first quality-related innovations contained in legislation and one of the most straightforward. In essence, the IQR program asks hospitals to submit quality data at regular intervals to the Centers for Medicare & Medicaid Services (CMS). That by itself was a major step forward in the early years of the quality improvement effort. The vast majority of hospitals have successfully complied with the rule and are avoiding the penalties that Medicare imposes for nonparticipation.

1.2.1 Rationale

The hospital IQR program proceeds from the belief that more transparency and accountability will enhance awareness of quality metrics among both hospitals and their patients and drive quality improvement. The program was initiated after the Institute of Medicine's (IOM) 1999 report, "To Err is Human," sent a shock wave through the US health care system. That report made clear that hospital safety and quality had never been at the level assumed. Many concerned stakeholders came to believe that the medical establishment would not take the steps necessary to alter this situation by itself—change would have to be imposed from the outside.

Congress took up the challenge in 2003 when it passed the Medicare Prescription Drug, Improvement, and Modernization Act of 2003 (MMA). This is the law that created the pharmaceutical benefit for Medicare beneficiaries, and naturally, that development received most of the attention. Yet, the law also set in motion the concept that hospitals would not be entitled to receive their full annual payment update (APU) unless they submitted quality-of-care data to CMS—a radical notion at the time.

The hospital IQR program "was the first step that CMS put in place to get everybody on board with what it meant to report quality measures," said Eric Fontana, practice manager of the data and analytics group at The Advisory

Board Company in Washington, DC. As a prerequisite to developing a more rigorous quality agenda, first "you have to get organizations to standardize the way they report and their various options for reporting."[10]

In the early years of the program, hospitals that didn't comply with the quality requirement saw their annual Medicare market basket update reduced by 0.4 percent. By FY2007, that penalty was increased to 2.0 percent for the market basket portion of their annual payment update, where it stands today. The vast majority of hospitals are in good standing with IQR. However, the penalty increases dramatically in CY2014. Hospitals that remain non-reporters will forfeit 25 percent of their total Medicare annual payment update in FY2016—a severe penalty that is almost sure to boost compliance close to the 100 percent mark.

1.2.2 Summary

The hospital IQR program serves as a foundation for most of CMS's inpatient quality improvement efforts. Data collected through IQR are used to power the Hospital Compare website, where patients and consumers may view quality ratings of hospitals in their region. The data also form the base of the HVBP (see Chapter 2), which rewards or penalizes hospitals in their Medicare reimbursements for the level of quality they demonstrate. The platform further provides the basic reporting infrastructure for the HRRP (see Chapter 3) and the HAC reduction programs (see Chapter 4).

The program started modestly, with just ten measures in 2005. At that time, when electronic health records (EHRs) were less prevalent than they are today, there were no requirements to use them; hospitals could send in their results on a paper form.

Since then, the number of measures has gradually gone up. In CY2014, CMS has asked hospitals to choose from among sixty-three different process, outcome, and survey measures. Some of those may be reported through an EHR; others require extraction from medical charts. CMS can pull an additional seventeen measures from claims.

---

[10] *Eric Fontana, telephone interview, November 27, 2013.*

Hospitals collect and submit data to CMS as much as eighteen months before the results of those data affect their Medicare payments. Thus, data reporting for the 2014 program year (and payment year) ended on May 15, 2013. The reporting period for the 2015 payment year will end on May 15, 2014.

1.2.3 Current State

The consistent effort to build out the quality reporting system during the past ten years has positioned hospitals well ahead of physicians' practices in their level of participation and sophistication. Almost all hospitals have engaged with this program and attained full compliance. Engagement with quality reporting by physicians has fallen considerably short of this level, and there are almost 150 times as many doctors who send claims to Medicare as there are hospitals.[11]

According to CMS, 3,296 hospitals successfully submitted quality data and will receive the full payment update for the 2014 program year. Only forty hospitals didn't qualify, many of which are rural hospitals, specialty facilities, or hospitals in the Indian Health Service. Of those forty, thirteen are in Texas. Another thirty-six hospitals declined to participate and will have 2.0 percent deducted from their APU.

"Frankly, the number is tiny, a fraction of a percent of organizations that don't meet the quality reporting standard," Fontana said. "I don't know why or what the barriers are to doing it. It's pretty much a given that any organization is going to meet this."

Although they're on the hook for the results, hospitals by themselves can't deliver the results that CMS is looking for; they need the cooperation of doctors.

"As hospital care has become more complex and sophisticated, both outcomes and efficiency are increasingly linked to the quality of teamwork, not only between various types of physicians but between physicians and the other professionals they depend on, including nurses, pharmacists, and technicians," wrote Robert Wachter, MD, renowned patient safety expert and associate chair of the Department of Medicine at the University of California, San Francisco, in a 2004

---

[11] *Alyna T. Chien, MD, and Meredith B. Rosenthal, "Medicare's Physician Value-Based Payment Modifier—Will the Tectonic Shift Create Waves?" New England Journal of Medicine 369:22. November 28, 2013.*

report on high-value hospitals.[12] "The successful medical center of the future will be marked by high levels of collaboration, a sense of shared mission, and recognition by both parties that one cannot possibly succeed without the other."

Bernd Wollschlaeger, MD, a family practice physician in Miami Beach, said, "This is a topic that is being drilled into physicians' minds at medical staff meetings. Administrators do care about it a lot. Margins at hospitals are not 10 percent or 5 percent; they're smaller—2 percent or 1.5 percent. When you talk about a 25 percent potential cut (in their annual Medicare update), that scares the bejesus out of the administrators. These statistics are being shown to physicians at staff meetings. How much this affects their behavior, we don't know." [13]

Wachter wrote that hospitals with physicians who are engaged as collaborators generally have leaders who manage to create a sense of shared mission. Other key ingredients, Wachter wrote, to achieving physician collaboration are site-based physicians—those physicians whose practice takes place mainly within the walls of the hospital. Hospitalists, he suggested, can play a key role in helping achieve high-quality care because, unlike other physicians who practice mostly in office-based settings, they are present and immersed in the hospital practice environment. In addition, unlike office-based physicians, hospitalists are often aligned with their hospital's financial incentives: In many cases, the physicians are employed by the hospital itself, but even when they are not, they often receive financial support from their institutions.

The need for greater hospital-physician collaboration hasn't escaped CMS, which in 2012 began a three-year demonstration project testing whether quality and cost improvements can be achieved by providing a single lump-sum payment for an episode of care rather than the separate fee-for-service (FFS) payments. The four models being examined in the Bundled Payments for Care Improvement Initiative will test whether bundled payments will encourage hospitals and physicians to work together to coordinate care and improve care transitions, to reduce rehospitalizations, and to ensure delivery of appropriate care following discharge.

---

[12] *http://www.commonwealthfund.org/usr_doc/Meyer_hopital_quality_commentary_wachter.pdf*

[13] *Bernd Wollschlaeger, MD, telephone interview, January 21, 2014.*

1.2.4 The Road Ahead

Over time, the preoccupation with measuring performance at a granular level, both within the hospital and without, is likely to become even more intense.

The measures that have been implemented so far tend to be "very process heavy," said Marcia Delk, MD, senior vice president for safety, quality, and credentialing and chief quality officer at WellStar, a five-hospital system in Atlanta.

Process measures, such as evaluating how many physicians prescribe beta-blockers to patients who suffered heart attacks, aim to evaluate whether patients are receiving timely and effective care. But while process measures are relatively easy to evaluate, critics say they are a proxy for what quality reporting strives to measure. Instead, many health care quality improvement experts advocate for shifting to an outcomes-based reporting system, touting the efficacy of measures such as mortality, hospital length of stay, and morbidity after certain procedures for evaluating the net result of a patient's health care experience.

Delk agrees. "The movement you need to see, to be looking at true value, would be from the patient's perspective," she says.[14] Patients want strong functional outcomes, with few complications and good success rates. The metrics contained in the hospital IQR program are not necessarily oriented toward that. As metrics evolve, they will need to include more direct outcome measurements that patients can connect with and understand.

Yet even those who advocate for shifting to a more outcomes-oriented approach to quality measurement say caution is warranted. One of the biggest concerns with outcomes measurement is risk-adjusting for confounding factors such as age and disease severity. This is critical for protecting providers from being unfairly penalized because of the unique characteristics of their patient population and ensuring that providers aren't incentivized to turn their backs on the oldest, sickest, and most complicated patients.

"What Medicare is doing is challenging us—to measure quality, to measure outcomes, to be more cost-effective, to be more mindful of the costs we incur, and to be more transparent and accountable," Wollschlaeger said. "All that is

---

[14] *Marcia Delk, MD, telephone interview, December 4, 2013.*

very new for physicians. Perhaps from the tradition of our training or the tradition of our practice or our profession, we feel intimidated. It is painful."

Yet there are significant numbers of administrators and physicians who are facing up to the changes in medicine. "We want to meet the challenge," Wollschlaeger said. "We will implement new modalities in our care and be more transparent. Therefore, I consider the changes positive—not easy, because it's going so fast—but positive."

Section 1.3: Technical Appendix: Inpatient Quality Reporting (IQR)

1.3.1 Overview

The hospital IQR program was created under provisions contained in Section 505(b) of the MMA of 2003. The hospital IQR program is designed to combine chart-abstracted data, reported by individual subsection (d) hospitals, with claims information extracted by the CMS to calculate hospital-specific measures of inpatient care.

The hospital IQR program data is reported for Medicare FFS patients over age sixty-five and, once collected and analyzed, the resulting performance measures results are used to:

- determine the application of a reimbursement adjustment made to an individual hospital's APU

- provide consumer information on hospital care quality via public posting on the Hospital Compare website

- provide feedback to participating hospitals to encourage quality of care improvements

- establish a data platform to support specific value-based reimbursement initiatives contained in the ACA of 2010, including:

  - the HVBP program
  - the HRRP program
  - the HAC reduction program

Given the broad utilization of the data collected as part of the IQR, it is not surprising that well over 99 percent of applicable hospitals participate in this voluntary program. Of eligible hospitals for the FY2014 program year, only seventy-seven failed to successfully meet reporting requirements. For FY2013–FY2014, CMS has provided a significant incentive for successful IQR participation in the form of a -2 percent adjustment in the APU for nonparticipating/unsuccessful reporting hospitals. Beginning with the FY2015 program year, non-IQR participating or unsuccessful reporting hospitals will have their *total* APU reduced by one-fourth.

Beginning with required reporting on a "starter set" of ten clinical measures for the FY2005 program year, IQR reporting requirements have undergone successive modifications in advance of the implementation of the value-based reimbursement initiatives. For the reporting year CY2014 (program year FY2016), the IQR contains sixty-two individual measures, including: chart-abstracted measures (e.g., Heart Attack, Heart Failure, Pneumonia, and Surgical Care Improvement); claims-based measures (e.g., mortality and readmissions measures for Heart Attack, Heart Failure, and Pneumonia); Agency for Healthcare Research and Quality (AHRQ) Patient Safety Indicators and Inpatient Quality Indicators; HAC measures; one survey-based measure (e.g., Patient Experience of Care); immunization measures; and structural measures.[15]

1.3.2 Timeline of IQR Developmental Events

1960s:

- Public and legislative concern about the quality of care in the Medicare program began with its approval on July 30, 1965, as President Lyndon B. Johnson signed the Medicare Bill into law.

- Within a year of its enactment, efforts were under way to understand and improve the quality of care provided by Medicare. These earliest attempts were significantly influenced by a model advanced by Avedis Donabedian, a physician and health services researcher at the University of Michigan. His 1966 article, "Evaluating the Quality of Medical Care," has become one of the most frequently cited public health-related articles of the twentieth century.[16]

---

[15] http://www.cms.gov/Newsroom/MediaReleaseDatabase/Press-Releases/2004-Press-Releases-Items/2004-05-20.html

[16] Donabedian A., "Evaluating the Quality of Medical Care." 1966, www.ncbi.nlm.nih.gov/pubmed/16279964

- Donabedian's model dealt almost exclusively with the *evaluation* of the medical care process at the level of *physician-patient* interaction. It excluded processes primarily related to the effective delivery of medical care at the *community* level—and "the difficult problem of economic efficiency as a measurable dimension of quality" was ignored.

- Despite these acknowledged shortcomings, the Donabedian Model, with its focus on three core dimensions (structure, process, and outcome), would significantly influence health care quality improvement philosophy for the next three decades.

1970s–1980s:

- Medicare legislative quality improvement efforts during the 1970s and 1980s reflected Donabedian's central focus around the *evaluation* of the medical care process through the creation of organizations focused on ensuring that care met professional standards of quality.

- The establishment of three in particular—The Experimental Medical Care Review Organization, The Professional Standards Review Organization, and The Utilization and Quality and Control Peer Review Organizations Program—are reflective of this approach.[17]

1990s:

1990:

- In an evaluation of the effectiveness of previous efforts in enhancing Medicare health care quality, the IOM observed in its 1990 report titled *Medicare: A Strategy for Quality Assurance, Volume 1*: "Despite these efforts, Medicare quality assurance to date has been insufficient, in large

---

[17] A. Bhatia et.al., *Evolution of Quality Review Programs for Medicare: Quality Assurance to Quality Improvement, Health Care Financing Review/Fall 2000/Volume 22, Number 1*, https://www.cms.gov/Research-Statistics-Data-and-Systems/Research/HealthCareFinancingReview/Downloads/00Fallpg69.pdf

measure because the programs were also heavily charged to control utilization and costs."[18]

- An additional key finding was that "different approaches to quality assurance may be necessary for different sites of care (e.g., hospital, home care, and ambulatory settings) and for different organizational structures, such as health maintenance organizations (HMOs) and fee-for-service practices."

1996: Executive Order 13017:

- As amended by EO 13040, President Clinton created the Advisory Commission on Consumer Protection and Quality in the Health Care Industry.

- This commission was charged to advise the president on changes occurring in the health care system and, where appropriate, to make recommendations on how best to promote and assure consumer protection and health care quality.[19]

1997: President's Commission on Consumer Protection and Quality in the Health Care Industry:

- November 20, 1997: The commission delivered its interim report to the president, titled, "A Consumer Bill of Rights and Responsibilities."[20]

1998: President's Commission on Consumer Protection and Quality in the Health Care Industry:

- The commission's final report was submitted on March 12, 1998.[21]

---

[18] *Medicare: A Strategy for Quality Assurance, Volume I (1990), The National Academies Press, http://www.nap.edu/catalog.php?record_id=1547*

[19] *President's Commission on Consumer Protection and Quality in the Health Care Industry, http://archive.ahrq.gov/hcqual/*

[20] *Consumer Bill of Rights & Responsibilities (11/20/97), http://govinfo.library.unt.edu/hcquality/press/cbor.html*

[21] *http://archive.ahrq.gov/hcqual/*

- The commission recommended that all segments of the health care industry embrace quality improvement and support clearly established aims for this improvement.

- The commission asserted that all sectors of the health care industry needed to be accountable for improving quality.

- The commission cited the lack of a systematic approach as hindering the industry's ability to sustain quality and stated that quality improvement should be demonstrated by providing information on performance using standardized quality measures.

- The commission made a recommendation to ensure the wide availability of valid, comprehensive, and comparative data that could be used to evaluate effectiveness for improving health.

1999: Institute of Medicine (IOM) Report: "To Err is Human: Building a Safer Health System":[22]

- The IOM report was an assessment report on the national aim of patient safety (as included in the 1998 Presidential Advisory Commission Report).

- The report concluded that tens of thousands of Americans die each year from errors in their care and hundreds of thousands suffer or barely escape from nonfatal injuries that a truly high-quality care system would largely prevent.

- The IOM reframed medical error as a chronic threat to public health, as lethal as breast cancer, motor vehicle accidents, or AIDS.

- A comprehensive strategy was described by which government, health care providers, industry, and consumers could reduce medical errors.

- Many of the IOM patient-safety recommendations are now reflected in the current HAC reduction initiatives and findings remain relevant today.

---

[22] *http://www.iom.edu/Reports/1999/to-err-is-human-building-a-safer-health-system.aspx*

2000–2005

2001: The CMS Quality Initiative:

- Health and Human Services (HHS) Secretary Tommy Thompson announced the CMS Quality Initiative, a commitment to ensuring high-quality health care through published consumer information on the performance of health care providers, coupled with health care quality improvement support through Medicare QIOs. The aims of the Quality Initiative were to:

    o empower consumers with quality of care information to make more informed decisions about their health care

    o to stimulate and support providers and clinicians to improve the quality of health care

2002: Nursing Home Quality Initiative (NHQI)

- This first Quality Initiative was launched nationally as the **Nursing Home Quality Initiative (NHQI)**:[23]

    o NHQI measures assess a resident's physical and clinical conditions and abilities, as well as preferences and life-care wishes.

    o Assessment data have been converted to develop quality measures that give consumers another source of information that shows how well nursing homes are caring for their residents' physical and clinical needs.

2002: Hospital Consumer Assessment of Healthcare Providers and Systems Survey (HCAHPS):[24]

- HCAHPS (pronounced "H-caps") is a survey instrument and data collection methodology for measuring patients' perceptions of their hospital experience.

---

[23] http://www.cms.gov/Medicare/Quality-Initiatives-Patient-Assessment-Instruments/NursingHomeQualityInits/index.html

[24] HCAHPS Fact Sheet, http://www.hcahpsonline.org/files/August%202013%20HCAHPS%20Fact%20Sheet2.pdf

- HCAHPS was developed as the first national, standardized, publicly reported survey of patients' perspectives of hospital care, which allows consumers to compare patient perspectives at different hospitals.

- In 2002, CMS partnered with the AHRQ to develop and pilot the HCAHPS.

- HCAHPS was designed to allow valid comparisons to be made across hospitals locally, regionally, and nationally.

- HCAHPS was endorsed in May 2005 by the National Quality Forum (NQF), a national organization that represents the consensus of many health care providers, consumer groups, professional associations, purchasers, federal agencies, and research and quality organizations.

- The federal Office of Management and Budget (OMB) endorsed the use of HCAHPS in December 2005 and specified HCAHPS use as part of the hospital IQR program in the Deficit Reduction Act (DRA) of 2005. CMS first implemented the HCAHPS survey in October 2006.

- The first reporting of HCAHPS results occurred in March 2008.

2002: Hospital Compare:[25]

- Initial development began in 2002 of the Hospital Compare website tool, created to publicly report credible and user-friendly information about the quality of care delivered in the nation's hospitals.

- The first Hospital Compare report was posted on April 1, 2005, and consisted of reporting on the starter set of ten NQF measures of the Hospital Quality Alliance (HQA).

2003: The Hospital Quality Initiative (HQI):

- As a more complex initiative than the NHQI, the HQI used a variety of tools to stimulate and support a significant improvement in the quality of hospital care.

---

[25] *http://www.cms.gov/Center/Special-Topic/Quality-of-Care-Center.html*

- The primary aim of the HQI was to refine and standardize hospital data, data transmission, and performance measures in order to construct a single robust, prioritized, and standard quality measure set for hospitals.

- The ultimate HQI goal was that "all private and public purchasers, oversight, and accrediting entities, and payers and providers of hospital care would use the same measures in their public reporting activities."

- The collected information would serve to inform providers, as well as consumers, about relative quality of care.

2003: Establishment of the National Voluntary Hospital Reporting Initiative (NVHRI):[26]

- The NVHRI was launched as part of the HQI. Renamed the HQA in 2004, this initiative represents a public-private collaboration to improve the quality of care provided by the nation's hospitals by measuring and publicly reporting on that care.

- The NVHRI/HQA was created as a consortium of organizations, including the CMS, the Joint Commission on Accreditation of Healthcare Organizations (JCAHO), the American Hospital Association (AHA), and consumer groups such as the American Association of Retired Persons (AARP) and the AFL-CIO.

- The NVRI/HQA was established to provide useful and valid information about hospital quality to the public, standardize data and data collection, and foster hospital quality improvement:

  o Unlike previous quality initiatives, the HQI was not initially supported with well-studied and validated clinical data sets and standardized data transmission infrastructure for public reporting.

  o In order to establish an initial data set from which to develop pertinent quality measures for hospitals, the AHA, the Federation of American Hospitals (FAH), and the Association of American Medical Colleges (AAMC) approached the JCAHO, the AHRQ, the NQF, and CMS to explore voluntary public reporting of

---

[26] http://www.cms.gov/Newsroom/MediaReleaseDatabase/Press-Releases/2004-Press-Releases-Items/2004-05-20.html

hospital performance measures. The CMS contracted with the NQF to develop such a consensus-derived set of hospital quality measures appropriate for public reporting.

- o The HQA began with the voluntary, public reporting of ten quality measures related to treatment of acute myocardial infarction (AMI), heart failure (HF), and pneumonia (PN) patients. Under the HQA, hospitals nationwide report data to the CMS on indicators of the quality of care measures.[27]

2003: Medicare Prescription Drug, Improvement, and Modernization Act of 2003 (MMA):

- The Medicare Improvements for Patients and Providers Act (MIPPA) was signed into law in December 2003.[28]

- MIPPA Section 3003 expanded upon the HQA by adding Section 1886(b)(3)(B)(vii) to the Social Security Act (SSA). This section established the authority for the Reporting Hospital Quality Data for Annual Payment Update Program (RHQDAPU) (now known as the Inpatient Quality Reporting Program (IQR)) and revised the mechanism used to update the standardized payment amount for inpatient hospital operating costs.

- The law established for FY2005–FY2007 that any subsection (d) hospital that did not submit data on the set of ten quality indicators established by the HHS secretary as of November 1, 2003, would have a reduction of 0.4 percentage points applied to their annual update percentage increase (also known as the "market basket" update).

- It also provides that any reduction would apply only to the fiscal year involved and would not be taken into account in computing the applicable percentage increase for a subsequent fiscal year.

---

[27] http://www.nmmra.org/providers/hospitals_initiatives.php

[28] Public Law 108–173, December 8, 2003, http://www.gpo.gov/fdsys/pkg/PLAW-108publ173/pdf/PLAW-108publ173.pdf

2005: Deficit Reduction Act (DRA) of 2005:[29]

- DRA 2005 was passed on February 9, 2006.

- **Section 5001(a)(2)(B)**

    - Section 5001(a)(2)(B) of the DRA, Public Law 109–171, further amended Section 1886(b)(3)(B) of the act and modified Section 501(b) of the MMA of 2003 to revise the mechanism used to update the standardized payment amount for hospital inpatient operating costs.

    - Payment updates reductions for FY2007 and each subsequent fiscal year were to be increased from -.4 to -2.0 percentage points for any subsection (d) hospital that does not submit quality data in a "form and manner, and at a time, specified by the (HHS) secretary."

    - The HHS secretary was required to "make outcome and efficiency measures publicly available under the hospital IQR program through the introduction of the Hospital Compare website on April 1, 2005.

    - HHS was required for the first time to develop a plan to implement a value-based purchasing (VBP) program for Medicare payment for subsection (d) hospitals, beginning with FY2009. The Medicare HVBP program was to be built on the current hospital IQR program and be budget-neutral.

        Note: *This action was delayed until the ACA of 2010.*

    - Section 5001 directed adoption of a baseline set of quality measures set forth in a November 2005 report by the IOM, beginning in FY2007.

    - Section 5001 directed quality adjustments in diagnosis-related group (DRG) payments to be made for certain HACS, beginning with discharges occurring on or after October 1, 2008.

---

[29] *Deficit Reduction Act of 2005, http://www.gpo.gov/fdsys/pkg/PLAW-109publ171/pdf/PLAW-109publ171.pdf*

- o Section 5001 created an additional incentive for acute-care hospitals to participate in HCAHPS through inclusion in the hospital IQR program, beginning in 2007.

- o In December 2005, the OMB gave its final approval for the national implementation of HCAHPS for public reporting purposes. HCAHPS results were first collected in October 2006 and reported in 2008.

2006–2013

2006: August 26: President Bush Signs EO 13410:[30]

- EO 13410 directs federal agencies to provide health care quality and price information for consumers and "to make relevant information available to these beneficiaries, enrollees, and providers in a readily useable manner."

- CMS implemented the HCAHPS survey in October 2006.

2006: Incorporation of HCAHPS and Readmission Measures into IQR:

- CMS added readmissions measures for HA, (HF), and PN to IQR requirements.

- HCAHPS survey results are included in the requirement for public reporting of quality measures. The Inpatient Prospective Payment System (IPPS) hospitals that fail to publicly report the required quality measures, which include the HCAHPS survey, will receive an annual payment update that is reduced by 2.0 percentage points.

2008: Initial Discussion of VBP for Physicians and Other Professional Services:

- The first public reporting of HCAHPS results was posted on the Hospital Compare website in March.

---

[30] *EO 13410 Promoting Quality and Efficient Health Care in Federal Government Administered or Sponsored Health Care Programs, http://nodis3.gsfc.nasa.gov/displayEO.cfm?id=EO_13410_*

- MIPPA of 2008 Section 131(d) required HHS to develop a VBP transition plan for providers (other than hospitals) receiving Medicare payments. In December 2008, HHS submitted a draft blueprint for transitioning physicians and other provider services to a Medicare VBP program.[31]

2009: Readmissions Reporting:

- CMS included the reporting of hospital performance against readmission measures on the Hospital Compare website.

2010: Introduction of the ACA:[32]

- To further leverage the information collected as part of the hospital IQR program, the ACA mandates the staggered implementation of a variety of value-dependent reimbursement initiatives. In addition, reporting requirements for non-subsection (d) hospitals are specified, along with plans for similar value-based initiatives.

- Sections of the ACA supported by the IQR include:

  - **Section 3001: HVBP program:**

    - Beginning with FY2013, CMS is directed to include risk adjustment for quality measures for outcomes of care in order to provide incentives for hospitals to continue to provide care for costly/complex patients.

    - Section 3001 required "to the extent practicable" alignment of hospital quality measures applicable to physicians.

    - A validation process for reported measures was established that involves random sampling of participating hospitals.

---

[31] *Medicare Improvements for Patients and Providers Act of 2008, http://www.gpo.gov/fdsys/pkg/PLAW-110publ275/pdf/PLAW-110publ275.pdf*

[32] *Patient Protection and Affordable Care Act, http://www.gpo.gov/fdsys/pkg/PLAW-111publ148/pdf/PLAW-111publ148.pdf*

o **Section 3004: quality reporting for long-term care hospitals, inpatient rehabilitation hospitals, and hospice programs.**

o **Section 3005: quality reporting for PPS-exempt cancer hospitals.**

o **Section 3006: plans for a VBP program for skilled nursing facilities and home health agencies.**

o **Section 3008: payment adjustment for conditions acquired in hospitals.**

o **Section 3025: the HRRP program.**

- **Section 3401:**

    o Beginning in FY2015, hospitals failing to submit required quality data required as part of the RHQDAPU/hospital IQR program will have their total APU percentage reduced by one-quarter. (This replaces the fixed 2 percent reduction applied to the market basket portion of the APU established in the DRA 2005.) This reduction is to be "determined without regard to other reductions in the annual payment update."

    Note: *In September 2010, the RHQDAPU was redesignated as (IQR).*

2013: CMS lists specifications for quality reporting programs in multiple settings of care:[33]

- hospital inpatient services, under the hospital IQR program (formerly referred to as the RHQDAPU program)

- hospital outpatient services, under the **Hospital Outpatient Quality Reporting (OQR)** Program (formerly referred to as the Hospital Outpatient Quality Data Reporting Program (HOP QDRP))

---

[33] *Page 50774, Federal Register/Vol. 78, No. 160/Monday, August 19, 2013/Rules and Regulations, www.gpo.gov/fdsys/pkg/FR-2013-08-19/pdf/2013-18956.pdf*

- care furnished by physicians and other eligible professionals (EPs), under the **PQRS,** formerly referred to as the Physician Quality Reporting Program Initiative (PQRI))

- inpatient rehabilitation facilities, under the **Inpatient Rehabilitation Facility Quality Reporting Program (IRF QRP)**

- long-term care hospitals, under the **Long-Term Care Hospital Quality Reporting (LTCHQR) Program**

- prospective payment system (PPS)-exempt cancer hospitals, under the **PPS-Exempt Cancer Hospital Quality Reporting (PCHQR)** Program

- ambulatory surgical centers, under the **Ambulatory Surgical Center Quality Reporting (ASCQR)** Program

- inpatient psychiatric facilities, under the **Inpatient Psychiatric Facilities Quality Reporting (IPFQR)** Program

- home health agencies, under the **Home Health Quality Reporting Program (HH QRP)**

- hospices, under the **Hospice Quality Reporting Program (HQRP)**

- CMS has also implemented an end-stage renal disease (ESRD) quality improvement program that links payment to performance.

1.3.3 IQR Calendar Year (CY) Reporting Requirements

Key Terms and IQR-Related Organizations

Hospital IQR Program Year

- The year in which negative payment adjustments are made to the market basket portion of an applicable hospital's APU, based on CMS's determination of successful or unsuccessful participation in the hospital IQR program. For a given program year, data is collected eighteen to twenty-four months prior to the start of the program year, based on the measure and the CMS-specified method of data collection.

Applicable Hospital

- Applicable hospitals are classified as subsection (d) hospitals and are generally those facilities reimbursed under the IPPS. Hospitals not considered "applicable" include psychiatric hospitals, rehabilitation hospitals, long-term care hospitals, children's hospitals, cancer hospitals, hospitals located in the US territories, critical access hospitals (CAH), and Maryland hospitals operating under a CMS waiver. For the FY2014 hospital IQR program year, there are 3,296 applicable hospitals.[34]

Successful Participation

- Successful participation is a determination by CMS that applicable hospitals participating in the IQR have submitted all required IQR quality data for a given program year in a form and manner, and at a time, specified by the HHS secretary to avoid negative adjustments to their APU. For the FY2014 hospital IQR program year, of 3,296 applicable hospitals, 3,220 successfully participated and received their full APU.[35]

Annual Payment Update (APU)

- As part of its annual hospital reimbursement calculation, CMS assigns a payment adjustment for Medicare services provided by hospitals in order to account for cost increases (inflation) throughout the fiscal year. This payment adjustment is called the APU and is an adjustment made to the market basket for a given hospital. Annual hospital IPPS updates are determined, in part, by the projected increase in the hospital market basket:

---

[34] *https://www.qualitynet.org/*

[35]

http://www.qualitynet.org/dcs/ContentServer?cid=1138115987129&pagename=QnetPublic%2FPage%2FQnetTier2

- The FY2014 Annual Payment Update for hospitals successfully participating in IQR (after deductions mandated by the ACA and Sequestration) is a net +1.7 percent.

- Nonparticipating or unsuccessfully participating hospitals in the IQR during FY2012 will have their FY2014 APU reduced by 2.0 percent, for a net APU of -.3 percent.[36]

Market Basket

A primary component of the calculation of a hospital's APU, the market basket amount represents the estimated change in price of goods and services used to furnish inpatient hospital care. The intent is to provide a payment increase to account for inflation that can cause increases in the cost of health care services. In order to receive their full market basket update, a hospital must submit valid IQR data on a set of predefined quality measures for a given year.

IQR Payment Adjustment

This is a negative adjustment made to an individual hospital's APU for unsuccessful or nonparticipation in IQR reporting for a given program year:

- For program years FY2013 and FY2014, the adjustment is -2.0 percent applied to the applicable market basket amount.

- For program years FY2015 onward, the IQR payment adjustment will be a 25 percent reduction in an individual hospital's total APU.[37] (Example: A hospital is slated to receive a total APU of 4 percent. With the application of the IQR adjustment, its APU will be reduced by 1 percent, for a revised APU of 3 percent.)

---

[36] https://www.federalregister.gov/.../medicare-program-hospital-inpatient-...

[37] Page 5081, Federal Register/Vol. 78, No. 160/Monday, August 19, 2013/Rules and Regulations, www.gpo.gov/fdsys/pkg/FR-2013-08-19/pdf/2013-18956.pdf

- Of 3,296 IQR-applicable hospitals for the FY2014 program:[38]

    o 40 hospitals were determined to be unsuccessful and received a -2.0 percent adjustment

    o 36 hospitals elected nonparticipation and received a -2.0 percent adjustment

QualityNet

- CMS established the QualityNet website to provide health care quality improvement news, resources, and data-reporting tools and applications used by health care providers and others in support of selected quality reporting programs:

- QualityNet was initially introduced in 2003 as the **Quality Net Exchange** to transmit network information related to the ESRD program.

- QualityNet is the only CMS-approved website for secure communications and health care quality data exchange among QIOs, hospitals, physicians' offices, nursing homes, ESRD networks and facilities, and data vendors.

- QualityNet-supported programs include:

    o hospital IQR

    o hospital OQR

    o ASCQR

    o PQRS

    o ESRD

- Instructions for using QualityNet in reporting IQR measures may be viewed on the QualityNet home page at: Guide to CMS Hospital IQR Program.

---

[38]

http://www.qualitynet.org/dcs/ContentServer?cid=1138115987129&pagename=QnetPublic%2FPage%2FQnetTier2

Quality Improvement Organization (QIO)

- QIOs are private (mostly not-for-profit organizations) that are staffed by professionals (mostly doctors and other health care professionals) who are trained to review medical care and help beneficiaries with complaints about the quality of care and to implement improvements throughout the spectrum of care. QIO contracts are three years in length, with each three-year cycle referenced as a statement of work (SOW):

  - By law, the mission of the QIO program is to improve the effectiveness, efficiency, economy, and quality of services delivered to Medicare beneficiaries. Based on this statutory charge and CMS's program experience, CMS identifies the core functions of the QIO program as:

    - improving quality of care for beneficiaries

    - protecting the integrity of the Medicare Trust Fund by ensuring that Medicare pays only for services and goods that are reasonable and necessary and that are provided in the most appropriate setting

    - protecting beneficiaries by expeditiously addressing individual complaints, such as: beneficiary complaints; provider-based notice appeals; violations of the Emergency Medical Treatment and Labor Act (EMTALA); and other related responsibilities as articulated in QIO-related law[39]

QIO Clinical Data Warehouse:

- The QIO Clinical Data Warehouse contains data uploaded from hospitals across the nation to:

  - **reduce the burden of duplicate data collection and reporting:** The CMS and the Joint Commission have come together to reduce the burden of duplicate record requests related to the IOR. Any

---

[39] *Quality Improvement Organizations, http://www.cms.gov/Medicare/Quality-Initiatives-Patient-Assessment-Instruments/QualityImprovementOrgs/index.html?redirect=/QualityImprovementOrgs/*

records requested by CMS will not be re-requested if they have already been uploaded to the QIO Clinical Data Warehouse.

- **provide comparative data on a state and national level:** The reports generated from the warehouse provide hospitals with more robust data allowing performance comparison with other hospitals. Such reports are available via QualityNet.

- **assist hospitals in preparing for national initiatives that are under way for quality information reporting:** The current public and nonpublic reporting initiatives that use QualityNet and the QIO Clinical Data Warehouse help prepare hospitals for any future public reporting initiative.

- **process hospital IQR program data:** Hospital data submitted via the QualityNet website is aggregated by the QIO warehouse prior to being forwarded to CMS.

1.3.4 CY2014 IQR Measures Reporting (FY2016 Program Year)

General:[40]

- Measures and measure sets are carried over from year to year. They are modified to align with the value-reimbursement program year requirements and to reflect changes in the assessed applicability of measures in providing quality care. CMS will suspend or retire measure sets or specific measures from the hospital IQR program and include additional reporting methods as necessary.

- For CY2014 reporting, there are sixty-two individual measures for which CMS requires data collection through the hospital IQR program. In addition, there is a data accuracy and completeness acknowledgement (DACA) requirement. As listed in the annual Final IPPS Rules, specific

---

[40] *QualityNet, Measure Comparison (Inpatient Hospital Quality Measures),*
http://www.qualitynet.org/dcs/ContentServer?pagename=QnetPublic%2FPage%2FQnetTier2&cid
=1141662756099

timelines are announced for the submission of data for three categories of measures sets, based on how information is obtained by CMS.

Chart-Abstracted Measure Overview:

- These are measures that require individual hospitals, or their authorized vendor, to enter data via the QualityNet website on a quarterly basis for a period two years in advance of a given program year.

Measures Requiring Web-Based Hospital Entry Overview:

- These are measures requiring either quarterly or annual reporting via the QualityNet website. Data entry is achieved through the secure side of QualityNet.org via an online tool available to authorized users.

Measures CMS-Extracted From Claims Overview:

- Hospitals are not required to report on these measures, as CMS will aggregate data from submitted claims during a specified period for an individual hospital. The time frame for extraction varies with measure sets.

1.3.5 Chart-Abstracted Measures

General:

Chart-abstracted IQR measures are directly reportable by hospitals or their authorized vendors. Measure data is submitted through the QualityNet website using the hospital's MyQualityNet account for aggregation and submission to CMS by the QIO Clinical Data Warehouse.

Note: Hospitals can authorize a third-party vendor to submit clinical data and HCAHPS data on behalf of the hospital.

- Hospitals participating in the hospital IQR program must continuously collect and report data quarterly for each of the quality measures in the measure sets (topic areas) that require chart abstractions, specifically: AMI, HF, PN, the Surgical Care Improvement Project (SCIP), ED, and immunizations (IMM). In addition, required population and sampling data is to be submitted for measures as outlined in the applicable year Specifications Manual:[41]

- o On a quarterly basis, hospitals submit aggregate population and sample size counts for Medicare and non-Medicare discharges for each of the topic areas that require chart-abstracted data.

- o Hospitals submit either a *complete population* of cases or a *random sample* for each of the measure sets covered by the quality measures (as required for each measure in the Specifications Manual). For discharges effective January 1, 2014, see: the Handbook IV: Specifications Manual for National Hospital Inpatient Quality Measures;) or the **Inpatient Specifications Manual**, Version 4.3.

- If a hospital has **five or fewer discharges in a quarter** for a measure set (AMI, HF, PN, ED, IMM, or the combined SCIP strata) the hospital:[42]

  - o may opt to submit the data for quality improvement efforts *only*, but is **not required to abstract and submit patient-level case data for measure set(s) with five or fewer discharges for that quarter**

  - o and must submit the required population and sampling data for all measure sets and strata, even when the data is zero.

- For CY2014 reporting, there are forty individual measures requiring chart-abstracted reporting by individual hospitals contained in ten measure sets related to:

  - o **Clinical Conditions** of AMI, HF, PN, STK, and VTE

  - o **SCIP**

  - o **ED**

---

[41] *Specifications Manual for National Hospital Inpatient Quality Measures, http://www.qualitynet.org/dcs/ContentServer?pagename=QnetPublic%2FPage%2FQnetTier2&cid =1141662756099*

[42] *Page 51641, Federal Register/Vol. 76, No. 160/Thursday, August 18, 2011/Rules and Regulations, http://www.cms.gov/Medicare/Medicare-Fee-for-Service-Payment/AcuteInpatientPPS/FY-2011-IPPS-Final-Rule-Home-Page.html*

- o **IMM**

- o **HAI**

- o **HCAHPS**

- With an average inpatient chart length in FY2014 estimated at some 412 pages, the chart-abstracted reporting process is labor-intensive and costly. (Since 2006, average chart length has increased from 140 to 412 pages and the average length of an HAI chart is 1,500 pages.)[43]

  - o For the forty CY2014-reportable chart-abstracted measures:

    - ▪ CMS estimates that each hospital will spend 1,900 hours annually submitting chart-abstracted data—or 47.5 hours per measure.[44]

    - ▪ At an estimated cost of $59 per hour, hospitals will spend approximately $112,100 annually to meet reporting requirements—or $2,802 per measure.

CY2014 Reportable Chart-Abstracted Measures:

- **Measures Set Summary:**

MEASURES SET	NUMBER OF INDIVIDUAL MEASURES
AMI	2
HF	1
STK	8
VTE	6
PN	1
SCIP	7
ED	7

---

[43] Page 50834, Federal Register/Vol. 78, No. 160/Monday, August 19, 2013/Rules and Regulations, www.gpo.gov/fdsys/pkg/FR-2013-08-19/pdf/2013-18956.pdf

[44] Pages 27749–27750, Federal Register/Vol. 78, No. 91/Friday, May 10, 2013/Proposed Rules http://www.cms.gov/Medicare/Medicare-Fee-for-Service-Payment/AcuteInpatientPPS/FY-2014-IPPS-Proposed-Rule-Home-Page-Items/FY-2014-IPPS-Proposed-Rule-CMS-1599-P-Regulations.html

IMM	1
HAI	6
HCAHPS	1

- **Individual Measures:**
  - As specified in the FY2014 Final IPPS Rule (Federal Register/Vol. 78, No. 160/Monday, August 19, 2013/Rules and Regulations), the following is a listing of hospital-reportable chart-abstracted measures for discharges occurring during CY2014 in support of the FY2016 program year.

    Note: *These same measures have been approved for program year FY2017, subject to change through the annual IPS rules.*

Table 1: List of CY2014 Chart-Abstracted Reportable Measures:[45]

MEASURES REQUIRING CHART ABSTRACTION AND SUBMISSION BY THE HOSPITAL OR ITS VENDOR FOR MEDICARE FFS DISCHARGES OCCURRING IN CY2014 TO BE APPLIED TO FY2016 PROGRAM YEAR	
Acute Myocardial Infarction (AMI)	
AMI 7a	Fibrinolytic Therapy Received Within 30 Minutes of Hospital Arrival
AMI 8a	Timing of Receipt of Primary Percutaneous Coronary Intervention (PCI)
Heart Failure (HF)	
HF-2	Evaluation of LVS Function
Stroke (STK)	
STK-1	Venous Thromboembolism (VTE) Prophylaxis
STK-2	Discharged on Antithrombotic Therapy
STK-3	Anticoagulation Therapy for Atrial Fibrillation/Flutter
STK-4	Thrombolytic Therapy
STK-5	Antithrombotic Therapy By End of Hospital Day 2
STK-6	Discharged on Statin Medication

[45] *QualityNet, Measure Comparison (Inpatient Hospital Quality Measures), http://www.qualitynet.org/dcs/ContentServer?pagename=QnetPublic%2FPage%2FQnetTier2&cid=1141662756099*

STK-8	Stroke Education
STK-10	Stroke Education
Venous Thromboembolism (VTE)	
VTE-1	Venous Thromboembolism Prophylaxis
VTE-2	Intensive Care Unit Venous Thromboembolism Prophylaxis
VTE-3	Venous Thromboembolism Patients with Anticoagulation Overlap Therapy
VTE-4	Venous Thromboembolism Patients Receiving Unfractionated Heparin with Dosages/Platelet Count Monitoring by Protocol or Nomogram
VTE-5	Venous Thromboembolism Warfarin Therapy Discharge Instructions
VTE-6	Hospital-Acquired Potentially Preventable Venous Thromboembolism
Pneumonia (PN)*	
PN-6	Initial Antibiotic Selection for Community-Acquired Pneumonia (CAP) in Immunocompetent Patient
Surgical Care Improvement Project (SCIP)	
SCIP-1	Prophylactic Antibiotic Received Within One Hour Prior to Surgical Incision
SCIP-2	Prophylactic Antibiotic Selection for Surgical Patients
SCIP-3	Prophylactic Antibiotics Discontinued Within 24 Hours After Surgery End Time
SCIP-4	Cardiac Surgery Patients With Controlled Postoperative Blood Glucose
SCIP-9	Urinary Catheter Removed on Postoperative Day 1 (POD 1) or Postoperative Day 2 (POD 2) with day of surgery being day zero
SCIP-CARD -2	Surgery Patients on Beta-Blocker Therapy Prior to Arrival Who Received a Beta-Blocker During the Perioperative Period
SCIP-VTE-2	Surgery Patients Who Received Appropriate Venous Thromboembolism Prophylaxis Within 24 Hours Prior to Surgery to 24 Hours After Surgery
Emergency Department (ED) (Listed in the Rule as "Emergency Department Throughput")	
ED-1a	Median Time from ED Arrival to ED Departure for Admitted ED Patients—Overall Rate
ED-1b	Median Time from ED Arrival to ED Departure for Admitted ED Patients—Reporting Measure
ED-1c	Median Time from ED Arrival to ED Departure for Admitted ED Patients—Observation Patients
ED-1d	Median Time from ED Arrival to ED Departure for Admitted ED Patients—Psychiatric/Mental Health Patients
ED-2a	Admit Decision Time to ED Departure Time for Admitted Patients—Overall Rate

ED-2b	Admit Decision Time to ED Departure Time for Admitted Patients—Reporting Measure
ED-2c	Admit Decision Time to ED Departure Time for Admitted Patients—Psychiatric/Mental Health Patients
Immunization (IMM) (Listed in the Rule as "Prevention: Global Immunization Measures")	
IMM-2*	Influenza Immunization
Healthcare-Associated Infection Measure (HAI) Submitted to CDC's NHSN	
	Central Line-Associated Bloodstream Infection (CLABSI)
	Surgical Site Infection (SSI-Colon, SSI-Abdominal Hysterectomy)
	Catheter-Associated Urinary Tract Infection (CAUTI)
	MRSA Bacteremia
	Clostridium Difficile (C. difficile)
	Health Care Personnel Influenza Vaccination
Hospital Consumer Assessment of Healthcare Providers and Systems Survey (HCAHPS)**	

*For CY2014 reporting of this measure, data for the period of October 1, 2013–March 31, 2014, must be submitted by May 15, 2014, for the FY2016 hospital IQR program year.

**Hospitals must obtain and submit at least 300 completed HCAHPS surveys in a rolling four-quarter period, unless the hospital is too small to obtain 300 completed surveys.[46]

Measures Validation Requirements:[47]

To ensure the accuracy of submitted IQR information, CMS has developed a validation process by which a number of hospitals each year are required to provide supporting charts for review:

- Hospitals selected for validation review are directed to submit a specified number of charts for a limited number of measures according to a published time frame.

- Selected hospitals pass IQR measure validation requirements by receiving a confidence interval of 75 percent or greater, based on the combined chart audit validations for a time period specified for an applicable program year.

---

[46] *Page 50819, Federal Register/Vol. 78, No. 160/Monday, August 19, 2013/Rules and Regulations, www.gpo.gov/fdsys/pkg/FR-2013-08-19/pdf/2013-18956.pdf*

[47] *Page 50833, Federal Register/Vol. 78, No. 160/Monday, August 19, 2013/Rules and Regulations, www.gpo.gov/fdsys/pkg/FR-2013-08-19/pdf/2013-18956.pdf*

- The current validation process involves:

  - an annual hospital validation sample size of 400 randomly selected hospitals and a supplemental sample of up to 200 hospitals to be selected for more targeted validation.

  - The supplemental sample of up to 200 hospitals will include all hospitals that fail validation in the previous year and a random sample of hospitals meeting certain targeting criteria:

    - any hospital with abnormal or conflicting data patterns

    - any hospital with rapidly changing data patterns

    - any hospital that submits data to NHSN after the hospital IQR program data submission deadline has passed

    - any hospital that joined the hospital IQR program within the previous three years and which has not been previously validated

    - any hospital that has not been randomly selected for validation in any of the previous three years

    - any hospital that passed validation in the previous year, but had a two-tailed confidence interval that included 75 percent

    - new for CY2014, any hospital that failed to report to NHSN at least half of the actual HAI events detected, as determined during the previous year's validation effort

- The validation period for FY2016 and beyond has been established in the FY2014 Final IPPS Rule to include the third and fourth calendar quarters of the year that occurs two years before the payment determination is made and the first and second quarters of the subsequent year.

- The confidence interval calculation is available on QualityNet.

- A full description of the IQR validation process is available in the FY2014 Final IPPS Rule.

Timeline for Chart-Abstracted Measures Reporting

Reporting Guidelines[48]

IQR reporting of specific measures sets must adhere to times and guidelines established in the applicable program year IPPS Final Rule. Varying submission dates have been established for measure set reporting, population and sampling submission, and measure validation requirements.

Population and Sample Size Counts:[49]

- Aggregate population and sample size counts for Medicare and non-Medicare discharges for each measure set are submitted quarterly via MyQualityNet.

- Hospitals that have five or fewer discharges (both Medicare and non-Medicare combined) within a measure set or the combined SCIP strata in a quarter are required to submit the aggregate population and sample size counts.

- Hospitals that have no discharges for a particular measure set are required to submit a zero in the application or XML.

  Note: Leaving the fields blank does not fulfill the requirement.

HCAHPS:

- Hospitals are required to continuously collect and submit HCAHPS survey data in accordance with the current HCAHPS Quality

---

[48] *Handbook II: CMS Hospital Inpatient Quality Reporting Program,* *https://www.qualitynet.org/dcs/BlobServer?blobkey=id&blobnocache=true&blobwhere=1228889674222&blobheader=multipart/octet-stream&blobheadername1=Content-Disposition&blobheadervalue1=attachment;filename%3DHndbkII_CMS-HosIQRprog_010912.pdf&blobcol=urldata&blobtable=MungoBlobs*

[49] *Handbook II: CMS Hospital Inpatient Quality Reporting Program,* *https://www.qualitynet.org/dcs/BlobServer?blobkey=id&blobnocache=true&blobwhere=1228889674222&blobheader=multipart/octet-stream&blobheadername1=Content-Disposition&blobheadervalue1=attachment;filename%3DHndbkII_CMS-HosIQRprog_010912.pdf&blobcol=urldata&blobtable=MungoBlobs*

Assurance Guidelines, which can be found on the HCAHPS website at: http://www.hcahpsonline.org

- Hospitals with five or fewer HCAHPS-eligible discharges in a month must submit the total number of HCAHPS-eligible cases to the QIO Clinical Data Warehouse for that month as part of its quarterly HCAHPS data submission.

- Hospitals with five or fewer HCAHPS-eligible discharges during a month are not required to submit HCAHPS surveys for that month. However, hospitals meeting the five or fewer exception may voluntarily submit the data for quality improvement purposes.

- When a hospital has no HCAHPS-eligible discharges in a given month, the hospital is still required to submit a zero for that month as part of its quarterly HCAHPS data submission.

- Hospitals and survey vendors must participate in all oversight activities conducted by the HCAHPS project team.

HAI Data:[50]

- During CY2014, hospitals will have until the hospital IQR program final submission deadline to submit their quarterly HAI data to the CDC NHSN for CLABSI, SSI, CAUTI, MRSA bacteremia, Clostridium difficile, and health care provider influenza vaccination.

- After the final hospital IQR program submission deadline has occurred for each calendar quarter of CY2014, CMS will obtain the hospital-specific calculations that have been generated by the NHSN for the hospital IQR program.

- Hospitals can request an HAI exception from submitting CLABSI, CAUTI, or SSI data when they meet the following:

  o Hospitals that do not have intensive care unit (ICU) locations or meet the CDC 80 percent rule (80 percent or more of the area's

---

[50] Page 50718, Federal Register/Vol. 78, No. 160/Monday, August 19, 2013/Rules and Regulations, www.gpo.gov/fdsys/pkg/FR-2013-08-19/pdf/2013-18956.pdf

patients are of a certain type (e.g., ICU patients)), the area is designated as that type of location—in this case, an ICU.

- o Hospitals that performed nine or fewer of any of the specified colon and abdominal hysterectomy procedures combined in the calendar year prior to the reporting year.

Complete Data Accuracy and Completeness Acknowledgement (DACA):

Hospitals must acknowledge by May 15, 2015, that all the information submitted as required by the hospital IQR program for FY2016 payment determination is complete and accurate to the best of its knowledge with respect to the time period of January 1, 2014, through December 31, 2014.

Disaster Waiver

CMS offers a process for hospitals to request and for CMS to grant extensions or waivers for the reporting of required quality data for one or more quarters when there are extraordinary circumstances beyond the control of the hospital:

- Waiver request forms must be submitted within thirty days of the date when the extraordinary circumstance occurred (forms may be submitted online).

- Hospitals are required to designate an appropriate, non-CEO contact as the contact for the extraordinary circumstances extensions or waivers requests.

- CMS may grant a waiver or extension to a hospital if it is determined that a systemic problem with one of the CMS data collection systems directly affected the ability of the hospital to submit data.

Established Timelines:

- IQR reporting of specific measures sets must adhere to timelines established in the applicable program year IPPS Final Rule.

- Varying submission dates have been established for measure set reporting, population and sampling submission, and measure validation requirements:

Table 2: CY2013-CY2014 IQR Reporting Timelines[51]

DISCHARGE QUARTERS	CLINICAL MEASURES AND HAI SUBMISSION	HCAHPS* SUBMISSION	POPULATION AND SAMPLING SUBMISSION	PERINATAL CARE (WEB-BASED MEASURE)	HAI VALIDATION TEMPLATES*	CDAC RECORD REQUEST*	ESTIMATED DATE RECORDS DUE TO CDAC*
1st Quarter 2013 1/1/13–3/31/13	08/15/13	07/08/13	08/01/13	once between: 07/01/13–08/15/13	N/A	09/05/13	10/17/13
2nd Quarter 2013 4/1/13–6/30/13	11/15/13	10/02/13	11/01/13	once between: 10/01/13–11/15/13	N/A	12/02/13	01/02/14
3rd Quarter 2013 7/1/13–9/30/13	02/15/14	01/02/14	02/01/14	once between: 01/01/14–02/15/14	N/A	02/28/14	03/31/14
4th Quarter 2013 10/1/13–12/31/13	05/15/14	04/02/14	05/01/14	once between: 04/01/14–05/15/14	05/01/14	05/30/14	06/30/14
1st Quarter 2014 1/1/14–3/31/14	08/15/14	07/12/14	08/01/14	once between: 07/01/14–08/15/14	08/01/14	08/28/14	09/29/14
2nd Quarter 2014 4/1/14–6/30/14	11/15/14	10/01/14	11/01/14	once between: 10/01/14–11/15/14	11/01/14	11/28/14	12/29/14
3rd Quarter 2014 7/1/14–9/30/14	02/15/15	to be determined	02/01/15	once between: 01/01/15–02/15/15	02/01/15	to be determined	to be determined
4th Quarter 2014 10/1/14–12/31/14	05/15/15	to be determined	05/01/15	once between: 04/01/15–05/15/15	05/01/15	to be determined	to be determined

* **For the FY2017 hospital IQR program, the HCAHPS data would be based on discharges from January 1, 2015, through December 31, 2015.**

Note: Data must be submitted no later than 11:59 p.m. PT on the submission deadline with the exception of validation medical records, which must be received by the CDAC no later than 4:30 p.m. ET.

---

[51] https://www.qualitynet.org/

IQR Feedback Reports to Confirm Reporting Accuracy:

- CMS provides two important feedback reports for IQR-participating hospitals to review for data submissions accuracy:

  - **Hospital IQR Program Provider Participation Report:** This report is sent out the day after the submitted file is processed, which includes a calculation of the number of hospital-submitted cases by topic, hospital self-reported aggregate population and sample size count, and Medicare FFS claims by clinical topic and SCIP surgical category:

    - Hospitals are able to use this report after submission to assess their patient-level data completeness and can submit additional patient-level cases before the quarterly patient-level deadline.

  - **QIO Clinical Data Warehouse Feedback Reports:** These reports illustrate submitted data to enable hospitals to ensure that their data were submitted on time and accepted into the QIO Clinical Data Warehouse.

1.3.6 Voluntary Electronic Health Records (EHRs) IQR Reporting Option for CY2014[52]

Overview:

- In the Final FY2014 IPPS Rule, CMS stated its future intention to "require hospitals to report electronically specified quality measures." Recognizing that a significant number of IQR-participating hospitals do not currently have EHR systems that are sufficiently constructed to allow submission of required information, CMS is providing a limited EHR reporting option for discharges occurring in CY2014. For the small number of hospitals that do not yet have an existing EHR system in

---

[52] *Page 50774, Federal Register/Vol. 78, No. 160/Monday, August 19, 2013/Rules and Regulations, www.gpo.gov/fdsys/pkg/FR-2013-08-19/pdf/2013-18956.pdf*

place, chart-abstracted reporting through QualityNet will continue be required.

- As a method to provide hospitals and CMS with the ability to test systems and adjust workflow in CY2014 in order to prepare for required electronic reporting, election of the EHR reporting option is "strongly recommended" by CMS.

- Hospitals participating in the voluntary EHR IQR reporting program must report on at least **one-quarter** of CY2014 quality measures data for each measure in at least one of four IQR measure sets: STK (with the exception of measure STK-1); VTE; ED; and PC:

  o Hospitals may select any, or all, of these measure sets for EHR reporting.

  o Hospitals may select any quarter for EHR reporting and reporting for all selected measures must be reported for that same time period.

- To encourage widespread use of the EHR reporting option in CY2014, CMS has created incentives for participating hospitals:

  o No other reporting for these measures would be required in CY2014:

    ▪ CMS estimates that the participation in the CY2014 EHR reporting option will save hospitals approximately 800 hours of labor required for manual chart-abstraction as part of the hospital IQR program. At an estimated cost of $59 per hour, hospitals could save approximately $47,200.[53]

  o Hospitals can elect to have the EHR reporting of IQR measures count toward qualification of their EHR Meaningful Use stage. For consideration of reporting toward Meaningful Use determination, hospitals must report IQR measures as follows:

    ▪ Hospitals in their first year of EHR reporting that desire EHR IQR reporting to count toward their Meaningful Use

---

[53] *Pages 50957, 51034, Federal Register/Vol. 78, No. 160/Monday, August 19, 2013/Rules and Regulations, www.gpo.gov/fdsys/pkg/FR-2013-08-19/pdf/2013-18956.pdf*

determination must report CYQ1 or CYQ2 2014 data by July 1, 2014.

- Hospitals beyond their first year of EHR reporting that desire EHR IQR reporting to count toward their Meaningful Use determination must report for any of the first three quarters of CY2014 (January 2, 2014–September 30, 2014) by November 30, 2014.

- Specific submission procedures are posted on the QualityNet website at: https://www.qualitynet.org/

    o CMS has stated that it will not publicly report the electronically reported data on the Hospital Compare website.

- Hospitals choosing to report one or more of the four measure sets (STK (with the exception of STK-1), VTE, ED, and PC) electronically during CY2014 will have applicable data extracted from their certified EHR technology (CEHRT) and submitted to CMS using the Health Level Seven (HL7) Quality Reporting Document Architecture (QRDA) Category I Revision 2 standard:

    o QRDA Category I specifies the framework for quality reporting, standardizes measure-defined data elements for interoperability between organizations, and is used to transmit clinical quality measure data needed to meet Meaningful Use (MU) requirements under the Medicare EHR incentive program.

Measures for CY2014 EHR Reporting Option:

- CMS requires EHR reporting of at least one-quarter of CY2014 quality measure data for each measure in each of four hospital IQR measure sets (STK (with exception of STK-1), VTE, ED, and PC). The individual measures include:

Table 3: CY2014 Measures for EHR Reporting Option[54]

Stroke (STK)	
STK-2	Discharged on Antithrombotic Therapy
STK-3	Anticoagulation Therapy for Atrial Fibrillation/Flutter
STK-4	Thrombolytic Therapy
STK-5	Antithrombotic Therapy By End of Hospital Day 2
STK-6	Discharged on Statin Medication
STK-8	Stroke Education
STK-10	Stroke Education
Venous Thromboembolism (VTE)	
VTE-1	Venous Thromboembolism Prophylaxis
VTE-2	Intensive Care Unit Venous Thromboembolism Prophylaxis
VTE-3	Venous Thromboembolism Patients with Anticoagulation Overlap Therapy
VTE-4	Venous Thromboembolism Patients Receiving Unfractionated Heparin with Dosages/Platelet Count Monitoring by Protocol or Nomogram
VTE-5	Venous Thromboembolism Warfarin Therapy Discharge Instructions
VTE-6	Hospital-Acquired Potentially Preventable Venous Thromboembolism
Emergency Department (ED) (Listed in the Rule as "Emergency Department Throughput")	
ED-1a	Median Time from ED Arrival to ED Departure for Admitted ED Patients—Overall Rate
ED-1b	Median Time from ED Arrival to ED Departure for Admitted ED Patients—Reporting Measure
ED-1c	Median Time from ED Arrival to ED Departure for Admitted ED Patients—Observation Patients
ED-1d	Median Time from ED Arrival to ED Departure for Admitted ED Patients—Psychiatric/Mental Health Patients
ED-2a	Admit Decision Time to ED Departure Time for Admitted Patients—Overall Rate
ED-2b	Admit Decision Time to ED Departure Time for Admitted Patients—Reporting Measure
ED-2c	Admit Decision Time to ED Departure Time for Admitted Patients—Psychiatric/Mental Health Patients
Perinatal Care	
PC-01	Elective Delivery Prior to 39 Completed Weeks Gestation: Percentage of Babies Electively Delivered Prior to 39 Completed Weeks Gestation

---

[54] *Pages 50806–50808, Federal Register/Vol. 78, No. 160/Monday, August 19, 2013/Rules and Regulations, www.gpo.gov/fdsys/pkg/FR-2013-08-19/pdf/2013-18956.pdf*

1.3.7 CY2014 Measures Requiring Web-Based Hospital Entry Reporting

- Data entry for specified measures is achieved through the secure side of QualityNet.org via an online tool available to authorized users.

- For the CY2014 reporting year, there are six individual measures contained in three measure sets that require web-based entry reporting:

MEASURE SET	NUMBER OF MEASURES
Structural Measures	4
DACA	1
Perinatal Care	1

Table 4: CY2014 Measures Requiring Web-Based Hospital Entry[55]

MEASURES REQUIRING WEB-BASED HOSPITAL ENTRY
Structural Measures
Participation in a Systematic Database for Cardiac Surgery
Participation in a Systematic Clinical Database Registry for Stroke Care
Participation in a Systematic Clinical Database Registry for Nursing Sensitive Care
Participation in a Systematic Clinical Database Registry for General Surgery
Data Accuracy and Completeness Acknowledgement
Data Accuracy and Completeness Acknowledgement
Perinatal Care
PC-01 Elective Delivery Prior to 39 Completed Weeks Gestation: Percentage of Babies Electively Delivered Prior to 39 Completed Weeks Gestation

*For reporting timeline, see Table 2 above.

---

[55] *QualityNet, Measure Comparison (Inpatient Hospital Quality Measures),
http://www.qualitynet.org/dcs/ContentServer?pagename=QnetPublic%2FPage%2FQnetTier2&cid=1141662756099*

CY2014 Web-Based Entry Reporting Timeline:

- Reporting for web-based entry measures is accomplished through tools provided on an individual hospital's MyQualityNet account.

- Web-based entry data is reported for a time period occurring two years prior to the program year and requires annual submission by May 15 of the year preceding the program year.

- CY2014 web-based entry reporting deadlines are as follows:

Table 5: CY2014 Web-Based Entry Measures Reporting Timeline:

MEASURE(S) REQUIREMENT	ANNUAL PAYMENT UPDATE FISCAL YEAR	DATES/ QUARTERS INCLUDED	SUBMISSION PERIOD/ DEADLINE
DACA	FY2016	January 1, 2014- December 31, 2014	April 1, 2015- May 15, 2015

1.3.8 CY2014 Measures CMS-Extracted From Claims

General:

CMS uses enrollment data as well as Medicare Parts A and B claims for Medicare FFS patients to calculate claims-based measures. No hospital data submission is required.

- For CY2014 reporting, CMS will extract data for six measures sets, including:

  - 30-Day Risk-Standardized Mortality (AMI, HF, PN, and COPD)

  - 30-Day Risk-Standardized Readmission (AMI, HF, COPD, STK, Hip/Knee Readmissions, PN, and Hospital-Wide All-Cause Unplanned Readmission (HWR)) o AHRQ Patient Safety Indicators (PSI) Composite Measures (PSI-90)

o AHRQ PSI and Nursing Sensitive Harmonized Measure

o Surgical Complications

o Cost Efficiency

Measures:

For CY2014, seventeen individual measures are CMS-extracted from claims data from different time periods, as specified in the IPPS Final Rules:

Table 6: CY2014 Measures CMS-Extracted From Claims[56]

MEASURES THAT ARE CMS-EXTRACTED FROM CLAIMS DATA FOR PROGRAM YEAR FY2016	
Mortality Measures (Medicare Patients)	
MORT-30-AMI	Acute Myocardial Infarction (AMI) 30-Day Mortality Rate
MORT-30-HF	Heart Failure (HF) 30-Day Mortality Rate
MORT-30-PN	Pneumonia (PN) 30-Day Mortality Rate
MORT-30-COPD	Chronic Obstructive Pulmonary Disease (COPD) 30-Day Mortality Rate
MORT-30-STK	Acute Ischemic Stroke (STK) 30-Day Mortality Rate
Readmission Measures (Medicare patients)	
READM-30-AMI	Acute Myocardial Infarction (AMI) 30-Day Readmission Rate
READM-30-HF	Heart Failure (HF) 30-Day Readmission Rate
READM-30-PN	Pneumonia (PN) 30-Day Readmission Rate
Hip/Knee Readmission	Hospital-Level 30-Day All-Cause Risk-Standardized Readmission Rate (RSRR) Following Elective Total Hip Arthroplasty (THA)/Total Knee Arthroplasty (TKA)
HWR	Hospital-Wide All-Cause Unplanned Readmission (HWR)
READM-30-COPD	Chronic Obstructive Pulmonary Disease (COPD) 30-Day Readmission Rate
READM-30-STK	Stroke (STK) 30-Day Readmission Rate
Agency for Healthcare Research and Quality (AHRQ) Measures	

---

[56] *QualityNet, Measure Comparison (Inpatient Hospital Quality Measures),
http://www.qualitynet.org/dcs/ContentServer?pagename=QnetPublic%2FPage%2FQnetTier2&cid
=1141662756099*

PSI-90	Complication/Patient Safety for Selected Indicators (PSI composite). PSIs in the composite display in the downloadable file on the Hospital Compare website: PSI-6 Latrogenic Pneumothorax PSI-12 Postoperative PE or DVT PSI-14 Postoperative Wound Dehiscence PSI-15 Accidental Puncture or Laceration
AHRQ PSI and Nursing Sensitive Care	
PSI-4	Death Among Surgical Patients with Serious Treatable Complications (Harmonized with Nursing Sensitive Care Measure, Failure to Rescue)
Surgical Complications	
Hip/Knee Complications	Hip/Knee Complications Hospital-Level Risk-Standardized Complication Rate (RSCR) Following Elective Primary Total Hip Arthroplasty (THA) and Total Knee Arthroplasty (TKA)
Cost Efficiency Measures	
	Medicare Spending per Beneficiary (MSPB)
	Acute Myocardial Infarction (AMI) Payment per Episode of Care

New for FY2016: Acute Myocardial Infarction (AMI) Payment per Episode of Care:[57]

- There is evidence of variation in payments at hospitals for AMI patients; mean thirty-day risk-standardized payment among Medicare FFS patients ages sixty-five or older hospitalized for AMI in 2008 was $20,207, and ranged from $15,521 to $27,317 across 1,846 hospitals. Because CMS already collects data on AMI mortality and readmissions, a determination of the association between AMI episode payments and quality/outcome measure is of great interest.

- CMS is seeking to align the AMI payment per episode of care measure with the existing AMI mortality and readmissions measures to capture payments for Medicare patients across all care settings, services, and supplies, except for Medicare Part D (that is, inpatient, outpatient, skilled nursing facility, home health, hospice, physician/clinical laboratory/ ambulance services, supplier Medicare Part B items, and durable medical equipment, prosthetics/orthotics, and supplies).

- The AMI payment measure assesses the hospital risk-standardized payment associated with a thirty-day episode of care for AMI for any non-

---

[57] Pages 50802–50805, Federal Register/Vol. 78, No. 160/Monday, August 19, 2013/Rules and Regulations, www.gpo.gov/fdsys/pkg/FR-2013-08-19/pdf/2013-18956.pdf

federal acute care hospital. The measure includes Medicare FFS patients ages sixty-five or older admitted for an AMI and calculates payments for these patients over a thirty-day episode of care, beginning with the index admission.

Time Periods for CMS Claims-Based Extracted Data Collection:

- Effectively determining performance for many of the CMS claims-extracted measures is made difficult when a small number of cases are reported. This is particularly problematic for smaller hospitals.

- To ensure an adequate number of cases for assessment of mortality, readmissions, surgical complication, and AHRQ patient safety measures, CMS uses a multiyear measurement period.

- By collecting a larger number of cases, CMS hopes to improve the precision of the estimation of each hospital's mortality, readmission, and complication measure results and thus identify outliers in hospital performance.

- Based on CMS assessment of a reasonable time period needed to gather a sufficient number of cases for each measure set to determine accurate measure performance across a range of participating hospitals, different measure set reporting time periods have been established:

  o The Thirty-Day Mortality and Thirty-Day Readmissions data for individual clinical conditions use a thirty-six-month reporting period ending prior to January 1 of the program year.

  o The AHRQ has determined that a twenty-four-month reporting period is sufficient for determination of the PSI data.

  o Surgical Complications are assessed using a thirty-three-month reporting period.

- Because the HWR measure is calculated using almost all Medicare FFS admissions, an adequate number of cases may be obtained in a single year and the data collection period is limited to twelve months.

- Data for the MSPB cost efficiency measure is reported for the twelve-month period immediately preceding the program year.

- The cost efficiency measure of AMI Cost per Episode of Care is aligned with the Thirty-Day Mortality and Readmissions measures and a thirty-six-month reporting period is also used, ending prior to January. 1 of the program year.

- The collection periods for CMS claims-extracted data supporting program years FY2014, FY2015, and FY2016 are as follows:

Table 7: CMS Claims-Extracted Data[58] Time Periods for Program Years FY2014–FY2016[59]

MEASURE SET	PROGRAM YEAR	DATA TIME FRAME
READMISSIONS, MORTALITY	FY2014	July 1, 2010–June 30, 2013
	FY2015	July 1, 2011–June 30, 2014
	FY2016	July 1, 2012–June 30, 2015
HOSPITAL-WIDE READMISSIONS (HWR)	FY2014	July 1, 2012–June 30, 2013
	FY2015	July 1, 2013–June 30, 2014
	FY2016	July 1, 2014–June 30, 2015
SURGICAL COMPLICATIONS	FY2014	July 1, 2010–March 31, 2013
	FY2015	July 1, 2011–March 31, 2014
	FY2016	July 1, 2012–March 31, 2015
AHRQ MEASURES	FY2014	July 1, 2011–June 30, 2013
	FY2015	July 1, 2012–June 30, 2014
	FY2016	July 1, 2013–June 30, 2014
COST EFFICIENCY MEASURES:		
Medicare Spend Per Beneficiary	FY2014	Jan. 1, 2013–Dec. 31, 2013
	FY2015	Jan. 1, 2014–Dec. 31, 2014
	FY2016	Jan. 1, 2015–Dec. 31, 2015
AMI Payment per Episode	FY2016	July 1, 2012–June 30, 2015

[58] http://www.cms.gov/Medicare/Quality-Initiatives-Patient-Assessment-Instruments/HospitalQualityInits/Measure-Methodology.html

[59] Medicare Hospital Quality Chartbook 2012, http://cms.gov/Medicare/Quality-Initiatives-Patient-Assessment-Instruments/HospitalQualityInits/Downloads/MedicareHospitalQualityChartbook2012.pdf

1.3.9 IQR Conclusion

- In the FY2014 Final IPPS Rule, CMS implemented changes that were aimed at improving the timelines and efficiency of the hospital IQR program. Through suspension, removal, or refinement of measures, CMS continues to demonstrate a commitment to ensuring that reported measures are relevant to the provision of quality care. In addition, as part of an ongoing effort to streamline administrative processes, CMS is allowing hospitals the option of reporting up to four measures sets through their EHR systems for CY2014.

- It is clear that the future direction of the hospital IQR program will involve greater utilization of electronic reporting to further reduce the labor-associated reporting burden on hospitals. Such a progression will, no doubt, be accompanied by increased data reporting requirements and shortened time frames.

- The resulting information will provide more timely feedback to providers and be utilized to create more robust value-based reimbursement programs. Through public reporting of captured metrics on the Hospital Compare website, consumers will be provided with an ever-expanding view of hospital health care quality.

Section 1.4: Appendix

1.4.1 Acronym Guide

ACA.............................Affordable Care Act of 2010

AHA.............................American Hospital Association

AHRQ ....Agency for Healthcare Research and Quality

AIDS............................Acquired Immune Deficiency Syndrome

AMI.............................Acute Myocardial Infarction

APU.............................Annual Payment Update

ASCQR ....Ambulatory Surgical Center Quality Reporting

CAH ....Critical Access Hospitals

CAP.............................Community-Acquired Pneumonia

CAUTI ....Catheter-Associated Urinary Tract Infection

CDAD..........................Clostridium Difficile-Associated Disease

CDC ....Centers for Disease Control and Prevention

CEO ....Chief Executive Officer

CLABSI ....Central Line-Associated Bloodstream Infection

CMS ....Centers for Medicare & Medicaid Services

COPD..........................Chronic Obstructive Pulmonary Disease

CY ....Calendar Year

DACA ....Data Accuracy and Completeness Acknowledgement

DRA ....Deficit Reduction Act of 2005, Public Law 109–171

DRG ....Diagnosis-Related Group

ED ....Emergency Department

EHR ....Electronic Health Record

EMTLA.......................Emergency Medical Treatment and Labor Act

EO ....Executive Order

FY...............................Fiscal Year

HAC ....Hospital-Acquired Conditions Reduction Program

HC ....Hospital Compare

HCAHPS....................Hospital Consumer Assessment of Healthcare Providers and Systems

HF ....Heart Failure

HH QRP	Home Health Quality Reporting Program
HHS	Department of Health and Human Services
HIQR	Hospital Inpatient Quality Reporting
HMO	Health Maintenance Organizations
HOP QDRP	Hospital Outpatient Quality Data Reporting Program (now OQR)
HQA	Hospital Quality Alliance
HQI	Hospital Quality Initiative
HQRP	Hospice Quality Reporting Program
HRRP	Hospital Readmission Reduction Program
HVBP	Hospital Value-Based Purchasing Program
HWR	Hospital-Wide Readmission (Hospital-Wide All-Cause Unplanned Readmission)
ICU	Intensive Care Unit
IMM	Immunizations
IOM	Institute of Medicine
IPF	Inpatient Psychiatric Facility
IPFQR	Inpatient Psychiatric Facility Quality Reporting
IPPS	Inpatient Prospective Payment System [Acute Care Hospital]
IQI	Inpatient Quality Indicators
IQR	Inpatient Quality Reporting
IRF	Inpatient Rehabilitation Facility
IRF QRP	Inpatient Rehabilitation Facility Quality Reporting Program
LTCH	Long-Term Care Hospital
LTCHQR	Long-Term Care Hospital Quality Reporting
MIPPA	Medicare Improvements for Patients and Providers Act of 2008, Public Law 110–275
MMA	Medicare Prescription Drug, Improvement, and Modernization Act of 2003
MRSA	Methicillin-Resistant Staphylococcus Aureus
NCQA	National Committee for Quality Assurance
NHQI	Nursing Home Quality Initiative
NHSN	National Health Safety Network
NQF	National Quality Forum
NQS	National Quality Strategy
NVHRI	National Voluntary Hospital Reporting Initiative

OMB......................... Executive Office of Management and Budget

OQR......................... Outpatient Quality Reporting (formerly HOP QDRP)

PC .... Perinatal Care

PCH .... PPS-Exempt Cancer Hospital

PN .... Pneumonia

PPS .... Prospective Payment System

PQRS....................... Physician Quality Reporting System

PSI .... Patient Safety Indicators

PTCA .... Percutaneous Transluminal Coronary Angioplasty

QIO .... Quality Improvement Organization

RHQDAPU .... Reporting Hospital Quality Data for Annual Payment Update
(now known as IQR)

SCIP......................... Surgical Care Improvement Project

SOW .... Statement of Work

SSI .... Surgical Site Infection

STK .... Stroke

TBD.......................... To Be Determined

THA.......................... Total Hip Arthroplasty

TKA .... Total Knee Arthroplasty

VBP.......................... Value-Based Purchasing

VTE .... Venous Thromboembolism

CHAPTER 2

The Hospital Value-Based Purchasing (HVBP) Program

Section 2.1: Flash Read!

For years, the Centers for Medicare & Medicaid Services (CMS) has been encouraging hospitals to report data on selected measures of quality. In the early 2000s, hospital quality reporting was voluntary; by 2004, CMS made data reporting mandatory, and hospitals that failed to comply received financial penalties. Starting in October 2012, as a result of the Affordable Care Act (ACA), CMS launched the new Hospital Value-Based Purchasing (HVBP) Program. Through this program, Medicare ties hospitals' Medicare reimbursement not only to quality reporting, but to hospital performance as well. The HVBP program is designed to assess the *value* (quality+cost) of inpatient care provided to Medicare beneficiaries.

- The HVBP program is mandated to be "budget-neutral." To ensure that anticipated incentives are fully offset by penalty amounts, each year CMS deducts a percentage of a participating hospital's per-discharge base operating Diagnosis-Related Group (DRG) rate to fund a national HVBP incentive pool. This "withhold" percentage is 1.25 percent for

FY2014 and escalates at .25 percent per year to a maximum of 2 percent by FY2017. Poor HVBP performance can result in the loss of some or all of the withheld reimbursement.

- Using information reported through the hospital Inpatient Quality Reporting (IQR) program, hospital performance is evaluated against specific metrics. Based on their performance, hospitals may earn positive or negative adjustments to their per-discharge base operating DRG rates, which are applied during a given HVBP program year.

- HVBP payments for FY2014 are determined by how hospitals scored on three sets of measures:

   1. The first set included thirteen "process" measures that rate how often hospitals adhered to clinical guidelines for activities such as selecting the correct antibiotic for pneumonia patients, controlling blood sugar in heart surgery patients, and averting catheter infections.

   2. The second set included eight measures selected from satisfaction surveys of patients who had recently left the hospital. For these measures, CMS only looked at the percent of patients who said they "always" had a favorable experience in certain areas, such as how well doctors and nurses communicated with patients, how well caregivers managed patients' pain, and how clean and quiet the hospital room and hall were.

   3. The third set evaluated mortality rates among Medicare patients admitted for heart attack, heart failure, or pneumonia. For each, CMS determined a hospital's risk-adjusted mortality rate for patients who died while in the hospital or within thirty days after leaving.

- The HVBP scoring methodology involves awarding "**achievement**" (performance against targeted benchmarks) or "**improvement**" points for each measure within the domains. For determining the total domain scores, CMS will use the higher of the achievement or improvement score. Such points are earned by comparing performance against specific measures during a **baseline** reporting period to a specific performance reporting period.

- A **Total Performance Score (TPS)** is obtained by summing total weighted domain scores. This score is then converted to a **Payment Adjustment Factor (PAF)** through the use of an annually established conversion factor.

- CMS simultaneously applies the annual HVBP withhold percentage and the HVBP PAF to a hospital's base operating DRG rate in determining the net FY2014 per-discharge rate. This calculation is made without regard to other pay-for-performance initiatives, such as the Hospital Readmissions Reduction Program (HRRP).

- HVBP participating hospitals receive a **Percentage Payment Summary Report** sixty days prior to the start of the fiscal year identified as a HVBP program year. This report contains detailed scoring data, as well as the TPS and PAF. However, participants *are not* provided information on the actual dollar amount of earned incentives or assessed penalties.

- →TAKE NOTE! Performance measures reported under the IQR for CY2014 will be included in HVBP program years FY2016–FY2019 for measures in either the baseline or performance reporting periods.

- By statute, CMS cannot add measures to the HVBP program until they have been reportable in the IQR program and posted on the Hospital Compare website for at least one year. The following CMS claims-extracted measures have been added to the IQR program for reporting in CY2014 and could be added to the HVBP program as early as FY2017:

MEASURES	EXTRACTED FROM CLAIMS
30-day mortality for stroke and chronic obstructive pulmonary disease (COPD)	7/1/12–6/30/15
Acute myocardial infarction (AMI) payment per episode of care	7/1/12–6/30/15

FY2014 HVBP Program Year Summary

- 2,730 hospitals received per-discharge HVBP PAFs:
  - ↑1,255 (46 percent) received a PAF>1.0, indicating a net increase (incentive) in per-discharge rates.

- With the conversion of the PAF into a per-discharge incentive payment, the Arkansas Heart Hospital received the largest positive adjustment at +.88 percent per discharge.

  o ↓1,473 (54 percent) received a PAF<1.0, indicating a net decrease (penalty) in per-discharge rates.

  - The largest per-discharge penalty was assessed against the Gallup Indian Medical Center at -1.14 percent.

FINANCIAL ESTIMATES BASED ON FY2014 HVBP PAF	
$1.1 billion	CMS estimate of the national HVBP incentive pool
$400,000	average HVBP per hospital withhold amount
$1.7 million	largest estimated HVBP increase for one hospital
$545,000	largest estimated HVBP decrease for one hospital

Section 2.2:
Provider Perspectives

After many decades as a largely passive payer of medical services for its beneficiaries, Medicare is in the process of pivoting toward a policy of obtaining more value for the dollars it spends. The National Quality Strategy (NQS) of the Department of Health and Human Services (HHS) directs CMS to simultaneously improve outcomes for individuals and populations while lowering costs. Of the numerous tools that Congress has granted CMS during the past eight years, value-based purchasing has the potential to be among the most transformational.[60]

2.2.1 Rationale

In 2013, the United States spent $2,915 billion on national health expenditures, or 18 percent of gross national product, according to estimates by the CMS Office of the Actuary. Of that, $929 billion, or 31.9 percent of the total, was spent on hospitals. No other category of spending comes close. Physician and clinical services comprised $589 billion, prescription drugs were $262 billion, nursing homes cost $157 billion, and structures and equipment amounted to $114 billion.[61]

If the goal is to make health care more efficient, hospital care is the obvious place to start. Did the ACA set out to target hospitals specifically? "That's hard to say," said Robert Lazerow, of The Advisory Group. "But as Willie Sutton, the bank robber, used to say, 'that's where the money is.'"[62]

---

[60] Jordan VanLare and Patrick Conway, "Value-Based Purchasing—National Programs to Move from Volume to Value," New England Journal of Medicine, 367:4, July 26, 2012, http://www.nejm.org/doi/full/10.1056/NEJMp1204939

[61] Gigi A. Cuckler, et al., "National Health Expenditure Projections, 2012–22: Slow Growth Until Coverage Expands and Economy Improves," Health Affairs, October 2013, http://content.healthaffairs.org/content/32/10/1820

[62] Robert Lazerow, telephone interview, November 25, 2013

A world of avoidable costs is buried inside the US hospital industry. The regional variations in spending and practice patterns revealed in *The Dartmouth Atlas* are just one source of data on how much excess spending could be wrung out if CMS and commercial insurers got serious about the issue. It's widely understood that there is little oversight or control over hospital spending,[63] and that patients are probably over-tested and over-treated in many of the country's hospitals.[64]

The ACA required CMS to create the HVBP program, building on quality reporting programs already in place such as Inpatient Quality Reporting (IQR) and the Hospital Consumer Assessment of Healthcare Providers and Systems (HCAHPS). IQR, developed in 2003, was the first step to get all providers to report quality measures in a standard format. Most organizations have been reporting successfully for a number of years.

Because Congress insisted that most provisions of the ACA be budget-neutral (that is, not oblige any higher federal spending), the HVBP program takes with one hand and gives back with the other. CMS creates a national HVBP incentive pool by withholding a percentage of each participating hospital's per-discharge reimbursement. Using these funds, the best-performing hospitals will receive incentive reimbursements and those performing poorly stand to lose. In essence, hospitals compete for the total pool of HVBP incentive funds. Roughly half the hospitals will earn back all withheld funds, or more, and half will lose some or all of what they contributed to the national incentive pool.

2.2.2 Summary

Starting in FY2013, hospitals covered by prospective payment saw their base rates decline by 1 percent, to create a pool of $963 million, or $311,448 per hospital, that could be redistributed according to results of the value-based purchasing initiative. In the program's second year, starting October 1, 2013,

---

[63] Elizabeth Rosenthal, "As Hospital Prices Soar, a Stitch Tops $500," *The New York Times*, December 3, 2013, http://www.nytimes.com/2013/12/03/health/as-hospital-costs-soar-single-stitch-tops-500.html

[64] Shannon Brownlee, *Overtreated: Why Too Much Medicine is Making Us Sicker and Poorer.* Bloomsbury, 2007.

Medicare reduced payments to 1,451 hospitals and raised payments to 1,231 hospitals.

The withholds are scheduled to rise by .25 percent each year from 2014 through 2017, when the top rate of 2 percent will be reached.

The domains for scoring started with clinical process of care and patient experience of care for the FY2013 reimbursement period. In FY2014, an outcome measure, mortality, is being added. In FY2015, the array of domains will expand considerably. Measures of patient safety, as well as hospital-acquired infections (central-line associated bloodstream infections (CLABSI)) are being added to the Outcomes Domain. For the first time, CMS will consider efficiency (Medicare spending per beneficiary) as a key domain. Each successive year, additional measures will be added to each category of evaluation.

2.2.3 Current State

Hospitals are already well into the FY2016 HVBP program. The baseline period for reporting clinical process of care (IQR) and patient experiences of care (HCAHPS) began January 1, 2012 and ended December 31, 2012. Based on those results, CMS set benchmark standards as the mean of the top decile (tenth) of scores in that starting period.

Hospital attainment during a "performance period" for the FY2016 program year (January 1, 2014–December 31, 2014) is used to find out how much improvement over the baseline period has been achieved and to see how each hospital compares to its national cohort.

"We have gotten our data back" from CMS, said Marcia Delk, MD, senior vice president for safety, quality and credentialing, and chief quality officer at WellStar, a five-hospital system in Atlanta. "It's a mixed bag, depending on which hospital you're looking at. We're not yet where we want to be—in the top decile."

In 2005 and 2006, ahead of the federal government's quality and pay-for-value push, WellStar set itself a goal of delivering highly reliable, high-quality world-class care. It developed metrics associated with each priority area and decided to focus on eliminating preventable harm and on delivering evidence-based medicine. During the subsequent five years, it made enormous progress toward these goals.[65]

In that time, WellStar has seen the virtual elimination of hospital-acquired conditions (HACs), such as Stage III and Stage IV pressure ulcers (rate of zero at all hospitals) and health care-associated infections (HAIs), such as Central Line Associated Bloodstream Infections (CLABSI), ventilator-associated pneumonia (VAP), and methicillin-resistant staph bacteremia. Additionally, across the system there has been an 85 percent reduction in health care-associated clostridium difficile-associated disease (CDAD) infections and an 84 percent reduction in safety events, using Healthcare Performance Improvement's SSER (Serious Safety Event Rate) classification methodology. These improvements and others have resulted in a 20 percent reduction in the overall system mortality rate, which is equivalent to approximately 3,500 lives saved.[66]

WellStar's previous work prepared it to adapt to the new regime for Medicare reimbursement. "There is alignment there which should lead to delivering that value equation, of quality over cost," Delk said. "We should be in a position to be successful in the changing reimbursement system."

Based on the results from CMS, WellStar has been able to prioritize its efforts. "The patient experience component is an area where we recognize we have some more work to do," Delk said. We did some significant work on readmissions reduction, but it was not enough to avoid a penalty. With additional improvements, we essentially eliminated the penalty the second year."

The devil is in the details. A hospital's quality positioning within the new framework depends on which statistics CMS chooses to highlight and how it applies them. "We struggle with, is there accuracy in the administrative data, and are the metrics available currently relevant?" Delk said.

WellStar has found that clinical registries—databases of health information on specific clinical conditions, procedures or populations—often offer more actionable data than administrative data, which many of the CMS metrics are based on. With the clinical registries, "you're actually getting into the chart and

---

[65] *Marcia Delk, MD, telephone interview, December 4, 2013.*
[66] *Statistics provided by Marcia Delk, MD*

understanding the clinical condition of the patient and the risk adjustments, and a true value."

However, clinical data registries rely on the skills of a clinician who can dig into the chart and understand the terminology and decision-making. Administrative data is easier to accumulate, especially using an electronic health record that automatically scoops up the relevant data points and forwards them to CMS with minimal human intervention.

WellStar has been aided in its journey by James L. Reinertsen, MD, a veteran of the Institute for Healthcare Improvement who now works as a consultant with leadership teams at health systems around the country. Reinertsen believes US hospitals have made enormous strides on error prevention and quality enhancement since the 1990s, especially around process measures. "People have gotten better at them," he said.[67]

When the idea of measuring quality first gathered steam, most metrics were basic process measures—things such as whether aspirin was given on the first day after a heart attack or whether oxygen levels were checked in a pneumonia patient. In those days the average hospital scored around 50 percent. "Every hospital in America is close to 100 percent now," Reinertsen said.

With the HVBP program, CMS now is placing hospitals into ten ranked cohorts, or deciles. Only the highest-performing two deciles—the top 20 percent—win the claw-back in Medicare reimbursements. Yet from a scoring perspective, the top two deciles of hospitals now effectively attain between 95 percent and 100 percent on almost every measure; the bottom deciles are around 92 percent to 95 percent.

"Most clinicians would agree with this: that when hospitals went from 50 percent to 95 percent, it made a big difference in patient care. There is no evidence that going from 95 percent to 99 percent makes any clinical difference," even though that may traverse the distance from worst decile to best decile, Reinertsen said.

The most effective way to close the gap is to double down on coding and documentation, and to introduce extra checks, at high cost, to push toward 100 percent. If a major hospital system stands to gain a million dollars if it moves from the fourth decile to the second, then hospital administrators will move

---

[67] *James L. Reinertsen, MD, telephone interview, November 25, 2013.*

heaven and earth to grab that extra reimbursement, knowing full well it makes no difference in real patient-care quality.

"There is an enormous amount of effort to get into the top two deciles. That's the only place you get a kicker in the payment," Reinertsen said. "If I have a problem with the current formulation of these measures for value-based purchasing, it's that the gap between worst and best performers has closed so dramatically. All the improvement that is likely to occur on the clinical end from these measures has already occurred. At what point do we say, enough is enough, let's move on?"

The trouble with this misdirected attention on small degrees of meaningless improvement is that other things of greater importance are being ignored, Reinertsen said. Things that would really affect patient outcomes, such as complications from robotic surgery, are simply not being measured.

Robert A. Berenson, MD, is another health policy analyst who thinks CMS hasn't hit the target on what measures it requires hospitals to report. In a medical journal article, he decried "the misapplication of performance measurement" insofar as it has been imposed on physicians. The measures that doctors are obligated to report and be graded on don't necessarily reflect their diagnostic or therapeutic skill, he has argued.[68]

"I'm not throwing in the towel on measures, I just think we should use them more opportunistically and strategically," he said. "It doesn't mean we can't use measures to solve problems." For instance, there is good literature showing that patients in the hospital die more often on weekends. "That is unacceptable."[69]

Some of the measures are constructive, such as keeping track of the length of time from a cardiac patient's arrival in the emergency room to a balloon angioplasty, Berenson said. What is really needed, though, are more metrics of core competencies that affect outcomes. Those are harder to construct, collect and evaluate. It is very difficult to assess the technical skill of a surgeon, for example, even though that would be one of the main objectives of an outcomes-based quality regimen.

[68] Robert A. Berenson, MD, and Deborah R. Kaye, MD, "Grading a Physician's Value—The Misapplication of Performance Measurement," New England Journal of Medicine, 369:2079–2081, November 28, 2013, http://www.nejm.org/doi/full/10.1056/NEJMp1312287

[69] Robert A. Berenson, MD, telephone interview, September 17, 2013.

Recently, though, a study was published that did exactly that. John D. Birkmeyer, MD, and the Michigan Bariatric Surgery Collaborative invited twenty surgeons to submit videotapes of their best laparoscopic gastric bypass. A team of ten peer surgeons evaluated the tapes for technical proficiency. The scores of technical competency varied widely, from 2.6 to 4.8 on a 5-point scale. The evaluators found that the bottom quartile was associated with higher complication rates (14.5 percent vs. 5.2 percent) and higher mortality (0.26 percent vs. 0.05 percent). The lowest quartile of surgeons also took longer in the operating room (137 minutes vs. 98 minutes), had higher rates of reoperation (3.4 percent vs. 1.6 percent), and had higher rates of readmission (6.3 percent vs. 2.7 percent). The study concluded that "peer rating of operative skill may be an effective strategy for assessing a surgeon's proficiency."[70]

This is a big advance over "Did you give the patient an aspirin?" or "Did you administer pre-operative antibiotics?" As the health care quality movement goes forward, these kinds of studies may pave a road toward more precise measures linking physician and hospital performance to real patient outcomes, and may eventually be included in the CMS data sets.

For the time being, however, many hospitals are still stuck in the logjam of trying to demonstrate that they compare favorably to most of their peer group, in quality, patient satisfaction, and use of resources. "My view is that health care leaders waste far too much energy on 'How do we compare to others?'" Reinertsen said, likening it to the Bowl Championship Series for college football. "Patients would be better served if we all focused on measurements that asked two questions: 1) Are we getting better? and 2) What's the gap between our current performance and the theoretical ideal?" Hospitals should be encouraged to improve from their own baselines and stop worrying about what the other guys are doing, he thinks. The CMS strategy pushes in the other direction.

W. Edwards Deming, the father of the quality improvement movement, wrote that three ways exist to achieve a better number: 1) improve the system; 2) sub-optimize the system, that is, achieve the number at the cost of some other more important number that may or may not get measured; and 3) cheat.

---

[70] John D. Birkmeyer, MD, et al., "Surgical Skill and Complication Rates after Bariatric Surgery, New England Journal of Medicine 369:15. October 10, 2013, http://www.nejm.org/doi/full/10.1056/NEJMsa1300625

"I think the larger value-based purchasing measures will result in sub-optimization of the system—effort that doesn't improve anything," Reinertsen said.

Delk, of WellStar, is aware of which parts of the HVBP program may be subject to gaming and which are not. "The patient experience metrics are collected externally by a vendor, so there's little room to game that," she said. "Core measures are supported by electronic record, so you'd have difficulty there. Some of the added measures, such as patient safety indicators, those are currently a combination of care- and coding-dependent. That's where everybody is concerned about the risk of variation on how well are you documenting."

The lodestar for true value in health care would be to consider metrics from the patient's perspective, Delk continued. "They're looking for functional outcomes, where they have a high level of function, minimal complications, and good success rates. A lot of the metrics now being used on a national level are not being focused on that."

Keith M. Starke, MD, chairman of the department of medicine at Mercy Hospital in St. Louis, agrees that many of the data submission requirements don't really impact patient care. "A lot of it is claims-based data, related to how accurate is your coding. It's not particularly rigorous on what actually occurred in patients," he said.[71] Chasing down the nuances of fundamentally unimportant metrics is counterproductive and frustrating to the medical staff. He is looking forward to the day when CMS will allow more submissions from clinical registries, whose metrics are built around more meaningful measures. In December 2013, CMS did respond to these calls by partially opening the door to increased use of registries in reporting data.

2.2.4 The Road Ahead

So far hospitals have been evaluated on clinical processes of care, patient experiences of care, and mortality. Their reimbursement for FY2014 is already being affected by their data from 2009 to 2012. Their performance data from 2012–2013 is the basis for reimbursement in FY2015. An AHRQ composite score for patient safety indicators and CLABSI infections has been added, plus

---

[71] *Keith M. Starke, MD, telephone interview, September 12, 2013.*

a score for efficiency, based on Medicare spending per beneficiary. More measures will be added through FY2019. The weightings gradually tilt away from clinical processes of care and toward outcomes and efficiency.

Despite the misgivings of physicians, hospital leaders, and quality experts, pay-for-performance and value-based purchasing are likely to continue and be enhanced in the coming years. It has "enormous face validity and ideological support even if success to date has been modest and the optimal program configuration is unclear," wrote Arnold M. Epstein, MD, of the Harvard School of Public Health.[72]

Ralph E. Lawson, chief financial officer of Baptist Health South Florida, a $2.3 billion system of six hospitals in Miami, thinks his hospitals will do "extremely well" under value-based purchasing "or anything that rewards quality."

"We have thought a lot about this. We are a higher cost organization than most of our competitors, but we really do focus on patients' experience and quality," Lawson said. "You create a pool of money by taking money away from everybody, and the winners get more than their share back."[73]

What worries him is getting the system's costs down to a lower level. It takes money to focus on quality, which means "more talented labor forces, better machinery." He is working closely with private insurance companies to ensure that, as patient census declines in the coming years, the hospital shares in the savings. As the overall incentives from CMS convert from fee-for-service—a system in which more patients and procedures mean more revenue—to pay-for-value, in which admissions decline as primary care expands to keep people out of the hospital, Lawson is paying close attention to the actual financial rewards for the hospital system's investments in quality.

It will be a few years yet before we know whether HVBP will work as designed, said Harvard researcher Ashish K. Jha, MD. "But what we do know is that two years into the program, certain hospitals seem to be doing well and others, not so much," he wrote in a blog post.[74] Notably, public hospitals and safety-net hospitals—those with high disproportionate share payments—generally do

---

[72] Arnold M. Epstein, MD, "Will Pay for Performance Improve Quality of Care? The Answer Is in the Details," *New England Journal of Medicine*, 367:19. November 8, 2012, http://www.nejm.org/doi/full/10.1056/NEJMe1212133

[73] Ralph E. Lawson, telephone interview, November 7, 2013.

[74] Ashish K. Jha, MD, "An Update on Value-Based Purchasing: Year 2," November 19, 2013, at https://blogs.sph.harvard.edu/ashish-jha/an-update-on-value-based-purchasing-year-2/

worse. "We don't know why," Jha wrote, but he suspects that the difference is driven by differences in patient experience scores. "Is it that poorer or minority patients are just less likely to give high scores on patient experience? Or are safety-net hospitals not doing as good of a job on patient-centered care?"

Robert Wachter, MD, a hospitalist and quality expert at the University of California-San Francisco, wondered in a comment whether safety-net hospitals "should be compared only against each other rather than against all hospitals." We don't want to give them a pass, yet we also need to acknowledge that their patient population and lack of resources are creating "an unlevel playing field," he remarked.

These are the kinds of questions that will inevitably be raised as value-based purchasing gains a historical record and trendline. Many issues that were previously not visible to physicians, hospital leaders, and payers will gradually come into the light, and have to be addressed.

Section 2.3: Technical Appendix: Hospital Value-Based Purchasing Program (HVBP)

2.3.1 HVBP Background

- With the implementation of the Hospital Inpatient Quality Reporting (IQR) initiative in 2005, CMS began laying the groundwork for the HVBP program through a series of initiatives aimed at encouraging hospitals and physicians to improve patient care quality and to better inform consumers through quality of care data reporting.

- The HVBP program was mandated under section 3001 of the ACA of 2010 as a budget-neutral incentive program utilizing data collected through the IQR program to differentially reimburse hospitals based on the *value* of services provided.

- Embracing "value" as the combined consequence of quality and cost, the ACA mandated the implementation of a series of *value-based reimbursement initiatives* supporting the desired transformation of Medicare's traditional role as a *passive payer* of services to that of an *active purchaser* of "value."

- Value-based initiatives for hospitals contained in the ACA include the HRRP, the HAC program, and the HVBP program.

- In contrast to the HRRP and HAC programs, the essential framework of value-based purchasing consists of a much broader array of clinical and structural metrics, including:
  - consensus-driven clinical measures
  - metrics for effective resource utilization measurement
  - incorporation of consumer feedback
  - a methodology for payment system redesign

- Through a process of evaluation, comparison, and payment modification, the desired end result of the HVBP is to foster greater levels of clinical and financial responsibility in total health care delivery.

- The HVBP program promotes better clinical outcomes for hospital patients, as well as improvements in their experience of care during hospital stays. Specifically, HVBP seeks to encourage hospitals to improve the quality and safety of care that Medicare beneficiaries and all patients receive during acute-care inpatient stays by:

  o reducing or eliminating the occurrence of adverse events (health care errors resulting in patient harm)

  o encouraging the adoption of evidence-based care standards and protocols that result in the optimal patient outcomes

  o redesigning critical hospital processes that improve patients' experience of care

- Initiation of HVBP incentive payments began in the hospital environment in FY2013 and demonstration projects have been conducted, or are underway, in Skilled Nursing Facilities (SNFs), Home Health Agencies (HHAs), and Accountable Care Organizations.

- Over time, the HVBP value-based payment strategies are expected to be extended to facility-based providers, as well as individual provider groups and Accountable Care Organizations as part of a comprehensive strategy to promote joint accountability between providers.[75]

2.3.2 Overview

- The HVBP program is designed to assess health care value provided by individual hospitals through comparative analysis of selected IQR program-reported measures assigned to weighted HVBP domains, against national standards, over time.

---

[75] http://www.cms.gov/Medicare/Quality-Initiatives-Patient-Assessment-Instruments/HospitalQualityInits/index.html?redirect=/HospitalQualityInits

- Utilizing a clearly defined scoring model, hospitals are evaluated on progress made between a baseline period and a performance period. Hospitals earn scoring points for demonstrating improvement or achievement against their own established baseline performance rates and in comparison to nationally established standards.

- Based on individual hospital performance, participants will receive differential per-discharge reimbursement rates during a program year. Such value-based reimbursement rates can significantly impact projected annual hospital earnings.

- Based on their performance, HVBP participating hospitals have the potential to:

  o WIN: Receive an **increased** per-discharge reimbursement rate resulting in annual revenue earnings in excess of the amount withheld to establish a national incentive pool.

  o LOSE: Receive a **reduced** annual per-discharge reimbursement rate resulting in a net loss of revenue.

  o DRAW: Have **no change** made to per-discharge rates, resulting in a hospital earning its full annual per-discharge reimbursement without modification.

    - For the FY2013 HVBP program year, 2,984 hospitals received HVBP scores and 1,557 (52 percent) earned increased per-discharge payment rates.

    - For the FY2014 HVBP program year, 2,730 hospitals received HVBP scores and 1,255 (46 percent) earned increased per-discharge rates.[76]

- The primary data source for the HVBP program is information collected through the hospital IQR process and includes hospital-reported chart-abstracted measures data, CMS claims-extracted information, and consumer experience of care survey data.

[76] http://www.cms.gov/Medicare/Quality-Initiatives-Patient-Assessment-Instruments/hospital-value-based-purchasing/

2.3.3 Budget Neutrality Requirement

Overview

- The ACA specifies that the HVBP incentive program is to be a "budget-neutral" program. This requires any financial incentives to be offset by equal reductions to reimbursements.

- To create an annual incentive pool of available funding, the ACA mandates that CMS prospectively apply annual percentage reductions to base operating amounts for each discharge in a given program year for HVBP participating hospitals. This establishes an annual "withhold" for an individual hospital, which is a product of the volume of Medicare discharges occurring in a program year and the application of an annual withhold percentage.

  *Note: The annual withhold percentage is also referred to as the **Base***

  Operating DRG Payment Amount Reduction.

- In FY2014, individual hospitals will have 1.25 percent deducted from the Base Operating DRG portion of each discharge to fund the HVBP incentive. CMS estimates that the resulting national amount available for value-based incentive payments for FY2014 discharges will be approximately $1.1 billion.[77]

  - For FY2014, 2,730 hospitals have received HVBP payment adjustment factors. The average withhold amount per participant equals $403,225 per hospital. This amount is almost $82,000 larger than the average estimated FY2013 withhold of $322,000 per hospital.

  - An estimate of annual withhold amounts for a given hospital can be seen in the following example:

EXAMPLE: HOSPITAL A	
FY2014 Wage-Adjusted Base Operating DRG rate	$5,370.28*
FY2014 withhold of 1.25 percent	$58.33 (per discharge)

---

[77] Page 50507, www.gpo.gov/fdsys/pkg/FR-2013-08-19/pdf/2013-18956.pdf

Estimated FY2014 Medicare Discharges	7,729
Estimated total withhold = $58.33 X 7,729	**$450,832**

*Assumes Wage Index (WI) = 1.0. For detailed discussion on wage-adjusted base operating DRG rates, see 4.15.2 below.

FY2014–FY2016 HVBP Annual Withhold Percentages[78]

- In years FY2014–FY2017, HVBP withhold percentages applied to base-operating DRG payments are scheduled to increase by .25 percent per year until a maximum of 2 percent is reached:

HVBP PROGRAM YEAR	% REDUCTION IN BASE OPERATING DRG
FY2014	1.25 percent
FY2015	1.50 percent
FY2016	1.75 percent
FY2017 and beyond	2.00 percent

- Performance against established metrics of the HVBP program will allow hospitals to earn back withheld amounts, earn more than the withheld funds, or receive less than withheld funding.

- The pool of available funds may not exceed an aggregate representing the sum of all participants' annual DRG withholdings.

2.3.4 HVBP Eligibility Requirements and Exclusions

Eligibility

- Participation in the HVBP program applies to **"subsection (d) defined hospitals"** in the fifty US states. Such hospitals may be broadly defined

---

[78] *FY2014 Value-based Incentive Payment Adjustment Factors, http://www.cms.gov/Medicare/Quality-Initiatives-Patient-Assessment-Instruments/hospital-value-based-purchasing/index.html?redirect=/Hospital-Value-Based-Purchasing/*

as those receiving payment under the Inpatient Prospective Payment System (IPPS).

- o Statutory definition of subsection (d) hospitals is contained in Section 1886 (o)(1)(C)(i) of the Social Security Act (SSA) **(See Appendix: Attachment C.)**

Exclusions:

Note: Hospitals that are excluded from the HVBP program will not have their base-operating DRG payments reduced to fund the national incentive pool (-1.25 percent for FY2014) and will not receive annual payment modifiers.

- Hospitals subject to payment reductions under the IQR program (i.e., non-reporting) are excluded.

- Hospitals and hospital units excluded from the IPPS. These include:[79]
    - o psychiatric hospitals
    - o rehabilitation hospitals
    - o long-term care hospitals
    - o children's hospitals
    - o cancer hospitals
    - o hospitals located in the US Territories
    - o critical access hospitals (CAH)

- Hospitals that are paid under Section 1814(b)(3) Outpatient Prospective Payment System (OPPS), but have received an exemption from the HHS secretary (Attachment B) are excluded:
    - o Hospitals located in Maryland receiving a waiver for the FY2014 program year are excluded. Such hospitals must undergo an annual resubmission of waiver process to continue exempt status.

---

[79] *http://www.ssa.gov/OP_Home/ssact/title18/1886.htm#act-1886-d-1-b*

- Hospitals cited for deficiencies during a defined performance period that pose immediate jeopardy to the health or safety of patients are excluded.

- In the FY2014 Final IPPS Rule, CMS established a process for hospitals to submit an HVBP program disaster/extraordinary circumstance waiver. Citing the impact of Hurricane Sandy on hospitals in the Northeast in 2012, this process would allow facilities to have a negatively impacted performance year excluded from HVBP evaluation.

- Hospitals without the minimum number of cases and measures specified for a given program year are excluded:

- As required by the ACA, CMS conducted an independent modeling analysis and established a minimum numbers of cases, measures, and surveys for hospitals to be eligible to participate in HVBP. Including hospitals that do not meet the minimum criteria could adversely skew results that would affect the overall program scoring.

2.3.5 HVBP Evaluation and Scoring Model

- In developing a methodology for evaluating hospital performance in the HVBP program, CMS sought to achieve six objectives:

  1. Performance scoring must be straightforward and transparent to hospitals, patients, and stakeholders.

  2. Scoring methodologies for all Medicare value-based purchasing programs should be aligned.

  3. Differences in performance scores should be reflective of true differences in performance.

  4. Scoring should appropriately measure *both* **quality achievement** *and* **improvement.**

  5. The scoring process should eliminate unintended consequences resulting from providing rewards for inappropriate hospital behaviors and outcomes.

6. Data collection must allow for a timely measurement of performance and use the most currently available information.[80]

Scoring Data Sources

- The HVBP program evaluates hospital performance against established consensus-based clinical measures and measures of consumer feedback for a baseline reporting period and an established performance period.

- Such data is collected through the IQR process and includes:

  o Hospital-Reported Chart-Abstracted and CMS Claims-Extracted Clinical Data

  o Hospital Consumer Assessment of Healthcare Providers and Systems (HCAHPS)

- Since 2005, the information provided by these data sources has greatly enhanced the responsiveness of hospitals in instituting changes, resulting in improved care quality and patient satisfaction. To further leverage the success of these programs and reward facilities for improved care quality, the ACA specified that selected data items from the IQR and HCAHPS serve as the basis for HVBP performance evaluation and comparison.

Inpatient Quality Reporting (IQR)

- In 2003, CMS began the National Voluntary Hospital Reporting Initiative (now known as the Hospital Quality Alliance) for all hospitals reimbursed through the federal IPPS (Attachment A). Through this public-private collaboration, measures of care quality have been reportable since 2005 and have been made publicly available. In 2005, this alliance resulted in the development of the Hospital Compare website to publicly report on care quality in the nation's hospitals. Through the establishment of

---

[80] *Pages 26491–26492 https://www.federalregister.gov/articles/2011/07/05/2011-16763/medicare-program-hospital-inpatient-value-based-purchasing-program-correction*

standard quality metrics, Hospital Compare allows for evaluation of patient care quality for a given institution.[81]

- Currently, hospitals that are paid under IPPS are incentivized to report data published on the Hospital Compare website through a quality data pay-for-reporting initiative known as the hospital IQR. For IQR program years FY2013–FY2015, hospitals that do not (or unsuccessfully) participate in the IQR program will receive a two–percentage-point reduction in the annual Hospital Market Basket portion of their Annual Payment Update (APU). Beginning with program year FY2016 (CY2014 reporting year) nonparticipation or unsuccessful participation in the IQR program will result in an individual hospital receiving a reduction equal to one-quarter of their total APU.[82]

Annual Hospital Market Basket

- The Hospital Market Basket is a calculated index to measure how much more or less it would cost, at a later time, to purchase the same mix of goods and services. Section 5201(c) of the Deficit Reduction Act (DRA) of 2005 requires an adjustment of the hospital basket percentage update for CY2007 and subsequent years based on the submission of quality data through IQR reporting.

- The index is updated against a fixed base period and provides Medicare with information on which to increase (adjust for inflation) or decrease (deflation) reimbursements. The impact of a 2 percent non-reporting reduction would be to continue to purchase goods and services at the prevailing prices and be reimbursed at a lower rate.

FY2016 IQR Reporting Requirements

- For CY2014 reporting (FY2016 program year), IQR requirements include reporting on a total of 63 quality measures related to heart attack,

---

[81] http://www.cms.gov/Medicare/Quality-Initiatives-Patient-Assessment-Instruments/HospitalQualityInits/index.html?redirect=/HospitalQualityInits

[82] Federal Register/Vol. 78, No. 160/Monday, August 19, 2013/Rules and Regulations, page 51034, www.gpo.gov/fdsys/pkg/FR-2013-08-19/pdf/2013-18956.pdf

heart failure, pneumonia, surgical care, indicators established by the Agency for Healthcare Research and Quality (AHRQ), mortality, readmissions, HACs, participation in systematic clinical database registries for various topics, efficiency, and patient satisfaction.[83]

- A subset of the measures collected under the IQR program is being used by CMS to implement three mandatory delivery system programs for hospitals mandated by the ACA—the HVBP program, the HRRP, and the HAC program.

    Note: For detailed information regarding the IQR program, see "Chapter 1: The Inpatient Quality Reporting Program."

HCAHPS

- Beginning in 2002, CMS partnered with the Agency for Healthcare Research and Quality (AHRQ) to develop and test a survey tool and data collection methodology for measuring patients' perceptions of their hospital experience. The result of that work was HCAHPS (pronounced "H-caps"), also known as the CAHPS Hospital Survey.

- As the first national, standardized, publicly reported survey of patients' perspectives on hospital care, HCAHPS was approved for use in December 2005 by the federal Office of Management and Budget (OMB). CMS implemented HCAHPS in 2006, and in 2008 made the first public report available on the Hospital Compare website, which allowed for local, regional, and national comparisons among hospitals from the consumer perspective.

- Through this survey, randomly administered to adult patients (Medicare and non-Medicare) between 48 hours and six weeks post-discharge, HCAHPS gathers information related to consumer satisfaction with hospital stays. Each day more than 28,000 patients are surveyed about their recent hospital experience utilizing HCAHPS and more than 8,400 patients each day complete the HCAHPS Survey.[84]

---

[83] *QualityNet: Measure Comparison,* http://www.qualitynet.org/dcs/ContentServer?pagename=QnetPublic%2FPage%2FQnetTier2&cid =1141662756099

[84] http://www.hcahpsonline.org/whatsnew.aspx#ExpandedSurvey

For FY2014, the HCAHPS survey (HCAHPS Expanded) contains thirty-two questions, including:

- eighteen core questions exploring critical aspects of the patient hospital experience (communication with nurses and doctors, the responsiveness of hospital staff, the cleanliness and quietness of the hospital environment, pain management, communication about medicines, discharge information, overall rating of hospital, and willingness of the patient to recommend the hospital)

- four items to direct patients to relevant questions

- three items to adjust for the mix of patients across hospitals

- two items that support Congressionally mandated reports

- three care transition items

- two "about you" items

- Hospitals must conduct surveys every month of the year and report results continuously on a quarterly basis.

- Data may be collected by the hospital or through use of an approved vendor using mail, telephone, mail with telephone follow-up, or active/interactive voice recognition (IVR).

- Publicly reported HCAHPS results are based on a compilation of the most recent four consecutive quarters of patient surveys and are posted on the Hospital Compare website quarterly.[85]

- Effective in July 2007, all hospitals paid under IPPS are required to collect and submit HCAHPS data in order to receive their full annual IPPS payment update as part of the IQR program. Failure to meet the IQR requirements for the HCAHPS measure will result in the application of IQR program penalties as described above.

- Non-IPPS hospitals, such as Critical Access Hospitals (CAHs), are not required to participate in HCAHPS, but many voluntarily administer the survey.

---

[85] *Page 26493, http://www.gpo.gov/fdsys/pkg/FR-2011-05-06/pdf/FR-2011-05-06.pdf*

o CAHs designated by Medicare as rural hospitals that have no more than twenty-five inpatient beds that can be used for inpatient services or swing-bed services. However, they may also operate up to ten beds for rehab or psychiatric care. Their average length of stay is 96 hours or less (not including swing beds or distinct rehab/psych units).

- The ACA mandated the utilization of specific HCAHPS feedback among the measures to be used to calculate value-based incentive payments in the HVBP program, beginning with discharges in October 2012 (FY2013).[86]

2.3.6 The Quality Domains HVBP Performance Scoring Model

Background

After conducting a review of alternative evaluation and scoring methodologies, CMS adopted the **Quality Domains Performance Scoring Model** to determine individual hospitals' performance under the HVBP program. This model compares hospital performance between a baseline period and a performance period for established metrics of defined Quality Domains of Care and awards points based on both achievement and improvement in determining a Total Performance Score (TPS). The TPS is then mathematically converted to an incentive payment percentage that is applied to each discharge occurring during a program year.

Quality Domain: a CMS-determined grouping of clinically or structurally related measures reported under the IQR program used for HVBP evaluation and scoring. Each domain is assigned a specific weighting, which is used to calculate the TPS for an individual hospital.

- Through its annual rule-making process, CMS may modify the included measures and the number of domains contained in the HVBP program. To the initial set of two domains used for the first year (FY2013) of the

---

[86] Page 617, Patient Protection and Affordable Care Act, http://www.gpo.gov/fdsys/pkg/BILLS-111hr3590enr/pdf/BILLS-111hr3590enr.pdf

HVBP program (Clinical Process of Care and Patient Experience of Care), CMS added "Outcomes" for FY2014 and "Efficiency" for FY2015. For years FY2015–FY2019, CMS will use four domains for scoring.[87]

DOMAIN	HVBP PROGRAM YEAR
Clinical Process of Care	FY2013–FY2017
Patient Experience of Care	FY2013–FY2017
Outcomes	FY2014–FY2017
Efficiency	FY2015–FY2017
Clinical Care	FY2017*
Safety	FY2017

*For FY2017, the Clinical Process of Care and Outcomes Domains will be included under a new domain titled "Clinical Care." This grouping allows for the maintenance of a four-domain model.

- Measures cannot be added to the HVBP program until they have been included in the IQR program and reported on Hospital Compare for at least one year.

Key Terms

- **Baseline Period:** The baseline period is a defined time frame for data collection to establish an initial period to determine current performance and improvement (when compared to a later time period called the performance period). Measures domains may have different baseline periods for a given HVBP program year. These periods are established and modified annually through the Final IPPS Rule.

- **Baseline Rate** (also referred to as the Improvement Threshold): The baseline rate is an individual hospital's performance for each measure during the baseline period, which is used as input for scoring improvement points. A minimum of ten cases (i.e., a baseline period denominator value greater than or equal to ten) is required to compute improvement points.

- **Benchmark:** A benchmark standard is a national standard determined for each measure to identify high levels of hospital performance during

---

[87] Pages 50700–50703 Federal Register/Vol. 78, No. 160/Monday, August 19, 2013/Rules and Regulations, www.gpo.gov/fdsys/pkg/FR-2013-08-19/pdf/2013-18956.pdf

the baseline period. These standards are established as the mean of the top decile (95th percentile) for all hospital scores achieved for each measure during the baseline period.

- **Achievement Threshold** (Achievement Performance Standard): The achievement threshold (or achievement performance standard) is a national standard that is established as the median (50th percentile) of hospital performance on a measure during a **baseline** period with respect to a fiscal year, with the *exception* of the Medicare spending per beneficiary (MSPB) measure. The MSBP achievement threshold is determined to be median (50th percentile) of hospital performance on a measure during the **performance** period with respect to a fiscal year.

- **Performance Period:** The performance period is a time frame during which data is collected to determine improvement over/above a participant's baseline performance and to determine comparative performance against national standards. CMS uses this comparison to determine achievement and improvement in quality. Measures domains may have different performance periods for a given HVBP program year. These periods are established and modified annually through the Final IPPS Rule.

- **Achievement Score:** The achievement score is a numeric score of 0–10 points assigned to each measure based on an individual hospital's measure attainment during the performance period as compared to the achievement threshold and the benchmark.

- **Improvement Score:** The improvement score is a numeric score of 0–9 points assigned to each measure for attainment during the performance period as compared to the individual hospital's baseline rate (improvement threshold).

- **Total Performance Score (TPS):** The TPS is calculated as the sum of weighted domain scores. The maximum TPS is a score of 100.

Scoring Methodology Overview

- The basic framework for HVBP program performance evaluation using the Quality Domain-Based Performance Scoring Model involves six steps:[88]

  - **Step 1:** Identify program year domains and measures.

  - **Step 2:** Establish performance benchmarks and thresholds for each domain.

  - **Step 3:** Score achievement *and* improvement for each domain.

  - **Step 4:** Apply the relative weighting for each domain.

  - **Step 5:** Calculate the Total Performance Score (TPS).

  - **Step 6:** Convert the TPS to a PAF.

2.3.7 Scoring Step 1: Identify Program Year Domains and Measures

Domain Weighting Overview

- For each HVBP program year, measures reported under the IQR program are grouped into related domains. Each domain is assigned an annual percentage weighting for calculation of a Total Performance Score (TPS).

- Domain weightings may change as specified in the annual Final IPPS Rule.

- HVBP program year FY2014 is comprised of three domains and hospitals must successfully meet reporting requirements for all three domains to receive an HVBP TPS.

---

[88] *Page 26514, Federal Register/Vol. 76, No. 88/Friday, May 6, 2011/Rules and Regulations*
http://www.gpo.gov/fdsys/pkg/FR-2011-05-06/pdf/FR-2011-05-06.pdf

- HVBP program years FY2015 and beyond require successful reporting for at least two of four domains.

  - **Reallocation of Domain Weightings:** Beginning with FY2015 and continuing forward, domains will be re-weighted proportionately if a hospital fails to achieve the minimum case/measures reporting requirements for all four domains. Hospitals must achieve requirements for at least two out of four domain scores to receive an HVBP TPS. The TPS will be scored out of a possible 100 points and the relative weights for the scored domains will remain equivalent.

  - **Domain Weighting Reallocation Example:** A hospital meets the minimum case and measure requirements for the Efficiency, Patient Experience of Care, and Outcome domains, but does not meet the minimum case requirements for the Clinical Process of Care domain:

    - With a weight of 20 percent for the Clinical Process of Care, the remaining weighting for the other three domains is 80 percent.

    - The 20 percent allocated to the Clinical Process of Care domain will be reallocated to the remaining applicable domains using the following formula:

      Original weight of each remaining domain ÷ total weight of remaining domains x 100. In this example, the reallocated weighting amounts for the remaining applicable domains are:

      - Clinical Process of Care = 25.0 percent

      - Patient Experience of Care = 37.5 percent

      - Outcome = 37.5 percent

      Note: The reallocated weights must total 100 percent.

FY2014–FY2016 Quality Domains

- For program year FY2014, there are three quality domains used for HVBP scoring. The Efficiency domain was added for FY2015 and FY2016. Individual measures within each domain are reported through the IQR system as hospital-reported chart-abstracted measures, CMS-extracted claims-based measures, or reported HCAHPS survey results.

- **Clinical Process of Care Domain:** Clinical Process of Care measures are chart-abstracted and are based on the rate at which a hospital provided the recommended process of care. Reflecting a greater emphasis on the results of care, process of care weighting is reduced over time. Beginning with a 70 percent weighting for FY2013, this weighting drops to 10 percent by FY2016.

- **Patient Experience of Care Domain:** This domain is composed of eight dimensions of the HCAHPS Survey. From FY2013–FY2015 the Patient Experience of Care domain comprises 30 percent of the total weighted performance score. Additionally, unlike other domains, the Patient Experience of Care Domain incorporates a consistency component in scoring methodology.

- **Outcome Domain:** This domain is composed of three claims-based mortality measures. As introduced in FY2014, the Outcomes domain was the lowest-weighted domain at 25 percent. In FY2016, the Outcomes domain is the highest-weighted domain at 40 percent.

- **Efficiency Domain (FY2015–FY2016):** CMS determines the Medicare Spending Per Beneficiary (MSPB) rate using claims-based information. First introduced as part of the FY2015 program, the Efficiency domain carries a weighting of 25 percent in FY2016.

Note: The MSPB reported for HVBP will differ from that reported on the Hospital Compare website due to the use of different comparison groups.

FY2014 Summary[89]

For program year FY2014 there are a total of twenty-four measures contained under three domains:

DOMAIN	MEASURES	DOMAIN WEIGHTING
Clinical Process of Care	13	45 percent

---

[89] *Page 53568, http://www.gpo.gov/fdsys/pkg/FR-2012-08-31/pdf/2012-19079.pdf*

Patient Experience of Care	8 (HCAHPS)	30 percent
Outcomes	3	25 percent

FY2014 Minimum Reporting Requirements:

- Clinical Process of Care: ten cases and four measures

- Patient Experience of Care: 100 completed surveys

- Outcome 30-Day Mortality: ten cases and two measures

Note: Hospitals must receive scores in all three FY2014 domains in order to receive a Total HVBP Performance Score. Hospitals unable to achieve this standard will be excluded from HVBP for FY2014.

FY2015 Summary[90]

For program year FY2015 there are a total of twenty-six measures contained under four domains:

DOMAIN	MEASURES	DOMAIN WEIGHTING
Clinical Process of Care	12	20 percent
Patient Experience of Care	8 (HCAHPS)	30 percent
Outcomes	5	30 percent
Efficiency	1	20 percent

FY2015 Minimum Reporting Requirements:

- Clinical Process of Care: ten cases and four measures

- Patient Experience of Care: 100 completed surveys

- Outcome Measures: Hospitals must report the applicable case minimum for at least two of the five measures for the Outcome domain:

---

[90] *Page 53584, http://www.gpo.gov/fdsys/pkg/FR-2012-08-31/pdf/2012-19079.pdf*

- o AMI 30-Day Mortality: twenty-five cases

- o HF 30-Day Mortality: twenty-five cases

- o PN 30-Day Mortality: twenty-five cases

- o AHRQ (PSI-90): three cases for any of the underlying indicators

- o HAI (CLABSI): one predicted infection

- o Efficiency (Medicare Spending Per Beneficiary): twenty-five cases

Note: Hospitals with sufficient data in at least two of the four domains will receive a TPS and domain weighting will be reallocated for unsuccessfully reported domains.

FY2016 Summary[91]

For program year FY2016 there are a total of twenty-five measures contained under four domains:

DOMAIN	MEASURES	DOMAIN WEIGHTING
Clinical Process of Care	8	10 percent
Patient Experience of Care	8 (HCAHPS)	25 percent
Outcomes	8	40 percent
Efficiency	1	25 percent

FY2016 Minimum Reporting Requirements:

- Clinical Process of Care: ten cases and four measures

- Patient Experience of Care: 100 completed surveys

- Outcome Measures: Hospitals must report the applicable case minimum for at least two of the five measures for the Outcome domain.

---

[91] *Page 50697, Federal Register/Vol. 78, No. 160/Monday, August 19, 2013/Rules and Regulations, www.gpo.gov/fdsys/pkg/FR-2013-08-19/pdf/2013-18956.pdf*

- o AMI 30-Day Mortality: twenty-five cases
- o HF 30-Day Mortality: twenty-five cases
- o PN 30-Day Mortality: twenty-five cases
- o AHRQ (PSI-90): three cases for any of the underlying indicators
- o HAI (CLABSI): one predicted infection
- o Efficiency (Medicare Spending Per Beneficiary): twenty-five cases

Note: Hospitals with sufficient data in at least two of the four domains will receive a TPS and domain weighting will be reallocated for unsuccessfully reported domains.

Table 1 FY2014–FY2016 Domains and Measures:

This listing is current with the publication of the FY2014 IPPS Final Rule dated August 19, 2013, and is subject to modification through subsequent annual rule-making.

Table 1: Measures Listing for FY2014–FY2016

Domain 1: Clinical Process of Care

ACUTE MYOCARDIAL INFARCTION (AMI)

MEASURE ID	MEASURE DESCRIPTION	FY2014	FY2015	FY2016
AMI-7a	fibrinolytic therapy received within 30 minutes of hospital arrival	Yes	Yes	Yes
AMI-8a	primary PCI received within 90 minutes of hospital arrival	Yes	Yes	No

HEART FAILURE (HF)

MEASURE ID	MEASURE DESCRIPTION	FY2014	FY2015	FY2016
HF-1	discharge instructions	Yes	Yes	No

PNEUMONIA (PN)

MEASURE ID	MEASURE DESCRIPTION	FY2014	FY2015	FY2016
PN-3b	blood cultures performed in the Emergency Department prior to initial antibiotic received in hospital	Yes	Yes	No
PN-6	initial antibiotic selection for CAP in immunocompetent patient	Yes	Yes	Yes

IMMUNIZATIONS (IMM)				
MEASURE ID	MEASURE DESCRIPTION	FY2014	FY2015	FY2016
IMM-2	influenza immunization	No	No	Yes

HEALTHCARE-ASSOCIATED INFECTION (HAI)				
MEASURE ID	MEASURE DESCRIPTION	FY2014	FY2015	FY2016
SCIP-Inf-1	prophylactic antibiotic received within one hour prior to surgical incision	Yes	Yes	No
SCIP-Inf-2	prophylactic antibiotic selection for surgical patients	Yes	Yes	Yes
SCIP-Inf-3	prophylactic antibiotics discontinued within 24 hours after surgery end time	Yes	Yes	Yes
SCIP-Inf-4	cardiac surgery patients with controlled 6AM postoperative serum glucose	Yes	Yes	No
SCIP-Inf-9	postoperative urinary catheter removal on postoperative Day 1 or 2	Yes	Yes	Yes

SURGICAL CARE IMPROVEMENT PROJECT (SCIP)				
MEASURE ID	MEASURE DESCRIPTION	FY2014	FY2015	FY2016
SCIP-Card-2	surgery patients on a beta-blocker prior to arrival that received a beta-blocker during the perioperative period	Yes	Yes	Yes
SCIP-VTE-1	surgery patients with recommended venous thromboembolism prophylaxis ordered	Yes	No	No
SCIP-VTE-2	surgery patients who received appropriate venous thromboembolism prophylaxis within 24 hours prior to surgery to 24 hours after surgery	Yes	Yes	Yes

Domain 2: Patient Experience of Care

HOSPITAL CONSUMER ASSESSMENT OF HEALTHCARE PROVIDERS AND SYSTEMS SURVEY (HCAHPS)				
MEASURE ID	MEASURE DESCRIPTION	FY2014	FY2015	FY2016
	communication with nurses	Yes	Yes	Yes
	communication with doctors	Yes	Yes	Yes
	responsiveness of hospital staff	Yes	Yes	Yes
	pain management	Yes	Yes	Yes
	communication about medicines	Yes	Yes	Yes
	cleanliness and quietness of hospital environment	Yes	Yes	Yes
	discharge information	Yes	Yes	Yes
	overall rating of hospital	Yes	Yes	Yes

Domain 3: Outcomes

MORTALITY (MORT) MEASURES

MEASURE ID	MEASURE DESCRIPTION	FY2014	FY2015	FY2016
MORT-30-AMI	acute myocardial infarction (AMI) 30-Day Mortality Rate	Yes	Yes	Yes
MORT-30-HF	heart failure (HF) 30-Day Mortality Rate	Yes	Yes	Yes
MORT-30-PN	pneumonia (PN) 30-Day Mortality Rate	Yes	Yes	Yes

AGENCY FOR HEALTHCARE RESEARCH AND QUALITY (AHRQ) MEASURES

MEASURE ID	MEASURE DESCRIPTION	FY2014	FY2015	FY2016
AHRQ PSI-90 Composite	complication/patient safety for selected indicators (Composite)	No	Yes	Yes

HOSPITAL-ACQUIRED INFECTIONS (HAI)

MEASURE ID	MEASURE DESCRIPTION	FY2014	FY2015	FY2016
CLABSI	central line-associated bloodstream infection	No	Yes	Yes
CAUTI	catheter-associated urinary tract infections	No	No	Yes

SURGICAL SITE INFECTIONS (SSI)

MEASURE ID	MEASURE DESCRIPTION	FY2014	FY2015	FY2016
SSI	colon	No	No	Yes
	abdominal hysterectomy	No	No	Yes

Domain 4: Efficiency

EFFICIENCY

MEASURE ID	MEASURE DESCRIPTION	FY2014	FY2015	FY2016
MSPB	Medicare spending per beneficiary	No	Yes	Yes

FY2017 Summary

- In the FY2014 Final IPPS Rule, CMS finalized assignment of HVBP measures to better align with the priorities of the NQS.[92]

- Also known as The National Strategy for Quality Improvement in Health Care, the NQS is a nationwide effort to align public and private interests to improve the quality of health and health care for all Americans. Part of the ACA, the National Quality Strategy is guided by three aims to provide better, more affordable care for the person and the community:

    o **Better care:** Improve the overall quality, by making health care more patient-centered, reliable, accessible, and safe.

    o **Healthy people/healthy communities**: Improve the health of the US population by supporting proven interventions to address behavioral, social, and environmental determinants of health in addition to delivering higher-quality care.

    o **Affordable care**: Reduce the cost of quality health care for individuals, families, employers, and government.

- This fundamental restructuring of HVBP domains and measures will assist in greater alignment among the hospital IQR program, the HVBP program, and the EHR Incentive Program.

    o The Clinical Care domain is to be added and includes both Outcomes and Process measures.

    o The Efficiency domain will include refined measures for Cost Reduction.

    o Care Coordination metrics will be added to the Patient and Caregiver Experience of Care domain.

- Using the same twenty-five individual measures approved for the FY2016 HVBP program, CMS has designated four new NQS-aligned domains for the FY2017 HVBP program:

---

[92] *Page 50703, Federal Register/Vol. 78, No. 160/Monday, August 19, 2013/Rules and Regulations, www.gpo.gov/fdsys/pkg/FR-2013-08-19/pdf/2013-18956.pdf*

DOMAIN	TOTAL MEASURES	DOMAIN WEIGHTING
Safety	5	15 percent
Clinical Care		35 percent
• Outcomes	3	• 25 percent
• Process	8	• 10 percent
Efficiency and Cost Reduction	1	25 percent
Patient and Caregiver Centered Experience of Care/Care Coordination	8 (HCAHP)	25 percent

- **FY2017 Minimum Reporting Requirements**

  As specified in the FY2014 Final IPPS Rule, CMS intends to address minimum reporting requirements for the NQS-aligned domains in future rule-making.

- As finalized in the FY2014 Final IPPS Rule, individual measures for the FY2017 HVBP have been aligned with NQS domains as follows:

Table 2: FY2017 NQS-Aligned HVBP Measures

Domain 1: Safety

CLABSI	central line-associated bloodstream infection
CAUTI	catheter-associated urinary tract infections
SSI	colon abdominal hysterectomy
AHRQ PSI-90 Composite	complication/patient safety for selected indicators (Composite)

Domain 2: Clinical Care

CLINICAL CARE: OUTCOMES:	
MORT-30-AMI	acute myocardial infarction (AMI) 30-Day Mortality Rate
MORT-30-HF	heart failure (HF) 30-Day Mortality Rate
MORT-30-PN	pneumonia (PN) 30-Day Mortality Rate

CLINICAL CARE: PROCESS:	
AMI-7a	fibrinolytic therapy received within 30 minutes of hospital arrival
IMM-2	influenza immunization
PN-6	initial antibiotic selection for CAP in immunocompetent patient
SCIP-Inf-2	prophylactic antibiotic selection for surgical patients
SCIP-Inf-3	prophylactic antibiotics discontinued within 24 hours after surgery end time
SCIP-Inf-9	postoperative urinary catheter removal on postoperative Day 1 or 2
SCIP-Card-2	surgery patients on a beta-blocker prior to arrival that received a beta-blocker during the perioperative period

Domain 3: Efficiency and Cost Reduction

CLINICAL CARE: OUTCOMES:	
MSPB	Medicare spending per beneficiary

Domain 4:
Patient and Caregiver Experience of Care/Care Coordination

HOSPITAL CONSUMER ASSESSMENT OF HEALTHCARE PROVIDERS AND SYSTEMS SURVEY (HCAHPS)
communication with nurses
communication with doctors
responsiveness of hospital staff
pain management
communication about medicines
cleanliness and quietness of hospital environment
discharge information
overall rating of hospital

2.3.8 Scoring Step 2: Benchmarks and Achievement Thresholds

Overview

Under the HVBP program, Medicare will make incentive payments to hospitals based on how well participants performed on each measure (achievement) or how much progress (improvement) was made on each measure, as compared to national benchmarks and achievement threshold standards. Comparative performance is measured between the defined baseline reporting period and performance reporting period for a given HVBP program year:

- **Benchmark:** A benchmark standard is a national standard determined for each measure to identify high levels of hospital performance during the baseline period. These standards are established as the mean of the top decile (95th percentile) for all hospital scores achieved for each measure during the baseline **period.**

- **Achievement Threshold (Achievement Performance Standard):** The achievement threshold is a national standard that is established as the median (50th percentile) of hospital performance on a measure during a baseline period with respect to a fiscal year, with the *exception* of the MSPB measure.*

  o The MSBP achievement threshold is determined to be median (50th percentile) of hospital performance on a measure during the performance period with respect to a fiscal year.

  *Finalized in FY2014 IPPS Final Rule.

- **Floor:** Used only for the HCAHPS domain, the floor standard is assigned to each HCAHPS measure and is established as the worst-performing hospital's performance rate during the baseline period, which defines the 0 percentile for this dimension.

- **Baseline Period:** The baseline period is a defined time frame for data collection to establish an initial period for determination of current performance and improvement (when compared to a later time period called the performance period). Measures domains may have different baseline periods for a given HVBP program year. These periods are established and modified annually through the Final IPPS Rule.

- **Performance Period:** The performance period is a time frame during which data is collected to determine improvement over a participant's baseline performance and to determine comparative performance against national standards. CMS uses this comparison to determine achievement and improvement in quality. Measures domains may have different Performance Periods for a given HVBP program year. These periods are established and modified annually through the Final IPPS Rule.

Baseline and Performance Reporting Periods

- Baseline and performance reporting periods are domain-specific and can range from a period of twelve to thirty-six months, with baseline periods ending up to four years prior to a program year and performance periods ending twelve to twenty-four months prior to a program year.

- In any given year, a HVBP participating hospital is simultaneously reporting in a baseline year and performance year for different HVBP program years:

  - During FY2014, hospitals are reporting information to be used for the baseline period of the FY2018 program year and within the performance periods for FY2016, FY2017, FY2018, and FY2019.

- The following domain-specific baseline and performance reporting periods for the HVBP program have been finalized:[93]

Table 3: FY2014 Baseline and Performance Periods

FY2014 Value-Based Purchasing Program:
Baseline and Performance Periods

DOMAIN	BASELINE PERIOD	PERFORMANCE PERIOD
Clinical Process of Care	April 1, 2010– December 31, 2010	April 1, 2012– December 31, 2012
Patient Experience of Care	April 1, 2010– December 31, 2010	April 1, 2012– December 31, 2012
Outcome (Mortality)	July 1, 2009– June 30, 2010	July 1, 2011– June 30, 2012

[93] *Hospital Value-Based Purchasing; Baseline and Performance Periods, https://www.qualitynet.org/*

Table 4: FY2015 Baseline and Performance Periods

FY2015 Value-Based Purchasing Program: Baseline and Performance Periods

DOMAIN	BASELINE PERIOD	PERFORMANCE PERIOD
Clinical Process of Care	January 1, 2011– December 31, 2011	January 1, 2013– December 31, 2013
Patient Experience of Care	January 1, 2011– December 31, 2011	January 1, 2013– December 31, 2013
OUTCOMES:		
Mortality	October 1, 2010– June 30, 2011	October 1, 2012– June 30 , 2013
AHRQ PSI-90 Composite	October15, 2010– June 30, 2011	October 15, 2012– June 30, 2013
CLABSI	January 1, 2011– December 31, 2011	February 1, 2013– December 31, 2013
Efficiency	May 1, 2011– December 31, 2011	May 1, 2013– December 31, 2013

Table 5: FY2016 Baseline and Performance Periods

FY2016 Value-Based Purchasing Program:
Baseline and Performance Periods

DOMAIN	BASELINE PERIOD	PERFORMANCE PERIOD
Clinical Process of Care:	January 1, 2012– December 31, 2012	January 1, 2014– December 31, 2014
Patient Experience of Care:	January 1,2012– December 31, 2012	January 1, 2014– December 31, 2014
OUTCOMES:		
Mortality	October 1, 2010– June 30, 2011	October 1, 2012– June 30, 2014
AHRQ Composite	October 15, 2010– June 30, 2011	October 15, 2012– June 30, 2014
Efficiency:	January 1, 2012– December 31, 2012	January 1, 2014– December 31, 2014

Table 6: FY2017 Baseline and Performance Periods

FY2017 Value-Based Purchasing Program:
Baseline and Performance Periods

DOMAIN	BASELINE PERIOD	PERFORMANCE PERIOD
Safety:	October 1, 2010– June 30, 2012	October 1, 2013– June 30, 2015
CLINICAL CARE:		
Clinical Care: Outcomes	October 1, 2010– June 30, 2012	October 1, 2013– June 30, 2015
Clinical Care: Process	January 1, 2013– December 31, 2013	January 1, 2015– December 31, 2015
Efficiency and Cost Reduction	January 1, 2013– December 31, 2013	January 1, 2015– December 31, 2015
Patient and Caregiver Centered Experience of Care/ Care Coordination	January 1, 2013– December 31, 2013	January 1, 2015– December 31, 2015

Table 7: FY2018 Baseline and Performance Periods

FY2018 Value-Based Purchasing Program:
Baseline and Performance Periods

DOMAIN	BASELINE PERIOD	PERFORMANCE PERIOD
Safety:	July 1, 2010–June 30, 2012	July 1, 2014–June 30, 2016
CLINICAL CARE:		
Clinical Care: Outcomes	October 1, 2009–June 30, 2012	October 1, 2013–June 30, 2016
Clinical Care: Process	January 1, 2014–December 31, 2014	January 1, 2016–December 31, 2016
Efficiency and Cost Reduction	January 1, 2014–December 31, 2014	January 1, 2016–December 31, 2016
Patient and Caregiver Centered Experience of Care/Care Coordination	January 1, 2014–December 31, 2014	January 1, 2016–December 31, 2016

Table 8: FY2019 Baseline and Performance Periods

FY2019 Value-Based Purchasing Program:
Baseline and Performance Periods

DOMAIN	BASELINE PERIOD	PERFORMANCE PERIOD
Safety:	July 1, 2010–June 30, 2012	July 1, 2015–June 30, 2017
CLINICAL CARE:		
Clinical Care: Outcomes	July 1, 2009–June 30, 2012	July 1, 2014–June 30, 2017
Clinical Care: Process	January 1, 2015–December 31, 2015	January 1, 2017–December 31, 2017
Efficiency and Cost Reduction	January 1, 2015–December 31, 2015	January 1, 2017–December 31, 2017
Patient and Caregiver Centered Experience of Care/Care Coordination	January 1, 2015–December 31, 2015	January 1, 2017–December 31, 2017

Finalized Achievement Thresholds and Benchmarks

- Benchmark and achievement threshold information for each measure in a given HVBP program year is published in the annual IPPS Final Rule as analysis for a baseline period is completed. In the FY2014 Final IPPS Rule published in August 2013, the FY2016 achievement thresholds and benchmarks were finalized for the baseline period ending December 31, 2012.

- Unlike domains or measures, which may remain the same from year to year, benchmarks and achievement thresholds are changed annually to reflect baseline period changes in care quality. For example, in comparing the achievement threshold and benchmark standard for the Clinical Process of Care measure AMI-7a: fibrinolytic therapy received within thirty minutes of hospital arrival for FY2014 to FY2016:

YEAR	ACHIEVEMENT THRESHOLD	BENCHMARK STANDARD
FY2014	.8066 (81 percent completion)	.9630 (96.3 percent completion)
FY2016	.8862 (89 percent completion)	1.000 (100 percent completion)

  - This indicates that between the baseline periods for FY2014 and FY2016:

    - The average hospital improved its ability to ensure administration of fibrinolytic therapy within thirty minutes of the arrival of a patient with an acute myocardial infarction from 81 percent to 88 percent of the time.

    - The highest-performing hospitals (95th percentile) improved from 96 percent to 100 percent on this same metric.

- Through previous rule-making, CMS finalized the benchmark and achievement threshold information for HVBP program years FY2014 and FY2015. In the Final FY2014 IPPS Rule published in August 2013, CMS finalized such data for the FY2016 HVBP year (analysis of baseline period ending December 31, 2012.)

- The applicable floor (HCAHPS only), achievement thresholds, and benchmarks for FY2014, FY2015, and FY2016 are as follows:

Table 9: FY2014 Program Year Measure Standards[94]

Clinical Process of Care Domain: 45 percent weighting

ACUTE MYOCARDIAL INFARCTION (AMI)			
MEASURE ID	MEASURE DESCRIPTION	ACHIEVMENT THRESHOLD	BENCHMARK
AMI-7a	fibrinolytic therapy received within 30 minutes of hospital arrival	0.8066	0.9630
AMI-8a	primary PCI received within 90 minutes of hospital arrival	0.9344	1.0

HEART FAILURE (HF)			
MEASURE ID	MEASURE DESCRIPTION	ACHIEVMENT THRESHOLD	BENCHMARK
HF-1	discharge instructions	0.9266	1.0

PNEUMONIA (PN)			
MEASURE ID	MEASURE DESCRIPTION	ACHIEVMENT THRESHOLD	BENCHMARK
PN-3b	blood cultures performed in the Emergency Department prior to initial antibiotic received in hospital	0.9730	1.0
PN-6	initial antibiotic selection for CAP in immunocompetent patient	0.9446	1.0

HEALTHCARE-ASSOCIATED INFECTIONS (HAI)			
MEASURE ID	MEASURE DESCRIPTION	ACHIEVMENT THRESHOLD	BENCHMARK
SCIP-Inf-1	prophylactic antibiotic received within one hour prior to surgical incision	0.9807	1.0
SCIP-Inf-2	prophylactic antibiotic selection for surgical patients	0.9813	1.0
SCIP-Inf-3	prophylactic antibiotics discontinued within 24 hours after surgery end time	0.9663	0.9996
SCIP-Inf-4	cardiac surgery patients with controlled 6AM postoperative serum glucose	0.9634	1.0
SCIP-Inf-9	postoperative urinary catheter removal on postoperative Day 1 or 2	0.9286	0.9989

---

[94] Page 74538, Federal Register/Volume 76/Issue 230/Wednesday, November 30, 2011, http://www.gpo.gov/fdsys/pkg/FR-2011-11-30/pdf/2011-28612.pdf

SURGERIES			
MEASURE ID	MEASURE DESCRIPTION	ACHIEVMENT THRESHOLD	BENCHMARK
SCIP-Card-2	surgery patients on a beta-blocker prior to arrival that received a beta-blocker during the perioperative period	0.9565	1.0
SCIP-VTE-1	surgery patients with recommended venous thromboembolism prophylaxis ordered	0.9462	1.0
SCIP-VTE-2	surgery patients who received appropriate venous thromboembolism prophylaxis within 24 hours prior to surgery to 24 hours after surgery.	0.9492	0.9983

MORTALITY OUTCOMES*: 25 PERCENT WEIGHTING			
MEASURE ID	MEASURE DESCRIPTION	ACHIEVMENT THRESHOLD	BENCHMARK
Mort-30-AMI	acute myocardial infarction (AMI) 30-Day Mortality Rate	0.8477	0.8673
Mort-30-HF	heart failure (HF) 30-Day Mortality Rate	0.8861	0.9042
Mort-30-PN	pneumonia (PN) 30-Day Mortality Rate	0.8818	0.9021

*Mortality Outcome measures are expressed as survival rates

These percentages represent the number of "always" answers for each question. No other answers are reported.

FY2014 table: http://www.gpo.gov/fdsys/pkg/FR-2011-11-30/pdf/2011-28612.pdf

FY2014 PATIENT EXPERIENCE OF CARE MEASURES: 30 PERCENT WEIGHTING			
SELECTED DIMENSIONS FROM THE HCAHPS SURVEY	FLOOR MINIMUM	ACHIEVMENT THRESHOLD	BENCHMARK
communication with nurses	42.84 percent	75.79 percent	84.99 percent
communication with doctors	55.49 percent	79.57 percent	88.45 percent
responsiveness of hospital staff	32.15 percent	62.21 percent	78.08 percent
pain management	40.79 percent	68.99 percent	77.92 percent
communication about medicines	36.01 percent	59.85 percent	71.54 percent
cleanliness and quietness of hospital	38.52 percent	63.54 percent	78.10 percent

| discharge information | 54.73 percent | 82.72 percent | 89.24 percent |
| overall rating of hospital | 30.91 percent | 67.03 percent | 82.55 percent |

Federal Register/Vol 76, No. 230/Wednesday, November 30, 2011/Rules and Regulations

Table 10: FY2015 Program Year Measure Standards[95]

Clinical Process of Care Measures: 20 percent weighting

ACUTE MYOCARDIAL INFARCTION (AMI)			
MEASURE ID	MEASURE DESCRIPTION	ACHIEVMENT THRESHOLD	BENCHMARK
AMI-7a	fibrinolytic therapy received within 30 minutes of hospital arrival	0.80000	1.0
AMI-8a	primary PCI received within 90 minutes of hospital arrival	0.95349	1.0

HEART FAILURE (HF)			
MEASURE ID	MEASURE DESCRIPTION	ACHIEVMENT THRESHOLD	BENCHMARK
HF-1	discharge instructions	0.94188	1.0

PNEUMONIA (PN)			
MEASURE ID	MEASURE DESCRIPTION	ACHIEVMENT THRESHOLD	BENCHMARK
PN-3b	blood cultures performed in the Emergency Department prior to initial antibiotic received in hospital	0.97783	1.0
PN-6	initial antibiotic selection for CAP in immunocompetent patient	0.95918	1.0

[95] Pages 53601–53602, Federal Register/Vol. 77, No. 170/Friday, August 31, 2012/Rules and Regulations, http://www.gpo.gov/fdsys/pkg/FR-2012-08-31/pdf/2012-19079.pdf

HEALTHCARE-ASSOCIATED INFECTIONS (HAI)

MEASURE ID	MEASURE DESCRIPTION	ACHIEVMENT THRESHOLD	BENCHMARK
SCIP-Inf-1	prophylactic antibiotic received within one hour prior to surgical incision	0.98639	1.0
SCIP-Inf-2	prophylactic antibiotic selection for surgical patients	0.98637	1.0
SCIP-Inf-3	prophylactic antibiotics discontinued within 24 hours after surgery end time	0.97494	1.0
SCIP-Inf-4	cardiac surgery patients with controlled 6AM postoperative serum glucose	0.95798	0.99767
SCIP-Inf-9	postoperative urinary catheter removal on postoperative Day 1 or 2	0.94891	0.99991

SURGERIES

MEASURE ID	MEASURE DESCRIPTION	ACHIEVMENT THRESHOLD	BENCHMARK
SCIP-Card-2	surgery patients on a beta-blocker prior to arrival that received a beta-blocker during the perioperative period	0.97175	1.0
SCIP-VTE-2	surgery patients who received appropriate venous thromboembolism prophylaxis within 24 hours prior to surgery to 24 hours after surgery.	0.97403	0.99998

MORTALITY OUTCOMES*: 30 PERCENT WEIGHTING

MEASURE ID	MEASURE DESCRIPTION	ACHIEVMENT THRESHOLD	BENCHMARK
Mort-30-AMI	acute myocardial infarction (AMI) 30-Day Mortality Rate	0.847472	0.862371
Mort-30-HF	heart failure (HF) 30-Day Mortality Rate	0.881510	0.900315
Mort-30-PN	pneumonia (PN) 30-Day Mortality Rate	0.882651	0.904181
PSI-90	patient safety for selected indicators (composite)	0.622879	0.451792
CLABSI	central line-associated bloodstream infections	0.437000	0.00000

*Mortality Outcome measures are expressed as survival rates

EFFICIENCY MEASURES: 20 PERCENT WEIGHTING			
MEASURE ID	**MEASURE DESCRIPTION**	**ACHIEVMENT THRESHOLD**	**BENCHMARK**
MSPB-1	Medicare spending per beneficiary	median Medicare spending per beneficiary ratio across all hospitals during the performance period	mean of the lowest Medicare spending per beneficiary rations across all hospitals during the performance period

Note: *During the period of May 1, 2011 through December 31, 2011, the achievement threshold would have been an MSPB ratio of 0.99, which corresponds to a standardized, risk-adjusted MSPB amount of $18,079, and the benchmark would have been 0.82, which corresponds to an MSPB amount of $14,985.*[96]

FY2015 PATIENT EXPERIENCE OF CARE MEASURES: 30 PERCENT WEIGHTING			
SELECTED DIMENSIONS FROM THE HCAHPS SURVEY	**FLOOR (MINIMUM)**	**PERFORMANCE STANDARD (ACHIEVMENT THRESHOLD)**	**BENCHMARK**
communication with nurses	47.77 percent	76.56 percent	85.70 percent
communication with doctors	55.62 percent	79.88 percent	88.79 percent
responsiveness of hospital staff	35.10 percent	63.17 percent	79.06 percent
pain management	43.58 percent	69.46 percent	78.17 percent
communication about medicines	35.48 percent	60.89 percent	71.85 percent
cleanliness and quietness of hospital	41.94 percent	64.07 percent	78.90 percent
discharge information	57.67 percent	83.54 percent	89.72 percent
overall rating of hospital	32.82 percent	67.96 percent	83.44 percent

[96] *Page 27614, Federal Register/Vol. 78, No. 91/Friday, May 10, 2013/Proposed Rules*

Table 11: FY2016 Program Year Measure Standards[97]

Clinical Process of Care Measures: 10 percent weighting

ACUTE MYOCARDIAL INFARCTION (AMI)			
MEASURE ID	**MEASURE DESCRIPTION**	**ACHIEVMENT THRESHOLD**	**BENCHMARK**
AMI-7a	fibrinolytic therapy received within 30 minutes of hospital arrival	0.99154	1.0

IMMUNIZATIONS			
MEASURE ID	**MEASURE DESCRIPTION**	**ACHIEVMENT THRESHOLD**	**BENCHMARK**
IMM-2:	influenza immunization	0.90607	0.98875

PNEUMONIA (PN)			
MEASURE ID	**MEASURE DESCRIPTION**	**ACHIEVMENT THRESHOLD**	**BENCHMARK**
PN-6	initial antibiotic selection for CAP in immunocompetent patient	0.96552	1.0

HEALTHCARE-ASSOCIATED INFECTIONS (HAI)			
MEASURE ID	**MEASURE DESCRIPTION**	**ACHIEVMENT THRESHOLD**	**BENCHMARK**
SCIP-Inf-2	prophylactic antibiotic selection for surgical patients	0.98086	1.00000
SCIP-Inf-3	prophylactic antibiotics discontinued within 24 hours after surgery end time	0.97971	1.00000
SCIP-Inf-9	postoperative urinary catheter removal on postoperative Day 1 or 2	0.97059	1.00000

---

[97] *Page 50697, Federal Register/Vol. 78, No. 160/Monday, August 19, 2013/Rules and Regulations, www.gpo.gov/fdsys/pkg/FR-2013-08-19/pdf/2013-18956.pdf*

SURGERIES			
MEASURE ID	MEASURE DESCRIPTION	ACHIEVMENT THRESHOLD	BENCHMARK
SCIP-Card-2	surgery patients on a beta-blocker prior to arrival that received a beta-blocker during the perioperative period	0.97727	1.0
SCIP-VTE-2	surgery patients who received appropriate venous thromboembolism prophylaxis within 24 hours prior to surgery to 24 hours after surgery.	0.98225	0.99998

MORTALITY OUTCOMES: 40 PERCENT WEIGHTING			
MEASURE ID	MEASURE DESCRIPTION	ACHIEVMENT THRESHOLD	BENCHMARK
Mort-30-AMI	acute myocardial infarction (AMI) 30-Day Mortality Rate	0.847472	0.862371
Mort-30-HF	heart failure (HF) 30-Day Mortality Rate	0.881510	0.900315
Mort-30-PN	pneumonia (PN) 30-Day Mortality Rate	0.882651	0.904181
PSI-90	patient safety for selected indicators (Composite)	0.622879	0.451792
CAUTI	catheter-associated urinary tract infection	0.801	0.00000
CLABSI	central line-associated bloodstream infections	0.465	0.00000
SSI:	surgical site infections (colon, abdominal hysterectomy)	0.752	0.00000

*Mortality Outcome measures are expressed as survival rates

EFFICIENCY MEASURES: 25 PERCENT WEIGHTING			
MEASURE ID	MEASURE DESCRIPTION	ACHIEVMENT THRESHOLD	BENCHMARK
MSPB-1	Medicare spending per beneficiary	median Medicare spending per beneficiary ratio across all hospitals during the performance period	mean of the lowest decile of Medicare spending per beneficiary rations across all hospitals during the performance period

FY2016 PATIENT EXPERIENCE OF CARE MEASURES: 25 PERCENT WEIGHTING			
SELECTED DIMENSIONS FROM THE HCAHPS SURVEY	FLOOR (MINIMUM)	PERFORMANCE STANDARD (ACHIEVMENT THRESHOLD)	BENCHMARK
communication with nurses	53.99 percent	77.67 percent	86.07 percent
communication with doctors	57.01 percent	80.40 percent	88.56 percent
responsiveness of hospital staff	38.21 percent	64.71 percent	79.76 percent
pain management	48.96 percent	70.18 percent	78.16 percent
communication about medicines	34.61 percent	62.33 percent	72.77 percent
cleanliness and quietness of hospital	43.08 percent	64.95 percent	79.10 percent
discharge information	61.36 percent	84.70 percent	90.39 percent
overall rating of hospital	36.95 percent	69.32 percent	83.97 percent

2.3.9 Scoring Step 3: Scoring Hospitals on Achievement and Improvement[98]

Overview

Using individual measure data collected during the baseline and performance periods, CMS developed a scoring methodology that rewards initial achievement, improvement, and consistency over time.

Note: *The consistency component score is applicable only to the HCAHPS.*

---

[98] *Page 26526, Federal Register/Vol. 76, No. 88/Friday, May 6, 2011/Rules and Regulations*
http://www.gpo.gov/fdsys/pkg/FR-2011-05-06/pdf/FR-2011-05-06.pdf

Achievement Scoring

For a given performance period, a hospital's individual domain measure scores are compared to where they fell relative to the national achievement threshold (baseline threshold) and the national benchmark standard (established during the baseline period). Each measure is then assigned achievement points based on this comparison.

- **10 achievement points**: Hospital measure score at or above the national benchmark.

- **1–9 achievement points**: Hospital measure score is equal to or above the achievement threshold (baseline threshold) and less than the benchmark.

- **0 achievement points:** The hospital measure score is below the achievement threshold.

Improvement Scoring

- **Improvement threshold** is an individual hospital's performance level on a measure during the baseline period with respect to a fiscal year.

- A hospital's individual domain measure scores attained during the performance period are compared to performance on the same measure during the baseline period. Improvement threshold and improvement points are awarded based on individual measure improvement.

  - **9 improvement points:** Hospital measure score at or above the national benchmark.

  - **1–9 improvement points**: Hospital measure score is between the baseline improvement performance standard and the benchmark.

  - **0 improvement points**: Hospital measure score is at or below the baseline improvement performance standard.

Consistency Scoring

- A consistency score is determined only for the HCAHPS domain and is based on the lowest score obtained in the eight HCAHPS measures during the performance period as defined by a mathematical formula involving comparison among a hospital's measure scores, the benchmark, baseline achievement threshold and a floor score:

   o The floor score is assigned to each HCAHPS measure and is the worst-performing hospital's performance rate during the baseline period, which defines the 0 percentile for this dimension.

   o The higher a hospital's lowest dimension score is above the "floor," the more consistency points the hospital will receive.

- Scoring:

   o **20 consistency points**: lowest measure score is above baseline achievement performance standard (50th percentile).

   o **1–19 consistency points**: awarded proportionately on scores between the floor and the achievement threshold.

   o **0 points**: lowest-measured score is below the floor standard.

2.3.10 Scoring Step 4: Assigning Relative Weights for Each Domain

FY2014–FY2016 Domains and Weightings

For the FY2014, FY2015, and F2016 HVBP program years, domain weightings are:

DOMAINS	FY2014	FY2015	FY2016
Clinical Process of Care	45 percent	20 percent	10 percent
Patient Experience of Care	30 percent	30 percent	25 percent
Outcome	25 percent	30 percent	40 percent
Efficiency	0 percent	20 percent	25 percent

FY2017 NQS-Aligned Domains and Weightings

For the FY2017 HVBP program year CMS is adopting NQS-aligned domains with the following weightings:

DOMAIN	DOMAIN WEIGHTING
Safety	15 percent
Clinical Care	35 percent
• Outcomes	25 percent
• Process	10 percent
Efficiency and Cost Reduction	25 percent
Patient and Caregiver Centered Experience of Care/Care Coordination	25 percent

2.3.11 Scoring Step 5: Calculating the Total Performance Score (TPS)[99]

Overview

- Determine individual measure scores for achievement and improvement:

    o **Achievement Score (0–10 possible points per measure):** based on how the hospital scored on a measure as compared to the national baseline standard for that measure and the national benchmark.

    o **Improvement Score (0–9 points possible):** determined by comparing scores achieved during the performance period with those achieved during the baseline period.

Calculate a Domain Measure Score

- For each measure, the *higher* of the Achievement or Improvement Score is totaled to determine a summed Measure Score for each domain.

---

[99] http://www.cms.gov/Medicare/Quality-Initiatives-Patient-Assessment-Instruments/hospital-value-based-purchasing/Downloads/NPCSlides071112.pdf

Through this process a hospital is rewarded for incremental progress made or a high level of overall achievement.

- For the Patient Care Experience domain, the consistency points are added to the Domain Measure Score total.

Calculate the TPS

- Each domain total is then multiplied by the domain weight and the weighted scores are added together to determine the Total Performance Score.

  Note: The maximum Total Performance Score is 100.

- These scores are communicated to hospitals as part of the Percentage Summary Report as shown below:

Communication via Percentage Payment Summary Report

TOTAL PERFORMANCE SCORE		
FACILITY	STATE	NATIONAL
72.850000000000	49.571719705914	46.525704094903

SCORES			
DOMAIN	UNWEIGHTED DOMAIN SCORE	WEIGHTING	WEIGHTED DOMAIN SCORE
Clinical Process of Care	96.0000000000	45%	43.2000000000
Patient Experience of Care	78.0000000000	30%	23.4000000000
Outcome	25.0000000000	25%	6.2500000000

2.3.12 Scoring Step 6: Convert the TPS to a Payment Adjustment Factor (PAF).

Linear Exchange Mathematical Model

- Once the Total Performance Score has been determined, CMS will use a "linear exchange" mathematical model to convert numeric scores to an incentive payment percentage. This model provides accelerated payments for higher scores and incentives for score improvement.

- The linear exchange value is used to construct a mathematical conversion "slope" along which a given TPS is converted to a specific incentive payment percentage. CMS will set the slope of the linear exchange function for each HVBP program year so that the estimated total value-based incentive payments to all participating hospitals are equal to the mandated national incentive pool for a program year.

- The slope of the exchange model is such that hospitals with scores above zero will receive incentive payments in a linear fashion.

- The slope will not be determined until CMS evaluates the performance period Total Performance Score distribution among participants.

- CMS publishes the linear slope conversion factor in the program year IPPS Rules. For the FY2014 program year the corrected slope published in the FY2014 IPPS Final Rule is: **2.0961880387**.

The Percentage Payment Summary Report (PPSR)[100]

- Upon determination of the TPS, CMS completes all payment adjustment calculations and uploads a PPSR to HVBP participating hospitals. This report illustrates summary scoring as well as individual measure performance.

- Section 1 of the PPSR is illustrated below and provides hospitals with the following HVBP program information:

---

[100] *Hospital Value-Based Purchasing; Reports, https://www.qualitynet.org/*

- o summary domain scoring information
- o the hospital TPS in comparison to state and national averages
- o annual withhold percentage (base operating DRG payment amount reduction)
- o the total value-based incentive payment percentage
- o the calculated HVBP net change to base operating DRG rates
- o the hospital-specific value-based incentive PAF to be applied to each Medicare discharge for the applicable program year
- o the Exchange Function Slope value Report Run Date: 09/20/2013

Hospital Value-Based Purchasing:

Value-Based Percentage Payment Report

Percentage Summary Report

Provider: 123456

Reporting Period: FY2014

Date as of 07/08/2013

TOTAL PERFORMANCE SCORE		
FACILITY	STATE	NATIONAL
72.850000000000	49.571719705914	46.525704094903

SCORES			
DOMAIN	UNWEIGHTED DOMAIN SCORE	WEIGHTING	WEIGHTED DOMAIN SCORE
Clinical Process of Care	96.0000000000	45%	43.2000000000
Patient Experience of Care	78.0000000000	30%	23.4000000000
Outcome	25.0000000000	25%	6.2500000000

VALUE-BASED PERCENTAGE PAYMENT SUMMARY FY2014				
BASE OPERATING DRG PAYMENT AMOUNT REDUCTION	VALUE-BASED INCENTIVE PAYMENT PERCENTAGE	NET CHANGE IN BASE OPERATING DRG PAYMENT AMOUNT	VALUE-BASED INCENTIVE PAYMENT ADJUSTMENT FACTOR	EXCHANGE FUNCTION SLOPE
1.250000000000%	1.9088412327%	+0.6588412327%	1.0065884123	2.0961880387

         [A]   [B]   [C]

Note: The base operating DRG payment amount reduction is also known as the annual HVBP withhold percentage.

2.3.13 Value-Based Payment Calculations of the Percentage Payment Summary Report

[A] **The Value-Based Incentive Payment Percentage[101]**

- The value-based incentive payment percentage represents the portion of the base operating DRG amount a hospital earned back (as compared to the annual withhold percentage) based on its performance in the HVBP program.

  - Win: If this number is greater than the base operating DRG reduction amount, the hospital earned back more than the base operating DRG reduction amount.

  - Lose: If this number is less than the base operating DRG reduction amount, the hospital did not earn back the full base operating DRG reduction amount. This value is rounded to 10 digits to the right of the decimal.

  - Draw: If this number is equal to the base operating DRG reduction amount, the hospital earned back the entire base operating DRG reduction amount.

---

[101] *Hospital Value-Based Purchasing; Reports, https://www.qualitynet.org/*

- The value-based incentive payment percentage is calculated as the product of the base operating DRG payment amount reduction, the quotient of the TPS divided by 100, and the Exchange Function.

- **Example: using the PPSR above:**

  (Annual Base Operating DRG Payment Amount Reduction in decimal form) x ((Total Performance Score/100)) x (Exchange Function Slope) = Value-Based Incentive Payment Percentage

  - For FY2014 HVBP Hospital #123456:

    - TPS = 72.85

    - The annual reduction to base operating DRG rates is 1.25 percent

    - The annual linear slope function is 2.0961880387

  - (.0125) x ((72.85/100)) x (2.0961880387) = .019088412327 or **1.9088412327%***

    > *The value-based incentive payment percentage is calculated as a decimal value instead of a percentage value. In order to convert the calculated decimal value to a percentage value matching the PPSR, multiply the value by 100 and round to 10 digits to the right of the decimal.

B | Net Change in Base Operating DRG Payment Amounts[102]

- The net change in base operating payment amounts represents the net amount a hospital's base operating DRG payments will be changed due to the HVBP program for a given program year.

- It is calculated as the difference between the calculated value-based incentive payment percentage and the annual withhold percentage:

  - a positive number means the hospital will have higher FY2014 payments because of its HVBP program performance.

---

[102] *Hospital Value-Based Purchasing; Reports, https://www.qualitynet.org/*

- A net amount of zero means there will be no change to the hospital's FY2014 payments as a result of the HVBP program.

  - A negative number means the hospital's payments will be lower due to the HVBP program. This value is rounded to 10 digits to the right of the decimal.

- **Example:** using the PPSR above:

  (Value-Based Incentive Payment Percentage – Annual Base Operating DRG Payment Amount Reduction) = Net Change in Base Operating DRG Payment Amounts

  (1.9088412327% – 1.25%) = +.6588412327% or +.66%

c Value-Based Incentive Payment Adjustment Factor[103]

- The value-based incentive PAF is a multiplier applied to the base operating DRG rate (as defined for the HVBP program) for each Medicare discharge during a HVBP program year.

- This factor determines whether a HVBP participating hospital will incur a HVBP "penalty" in the form of reduced DRG reimbursements or earn "incentive" amounts with higher DRG reimbursement rates:

  - If this value is greater than one, a hospital will receive higher DRG payments as a result of HVBP performance.

  - If this value is equal to one, a hospital's payments will not be changed due to the HVBP program.

  - If this value is less than one, a hospital's HVBP program year DRG payments will be lower due to the HVBP program.

  - This value is rounded to 10 digits to the right of the decimal.

  - For the FY2014 HVBP program year, HVBP incentive factors ranged from a low for the Gallup Indian Medical Center of .988600499 to a high of 1.00881776 for the Arkansas Heart Hospital.

---

[103] *Hospital Value-Based Purchasing; Reports, https://www.qualitynet.org/*

- The value-based incentive PAF for each discharge is determined by:

  - converting the net change in base operating DRG payment amounts percentage into decimal form by dividing it by 100 and adding the numerical result to 1.00.

- **Example:** using the PPSR above:
  (Net Change in Base Operating DRG Payment Amounts/100) + (1.000000000) = Value-Based Incentive Payment Adjustment Factor
  (+.6588412327/100) + 1.000000000 = 1.006588412327

- The wage-adjusted base operating DRG rate for each Medicare discharge occurring for Provider 123456 during the HVBP program year would be multiplied by the PAF. This increase represents a .66 percent increase to the wage-adjusted base operating DRG.

2.3.14 Value-Based Purchasing Reports Provided to Hospitals

Fiscal Year Baseline Measures Report

- The Baseline Measures Report is provided to hospitals upon calculation of the baseline period measures performance for the quality domains:

  - The Baseline Report for the FY2014 HVBP program year was released in December 2012.

    Note: The performance period for the Clinical Process of Care and Patient Experience of Care domains **ended** December 2012 and the performance period for Outcomes ended in June 2012.

- For each measure, the report displays hospital baseline performance and lists the applicable benchmarks and achievement thresholds for each measure.

- Floor rates for each HCAHPS item are also provided.

Percentage Payment Summary Report (PPSR)

- The PPSR is uploaded to hospitals at or near the start of a HVBP program year.

- This report informs hospitals of their TPS and information supporting calculation of the TPS, to include unweighted and weighted domain scoring.

- In addition, the following summary sections provide reimbursement rate information:

  o **Base operating DRG payment amount reduction:** the annual percentage reduction to a hospital's base operating DRG payment amounts used to fund the national incentive pool.

  o **Value-based incentive payment percentage:** the portion of the base operating DRG amount a hospital earned back, based on its performance in the HVBP.

  o **Net change in base operating DRG payment amount:** the amount a hospital's FY2014 base operating DRG payments will be changed due to the HVBP program.

  o **Value-based incentive PAF:** the value that is multiplied by the base operating DRG amount for each discharge at a hospital occurring in a HVBP program year.

- **A hospital's FY2014 PPSR is divided into four sections:**
  o Percentage Payment Summary
  o TPS
  o unweighted and weighted domain scores
  o weighting

- **Value-Based Percentage Payment Summary:**
  o base operating DRG payment amount reduction
  o value-based incentive payment percentage
  o net change in base operating DRG payment amount
  o value-based incentive PAF
  o exchange function slope

- **Clinical Process of Care Domain Summary:**
  - details on the thirteen Clinical Process of Care measures

- **Patient Experience of Care Domain Summary:**
  - details on the eight Patient Experience of Care dimensions

- **Outcome Domain Summary:**
  - details on the three Mortality measures

2.3.15 Process for Determining Financial Impact of HVBP Program

Overview

- All payment impact information resulting from the HVBP program is communicated to hospitals through the rule-making process or through hospital-specific reports uploaded to individual MyQualityNet accounts.

- Because such information is provided only as a percentage change to the base operating DRG rates, the total financial impact to an individual hospital is obscured and may not be fully understood or appreciated.

- The process for estimating the fiscal impact of an HVBP year is fairly straightforward and it is possible to model the net impact of the HVBP program on a participant's financial bottom line.

- Because the annual payment amount reduction (withhold) and the HVBP PAF are both percentage adjustments applied directly to the base operating DRG payment amount, an accurate determination of this hospital-specific rate is essential.

- To determine the base operating DRG amount for a given hospital, the following information is needed:
  - applicable year national adjusted operating standardized amounts (withhold percentage of base DRG amount)
  - individual hospital wage index (WI)*

- o transfer-adjusted case mix index for hospital*

- o annual new technology add-on payments (NTAP) **

- o number of Medicare fee-for-service discharges *

- o value-based purchasing PAF ***

*This data is available for FY2014 at CMS.gov under FY2014 Final Rules IPPS Impact Files or link: FY2014 FR Impact File: updated September 2013 [ZIP, 1MB]

**All other elements of information needed to calculate the base operating DRG can be found in CMS data tables. The annual NTAP amount must be provided by a hospital or estimated as a per-discharge amount.

***This data is available for FY2014 at CMS.gov or link: HVBP Table 16A (final rule and correction notice) and Table 16B [ZIP, 278KB]

Key Terms:

- **Base operating DRG rate**[104] "Section 1886(q)(2) of the Social Security Act clearly defines the base operating DRG payment amount **as the wage-adjusted DRG payment amount, plus any applicable new technology add-on payments, excluding adjustments or add-on payments for IME, DSH, outliers, and low-volume hospitals.**"

*(**Note:** See **Appendix: Attachment F** for a complete definition of base operating DRG.)*

[104] Pages 53382–533383, Federal Register/Vol. 77, No. 170/Friday, August 31, 2012/Rules and Regulations, http://www.gpo.gov/fdsys/pkg/FR-2012-08-31/pdf/2012-19079.pdf

o The DRG classification system groups similar clinical conditions (diagnoses) and the procedures furnished by the hospital during the stay. The beneficiary's principal diagnosis and up to twenty-four secondary diagnoses (indicating comorbidities and complication) determine the appropriate DRG assignment. Similarly, DRG assignment can be affected by up to twenty-five procedures furnished during the stay.

o CMS reviews the DRG definitions annually to ensure that each group continues to include cases with clinically similar conditions that require comparable amounts of inpatient resources. When the review shows that subsets of clinically similar cases within a DRG consume significantly different amounts of resources, CMS may assign them to a different DRG with comparable resource use or create a new DRG.

o DRG reimbursement begins with an annually established base operating rate that is then modified based on additional factors specific to treatment and the hospital environment.

o Although final reimbursement under the DRG system includes a number of other factors, the following components are excluded for the purpose of determining the base operating DRG amount used for the HVBP program:

- **Add-on payments for indirect medical education (IME):** the costs associated with a teaching institution

- **Payments to hospitals serving low-income populations:** disproportionate share hospitals (DSH)

- **"Outlier" payments:** additional payments made for the most expensive 1 percent of hospital stays

- **additional payments** made to low-volume hospitals

o The base operating DRG rate is the portion of per-discharge Medicare reimbursement impacted by application of the HVBP withhold and incentive payments.

- **Case Mix Index (CMI):** The CMI reflects the severity of inpatient cases and is the measure of the average DRG weight for cases paid under the IPPS. A higher CMI indicates more complex patient cases. Because the

DRG weight determines the prospective payment for each case, any percentage increase in the CMI corresponds to an equal percentage increase in hospital payments.

- **National adjusted operating standardized amounts (base DRG amount):** Composed of labor and non-labor portions, these annually established base DRG amounts reflect per-discharge amounts for hospitals successfully or unsuccessfully participating in the IQR reporting program. For FY2014 the total DRG for successful IQR participants is $5,370.28 and $5,264.67 for unsuccessful IQR participants.

- **New Technology Add-On Payments (NTAP):**[105]

  - DRG rates are recalculated annually, using two years of data. As a result, any newly introduced technology will not be reimbursed for at least two years.

  - To address this lag, CMS introduced New Technology Add-on Payments in 2001 to allow reimbursement for technologies that met three criteria:

    - the technology is considered "new" (within two to three years of FDA approval)

    - the average cost of a patient case using the technology is inadequately paid under the current DRG system

    - the new technology represents a "substantial clinical improvement" over the existing standard of care

  - New technology add-on payments are included as part of the HVBP program definition of the base operating DRG Rate. The aggregate amount reimbursed annually for new technology will be equally split over total Medicare discharges during a program year. This amount will be added to the per-discharge wage adjusted base operating DRG rate.

  - Approved new technology items are listed in the annual IPPS Final Rules along with fiscal year reimbursement rates. The

---

[105] Page 51023, Federal Register/Vol. 78, No. 160/Monday, August 19, 2013/Rules and Regulations, www.gpo.gov/fdsys/pkg/FR-2013-08-19/pdf/2013-18956.pdf

current listing of new technology items may be viewed in Appendix 2.4.6 Attachment E.

- **Transfer Adjustment:** The FY2014 Final IPPS Rule accepted a comment that transfer adjustments should be included in the definition of base operating DRG payment amount. The transfer adjustment is the reduction applied to the payment amount when a patient leaves the hospital before the average length of stay for their DRG and continues to receive treatment in either another acute hospital or a post- acute setting.

- **Transfer Adjusted Case Mix:** The Transfer Adjusted Case Mix reflects the revised average DRG case severity through the application of an adjustment to account for patients leaving the hospital before the average length of stay for their DRG.

- **Wage-Adjusted DRG Operating Payment:** For the HVBP program, the wage-adjusted DRG operating payment is defined as the applicable average federal rate adjusted for:

  - resource utilization by the applicable MS-DRG relative weight

  - differences in geographic costs by the applicable area WI (and by the applicable COLA for hospitals located in Alaska and Hawaii)

  - any applicable patient transfer adjustments (new for FY2014)

    Note: This definition is the same as the one adopted in this rule for the HRRP. The definition excludes adjustments for IME, DSH, low-volume hospitals, outliers, and the readmissions reduction program adjustment.

- **Wage-Adjusted Federal Standard Rate:** The wage-adjusted federal standard rate is established for an individual hospital by multiplying the applicable labor portion of the base DRG rate by a hospital's individual WI and adding this sum to the established non-labor portion of the base DRG.

- **Wage Index:**[106] The annual base DRG rate is calculated based on adjustments made to a "labor-related share" and a "nonlabor-related share." The percentage that each component contributes to the total

---

[106] *Wage Index Chart Pack, November 2011, American Hospital Association,* www.aha.org/content/11/11nov-wageindex.pdf

base DRG can vary based on the relative wage levels present for a given geographic area. CMS calculates a WI for specific geographical areas to reflect differences between "high-wage" and "low-wage" areas.

- o High-wage areas are associated with an assigned WI of greater than 1.0 and low-wage areas are indicated by a WI equal to or less than 1.0.

- o Hospitals are first grouped according to their location in a high-wage or low-wage area. Based on this designation, the amount of the assigned labor-related share portion of the base DRG is different, as shown below:

    - For FY2014: base DRG rate = $5,370.28

HIGH-WAGE AREA: (WI>1.00)	
labor-related share =	$3,737.71 or 69.6 percent of base DRG
nonlabor-related share =	$1,632.57 or 30.4 percent of base DRG
Total	**$5,370.28**

LOW-WAGE AREA: (WI<1.00)	
labor-related share =	$3,329.57 or 62 percent of base DRG
nonlabor-related share =	$2,040.71 or 38 percent of base DRG
Total	**$5,370.28**

- o These labor-related share amounts are further modified by the application of a hospital-specific WI, based on the geographic location of the hospital. The resulting amount may be higher or lower than the national base DRG rate:

Application of Hospital-Specific WI: Low-wage Area Hospital

- Hospital A is located in Mobile, Alabama, with a WI of .8106 (less than 1.0 indicating low-wage area DRG composition)

- (WI x Labor-Related Share for Low-Wage Area) + Nonlabor-Related Share for Low-Wage Area = Wage-Adjusted Federal Standard Rate

- (.8106 x $3,329) + $2040.71 = $4,739.20

Application of Hospital-Specific WI: High-wage Area Hospital

- Hospital B is located in San Francisco with a WI of 1.6269 (> than 1.0 indicating high-wage area DRG composition)

- (WI x Labor-Related Share for High-Wage Area) + Nonlabor-Related Share for High-Wage Area = Wage-Adjusted Federal Standard Rate

- (1.6269 x $3,737.71) + $1,632.57 = $7,713.45

Note: *The FY2014 assigned WI table for individual hospitals can be viewed at: http://www.cms.gov/Medicare/Medicare-Fee-for-Service-Payment/AcuteInpatientPPS/FY2014-IPPS-Final-Rule-Home-Page.html*

Determining the Base Operating DRG Rate

For all calculations in this section, data from a HVBP-participating hospital will be used. This data is contained in the FY2014 Final IPPS Rule Impact File. This file contains the following data sources:

- March 2013 update of FY2012 MEDPAR

- March 2013 update of provider specific file

- FY2010/FY2011 Cost Report data

As a result of the data sources used, the number of discharges and CMI listed through other data sources, such as the American Hospital Directory website, may differ slightly.

In addition, the data presented above in the PPSR for provider #123456 will be used to calculate revenue information.

General Information for Hospital A: Hospital A (provider #123456) is a large urban hospital located in a high-wage area in the Northeastern United States that successfully participated in the IQR program during FY2013 and received their full annual payment update.

Data From FY2014 FR Impact File, updated September 2013:

ITEM	FY2014 VALUE	COLUMN & HEADING LOCATION
Wage Index	1.3129	(column L; heading: FY2014 WAGE INDEX)
Case Mix	2.010166	(column AJ; heading: CMIV30)
Transfer Adjusted Case Mix Index	1.991461	(column AH; heading: TACMIV30)
Annual Medicare Discharges	10,140	(column AG; heading: BILLS)

Other:

- HVBP PAF 1.004976968

- average per-discharge amounts for NTAP = $10.00*

  This amount was assumed for the example based on assumed total spending on new technology of $101,140.00 ($101,140/10,140 discharges) = $10.00 per discharge.

Determine the Federal Standard Rate

- **Step 1:** Select the applicable average standardized DRG amount depending on whether the hospital submitted qualifying IQR program data from the FY2014 national adjusted operating standardized amounts table below: **Hospital A** successfully completed IQR reporting and received its full APU:

LABOR-RELATED	NONLABOR-RELATED
$3,737.71	$1,632.57

Table 12: FY2014 Final Rule DRG Table

High Wage Market: Hospital Wage Index >1.0

TABLE 1A. NATIONAL ADJUSTED OPERATING STANDARDIZED AMOUNTS; LABOR/NONLABOR (69.6% LABOR SHARE/ 30.4% NONLABOR SHARE IF WI GREATER THAN 1)			
Successful Submission of IQR Data: Full Update (1.7%)		Unsuccessful Submission of IQR Data: Reduced Update (-0.3%)	
Labor-related	Nonlabor-related	Labor-related	Nonlabor-related
$3,737.71	$1,632.57	$3,664.21	$1,600.46

Low Wage Market: Hospital Wage Index <1.0

TABLE 1B. NATIONAL ADJUSTED OPERATING STANDARDIZED AMOUNTS; LABOR/NONLABOR (62% LABOR SHARE/ 38% NONLABOR SHARE IF WI LESS THAN OR EQUAL TO 1)			
Full Update (1.7%)		Reduced Update (-0.3%)	
Labor-related	Nonlabor-related	Labor-related	Nonlabor-related
$3,329.57	$2,040.71	$3,264.10	$2,000.57

- **Step 2:** Multiply the labor-related portion of the standardized amount by the applicable WI for the geographic area in which the hospital is located. Hospital A: $3,737.71 X 1.3129 = $4,907.24

- **Step 3:** For hospitals in Alaska and Hawaii, multiply the nonlabor-related portion of the standardized amount by the applicable cost-of-living adjustment factor. Hospital A: not applicable.

- **Step 4:** Add the amount from Step 2 and the nonlabor-related portion of the standardized amount (adjusted, if applicable, under Step 3). Hospital A: $4,907.24 + $1,632.57 = $6,539.81 (wage-adjusted federal standard rate)

- **Determine Wage-Adjusted Base Operating DRG (WABO DRG) Payment.**

- o **Apply the Transfer Adjusted Case Mix Index:** The CMI provides the average severity of all hospital cases for an annual period. In the FY2014 Final IPS Rule, CMS agreed to include a transfer adjustment in the calculation of the WABO DRG payment to account for those patients who left the hospital earlier than their DRG specified. The net effect of the application of the transfer adjustment is a reduction in the CMI and lowered reimbursement. **Multiply the amount calculated in Step 4 by the Transfer Adjusted Case Mix Index** $6,539.81 x 1.991461 = $13,023.78 (WABO DRG Payment)

- **Complete calculation of Base Operating DRG Rate:**

  - o Add the average per-discharge amount of any **NTAP** to the WABO DRG to determine the Base Operating DRG Rate:

  - o $13,023.78 + $10.00* = **$13,033.78 (Base Operating DRG Rate for Hospital A)**

  - o *Amount assumed for example.

Calculate Fiscal Impact of HVBP Program

- o Base Operating DRG Amount = $13,033.78

- o Number of Annual Medicare Discharges = 10,140

Data from the Payment Summary Report for Hospital A (provider #123456)

VALUE-BASED PERCENTAGE PAYMENT SUMMARY FY2014				
BASE OPERATING DRG PAYMENT AMOUNT REDUCTION	VALUE-BASED INCENTIVE PAYMENT PERCENTAGE	NET CHANGE IN BASE OPERATING DRG PAYMENT AMOUNT	VALUE-BASED INCENTIVE PAYMENT ADJUSTMENT FACTOR	EXCHANGE FUNCTION SLOPE
1.250000000000%	1.9088412327%	+0.6588412327%	1.0065884123	2.0961880387

- Determine estimated annual withhold amount used to fund the national HVBP incentive pool:

    o **(Annual withhold expressed in decimal form* x Base Operating DRG rate) x Total Discharges**

    o (.0125 x $13,033.78) x 10,140 = **$1,652,031**

    o *also referred to as base operating DRG payment amount reduction.

    o **$1,652,031/10,140 = $162.00 withheld per discharge**

- Determine the total net gain or loss in annual revenue resulting from the application of the **Value-Based Incentive PAF** on a per-discharge basis:

    o **((Value-Based Incentive Adjustment Factor x Base Operating DRG Rate) x Annual Discharge Rate) – (Base Operating DRG Rate x Annual Discharge Rate) = Net Revenue Gain or Loss**

    o ((1.0065884123 x $13,033.78) x 10,140) – ($13,033.78 x 10,140) **= $870,758**

    o **$870,758/10,140 = $86.00 per discharge above the full base operating DRG rate**

2.3.16 Conclusion

- Based on an annual Medicare discharge rate of 10,140, Hospital A will have $1,652,031 withheld from their fiscal year revenues in the form of reductions made to per-discharge reimbursement rates (or $163.00 withheld per discharge). However, by achieving a TPS well above state and national averages, Hospital A received a positive HVBP PAF of 1.0065884123 above, which resulted in the hospital fully earning back its withhold amount and realizing an additional $86.00 per discharge. The overall result of HVBP performance is a net gain of $870,858.00 for Hospital A.

- Withhold amounts and incentive payments are applied simultaneously during a given HVBP program year. For Hospital A this means that for each Medicare discharge occurring in FY2014, CMS will:

  - deduct $163 for withhold

  - add back ($163 + $86) = $249.00

- The net impact of this reimbursement methodology is that Hospital A fully earned back all withhold amounts and was paid an incentive of $86.00 per discharge for HVBP performance.

Section 2.4: Appendix

2.4.1 Acronym Guide

ACA............................Affordable Care Act

AHRQ.........................Agency for Healthcare Research and Quality

AMI............................Acute Myocardial Infarction

APU............................Annual Payment Update

CAH ....Critical Access Hospital

CAUTI ....Catheter-Associated Urinary Tract Infection

CLABSI ....Central Line-Associated Bloodstream Infection

CMI ....Case Mix Index

CMS ....Centers for Medicare & Medicaid Services

COPD.........................Chronic Obstructive Pulmonary Disease

CY ....Calendar Year

DPP...........................Disproportionate Patient Percentage

DRA ....Deficit Reduction Act (of 2005)

DRG ....Diagnosis-Related Group

DSH ....Disproportionate Share Hospital

EHR ....Electronic Health Record

EMR ....Electronic Medical Record

FQHC ....Federally Qualified Health Center

FTE ....Full-Time Equivalent

FY..............................Fiscal Year

GME...........................Graduate Medical Education

HACs..........................Hospital-Acquired Conditions

HAI ....Healthcare-Associated Infection

HCAHPS ....Hospital Consumer Assessment of
 Healthcare Providers and Systems

HF ....Heart Failure

HHA ....Home Health Agency

HHS ....Department of Health and Human Services

HIS .... Health Information System

HIT .... Health Information Technology

HQA .... Hospital Quality Alliance

HQI .... Hospital Quality Initiative

HRRP .... Hospital Readmissions Reduction Program

HVBP .... Hospital Value-Based Purchasing Program

IME .... Indirect Medical Education

IPPS .... [Acute care hospital] Inpatient Prospective Payment System

IRF .... Inpatient Rehabilitation Facility

IVR .... Interactive Voice Recognition

IQR .... Inpatient Quality Reporting

LOS .... Length of Stay

LTC-DRG .... Long-Term Care Diagnosis-Related Group

LTCH .... Long-Term Care Hospital

LTCHQR .... Long-Term Care Hospital Quality Reporting

MedPAC .... Medicare Payment Advisory Commission

MedPAR .... Medicare Provider Analysis and Review File

MS-DRG .... Medicare Severity Diagnosis-Related Group

MS-LTC-DRG .... Medicare Severity Long-Term Care Diagnosis-Related Group

MSPB .... Medicare Spending per Beneficiary

NCQA .... National Committee for Quality Assurance

NQF .... National Quality Forum

NTAP .... New Technology Add-On Payment

NVHRI .... National Voluntary Hospital Reporting Initiative

OMB .... Executive Office of Management and Budget

OPPS .... Outpatient Prospective Payment System

PN .... Pneumonia

PAF .... Payment Adjustment Factor

PPS .... Prospective Payment System

QIG .... Quality Improvement Group, CMS

RHQDAPU .... Reporting Hospital Quality Data for Annual Payment Update

SCH .... Sole Community Hospital

SCIP .... Surgical Care Improvement Project

SNF .... Skilled Nursing Facility

TPS .... Total Performance Score

HVBP .... Hospital Value-Based Purchasing Program

WI .... Wage Index

2.4.2 Attachment A: Acute Care Inpatient Prospective Payment System (IPPS)

Overview

The Inpatient Prospective Payment System (IPPS) is the method by which facilities are reimbursed for inpatient care of Medicare patients. Facilities contract with Medicare to furnish acute hospital inpatient care and agree to accept predetermined acute rates as payment in full under IPPS guidelines.

The inpatient hospital benefit covers beneficiaries for ninety days of care per episode of illness with an additional sixty-day lifetime reserve. Illness episodes begin when beneficiaries are admitted and end after they have been out of the hospital or Skilled Nursing Facility (SNF) for sixty consecutive days.

Basis for Inpatient Prospective Payment System Payment

Generally, hospitals receive Medicare IPPS payment on a per-discharge or per-case basis for Medicare beneficiaries with inpatient stays. All outpatient diagnostic services and admission-related outpatient non-diagnostic services provided by the admitting hospital—or an entity that is wholly owned or operated by the admitting hospital on the date of a beneficiary's inpatient admission or within three days immediately preceding the date of a beneficiary's inpatient admission—must be included on the claim for the beneficiary's inpatient stay and must not be separately billed to Medicare Part B.

Discharges are assigned DRGs, a classification system that groups similar clinical conditions (diagnoses) and the procedures furnished by the hospital during the stay. The beneficiary's principal diagnosis and up to twenty-four secondary diagnoses that indicate comorbidities and complications will determine the DRG assignment. Similarly, DRG assignment can be affected by up to twenty-five procedures furnished during the stay. CMS reviews the DRG definitions annually to ensure that each group continues to include cases with clinically similar conditions that require comparable amounts of inpatient resources. When the review shows that subsets of clinically similar cases within a DRG consume significantly different amounts of resources, CMS may assign them to a different DRG with comparable resource use or create a new DRG.

For discharges occurring on or after October 1, 2007, CMS is using a new DRG system called Medicare Severity (MS)-DRG to better account for severity of illness and resource consumption for Medicare beneficiaries. Use of MS-DRGs was transitioned during a two-year period. For the period from October 1, 2007, through September 30, 2008, payment was based on a 50/50 blend of MS-DRGs and the previous DRG system. Beginning October 1, 2008 (FY2009), and after, payment is based solely on the MS-DRGs. There are three levels of severity in the MS-DRGs based on secondary diagnosis codes:

1. major complication/comorbidity, which reflects the highest level of severity

2. complication/comorbidity, which is the next level of severity

3. non-complication/comorbidity, which does not significantly affect severity of illness and resource use

Payment Rates

The IPPS per-discharge payment is based on two national base payment rates or "standardized amounts": one that provides for operating expenses and another for capital expenses. These payment rates are adjusted to account for:

- the costs associated with the beneficiary's clinical condition and related treatment relative to the costs of the average Medicare case (i.e., the DRG relative weight, as described in the "How Payment Rates Are Set" section below)

- market conditions in the facility's location relative to national conditions (i.e., the WI, as described in the "How Payment Rates Are Set" section below)

Additional Payment Adjustments:

- In addition to these adjusted per-discharge base payment rates, hospitals can qualify for outlier payments for cases that are extremely costly.

- Hospitals that train residents in approved Graduate Medical Education (GME) Programs also receive a payment separate from the IPPS for the direct costs of training residents.

- The operating and capital payment rates for these teaching hospitals are increased to reflect the higher indirect patient care costs of teaching hospitals relative to nonteaching hospitals or indirect costs of graduate medical education (Indirect Medical Education [IME]).

- Operating and capital payment rates are also increased for facilities that treat a disproportionate share of low-income patients.

- In addition, hospitals may be paid an additional amount for treating patients with certain approved technologies that are new and costly and offer a substantial clinical improvement over existing treatments available to Medicare beneficiaries.

- Finally, in some cases, payment is reduced when a beneficiary has a short length of stay (LOS) and is transferred to another acute care hospital or, in some circumstances, to a post-acute care setting.

The steps for determining an IPPS payment are:

- The hospital submits a bill to the Medicare Administrative Contractor (MAC) for each Medicare patient it treats. Based on the information on the bill, the MAC categorizes the case into a DRG.

- The base payment rate, or standardized amount (a dollar figure), includes a labor-related and nonlabor-related share. The labor-related share is adjusted by a WI to reflect area differences in the cost of labor. If the area WI is greater than 1.0000, the labor share equals 68.8 percent. The law requires that the labor share equal 62 percent if the area WI is less than or equal to 1.0000. The nonlabor-related share is adjusted by a cost-of-living adjustment (COLA) factor, which equals 1.0000 for all states except Alaska and Hawaii.

- The wage-adjusted standardized amount is multiplied by a relative weight for the DRG. The relative weight is specific to each of 751 DRGs (for FY2012) and represents the relative average costs associated with one DRG.

- If applicable, additional amounts will be added to the IPPS payment in the following situations:

  o the hospital engages in teaching medical residents to reflect the higher indirect patient care costs of teaching hospitals relative to non-teaching hospitals

  o the hospital treats a disproportionate share of low-income patients

  o the hospital has cases that involve certain approved new technologies

  o the hospital has high-cost outlier cases

  http://www.cms.gov/Outreach-and-Education/Medicare-Learning-Network-MLN/MLNProducts/downloads/AcutePaymtSysfctsht.pdf

2.4.3 Attachment B: Outpatient Prospective Payment System (OPPS)

Background

Since August 2000, Medicare has paid hospitals for most services furnished in their outpatient departments under the OPPS. Medicare currently pays more than 4,000 hospitals—including general acute-care hospitals, inpatient rehabilitation facilities, inpatient psychiatric facilities, long-term acute care hospitals, children's hospitals, and cancer hospitals—for outpatient services under the OPPS. Medicare also pays community mental health centers (CMHCs) under the OPPS for partial hospitalization program (PHP) services. The OPPS payments cover facility resources including equipment, supplies, and hospital staff, but do not pay for the services of physicians and non-physician practitioners who are paid separately under the Medicare Physician Fee Schedule (MPFS).

OPPS Payment Groups

Services under the OPPS are classified into payment groups called ambulatory payment classifications (APCs). Services in each APC are clinically similar and require the use of similar resources. A payment rate is established for each APC. The APC payment rates are adjusted for geographic cost differences, and payment rates and policies are updated annually through rule-making. The final rule becomes effective January 1 of the applicable year.

Required Copayments

Beneficiaries generally share in the cost of services furnished under the OPPS by paying either a 20 percent coinsurance or, for certain services, a copayment that under the Medicare law may not exceed 40 percent of the total payment for the APC. The statutory copayment is gradually being replaced by the 20 percent coinsurance as the composition of APC groups is updated in response to policy changes or new cost data. CMS estimates that the overall beneficiary share of the total payments for Medicare-covered outpatient services will be about 21.8 percent in CY2012.

http://www.cms.gov/apps/media/press/factsheet.asp?Counter=4145

2.4.4 Attachment C: Subsection (d) Hospital Designation

The definition of a subsection (d) hospital as defined in Section 1886(d)(1)(B) of the SSA is as follows:

"(B) As used in this section, the term 'subsection (d) hospital' means a hospital located in one of the fifty States or the District of Columbia other than—

 i. a psychiatric hospital (as defined in section 1861(f)),

 ii. a rehabilitation hospital (as defined by the Secretary),

 iii. a hospital whose inpatients are predominantly individuals under 18 years of age,

 iv.

   I. a hospital which has an average inpatient length of stay (as determined by the Secretary of greater than 25 days, or

II.   a hospital that first received payment under this subsection in 1986 which has an average inpatient length of stay (as determined by the Secretary) of greater than 20 days and that has 80 percent or more of its annual Medicare inpatient discharges with a principal diagnosis that reflects a finding of neoplastic disease in the 12-month cost reporting period ending in fiscal year 1997, or

v.

III.   a hospital that the Secretary has classified, at any time on or before December 31, 1990, (or, in the case of a hospital that, as of the date of the enactment of this clause, is located in a State operating a demonstration project under section 1814(b), on or before December 31, 1991) for purposes of applying exceptions adjustments to payment amounts under this subsection, as a hospital involved extensively in treatment for or research on cancer,

IV.   a hospital that was recognized as a comprehensive cancer center or clinical cancer research center by the National Cancer Institute of the National Institutes of Health as of April 20, 1983, that is located in a State which, as of December 19, 1989, was not operating a demonstration project under section 1814(b), that applied and was denied, on or before December 31, 1990, for classification as a hospital involved extensively in treatment for or research on cancer under this clause (as in effect on the day before the date of the enactment of this sub clause), that as of the date of the enactment of this sub clause, is licensed for less than 50 acute care beds, and that demonstrates for the 4-year period ending on December 31, 1996, that at least 50 percent of its total discharges have a principal finding of neoplastic disease, as defined in subparagraph (E), or

V.   a hospital that was recognized as a clinical cancer research center by the National Cancer Institute of the National Institutes of Health as of February 18, 1998, that has never been reimbursed for inpatient hospital services pursuant to a reimbursement system under a demonstration project under section 1814(b), that is a freestanding facility organized primarily for treatment of and research on cancer and is not a unit of another hospital, that as of the date of the enactment of this sub clause, is licensed for 162 acute care beds, and that demonstrates for the 4-year period ending on June 30, 1999, that at least 50 percent of its total discharges have a principal finding of neoplastic disease, as defined in subparagraph (E); and, in accordance with regulations of the Secretary, does not include a psychiatric or rehabilitation unit of the hospital which is a distinct part of the hospital (as defined by the Secretary). A hospital that was classified by the Secretary on or before September 30, 1995, as a hospital described in clause (iv) shall continue to be so classified notwithstanding that it is located in the same building as, or on the same campus as, another hospital."

Source: *http://www.ssa.gov/OP_Home/ssact/title18/1886.htm#act-1886-d-1-b*

2.4.5 Attachment D: HVBP Program Years FY2014–FY2019 Summary Information

FY2014: For program year FY2014 there are a total of twenty-four measures contained under three domains:

DOMAIN	MEASURES	DOMAIN WEIGHTING
Clinical Process of Care	13	45 percent
Patient Experience of Care	8 (HCAHPS)	30 percent
Outcomes	3	25 percent

FY2014 Minimum Reporting Requirements:

- Clinical Process of Care: ten cases and four measures

- Patient Experience of Care: 100 completed surveys

- Outcome 30-Day Mortality: ten cases and two measures

   Note: Hospitals must receive scores in all three FY2014 domains in order to receive a Total HVBP Performance Score. Hospitals unable to achieve this standard will be excluded from HVBP for FY2014.

FY2014 HVBP Baseline and Performance Periods

FY2014 Value-Based Purchasing Program: Baseline and Performance
Periods

DOMAIN	BASELINE PERIOD	PERFORMANCE PERIOD
Clinical Process of Care	April 1, 2010– December 31, 2010	April 1, 2012– December 31, 2012
Patient Experience of Care	April 1, 2010– December 31, 2010	April 1, 2012– December 31, 2012
Outcome (Mortality)	July 1, 2009– June 30, 2010	July 1, 2011– June 30, 2012

FY2015: For program year FY2015 there are a total of twenty-six measures
contained under four domains:

DOMAIN	MEASURES	DOMAIN WEIGHTING
Clinical Process of Care	12	20 percent
Patient Experience of Care	8 (HCAHPS)	30 percent
Outcomes	5	30 percent
Efficiency	1	20 percent

FY2015 Minimum Reporting Requirements:

- Clinical Process of Care: ten cases and four measures

- Patient Experience of Care: 100 completed surveys

- Outcome Measures: Hospitals must report the applicable case minimum
  for at least two of the five measures for the Outcome domain:

  o AMI 30-Day Mortality: twenty-five cases

  o HF 30-Day Mortality: twenty-five cases

  o PN 30-Day Mortality: twenty-five cases

  o AHRQ (PSI-90): three cases for any of the underlying indicators

  o HAI (CLABSI): one predicted infection

     o Efficiency (Medicare Spending Per Beneficiary): twenty-five cases

Note: Hospitals with sufficient data in at least two of the four domains will receive a TPS and domain weighting will be reallocated for unsuccessfully reported domains.

FY2015 HVBP Baseline and Performance Periods

FY2015 Value-Based Purchasing Program: Baseline and Performance Periods

DOMAIN	BASELINE PERIOD	PERFORMANCE PERIOD
Clinical Process of Care	January 1, 2011– December 31, 2011	January 1, 2013– December 31, 2013
Patient Experience of Care	January 1, 2011– December 31, 2011	January 1, 2013– December 31, 2013
OUTCOMES:		
Mortality	October 1, 2010– June 30, 2011	October 1, 2012– June 30 , 2013
AHRQ PSI-90 Composite	October15, 2010– June 30, 2011	October 15, 2012– June 30, 2013
CLABSI	January 1, 2011– December 31, 2011	February 1, 2013– December 31, 2013
Efficiency	May 1, 2011– December 31, 2011	May 1, 2013– December 31, 2013

FY2016: For program year FY2016 there are a total of twenty-five measures contained under four domains:

DOMAIN	MEASURES	DOMAIN WEIGHTING
Clinical Process of Care	8	10 percent
Patient Experience of Care	8 (HCAHPS)	25 percent
Outcomes	8	40 percent
Efficiency	1	25 percent

FY2016 Minimum Reporting Requirements:

- Clinical Process of Care: ten cases and four measures

- Patient Experience of Care: 100 completed surveys

- Outcome Measures: Hospitals must report the applicable case minimum for at least two of the five measures for the Outcome domain.

  - AMI 30-Day Mortality: twenty-five cases

  - HF 30-Day Mortality: twenty-five cases

  - PN 30-Day Mortality: twenty-five cases

  - AHRQ (PSI-90): three cases for any of the underlying indicators

  - HAI (CLABSI): one predicted infection

  - Efficiency (Medicare Spending Per Beneficiary): twenty-five cases

  Note: Hospitals with sufficient data in at least two of the four domains will receive a TPS and domain weighting will be reallocated for unsuccessfully reported domains.

FY2016 HVBP Baseline and Performance Periods

FY2016 Value-Based Purchasing Program: Baseline and Performance Periods

DOMAIN	BASELINE PERIOD	PERFORMANCE PERIOD
Clinical Process of Care:	January 1, 2012– December 31, 2012	January 1, 2014– December 31, 2014
Patient Experience of Care:	January 1,2012– December 31, 2012	January 1, 2014– December 31, 2014
OUTCOMES:		
Mortality	October 1, 2010– June 30, 2011	October 1, 2012– June 30, 2014
AHRQ Composite	October 15, 2010– June 30, 2011	October 15, 2012– June 30, 2014
Efficiency:	January 1, 2012– December 31, 2012	January 1, 2014– December 31, 2014

FY2017:

DOMAIN	TOTAL MEASURES	DOMAIN WEIGHTING
Safety	5	15 percent
Clinical Care		35 percent
• Outcomes	3	25 percent
• Process	8	10 percent
Efficiency and Cost Reduction	1	25 percent
Patient and Caregiver Centered Experience of Care/ Care Coordination	8 (HCAHP)	25 percent

FY2017 Minimum Reporting Requirements

As specified in the FY2014 Final IPPS Rule, CMS intends to address minimum reporting requirements for the NQS-aligned domains in future rule-making.

FY2017 HVBP Baseline and Performance Periods

FY2017 Value-Based Purchasing Program: Baseline and Performance Periods

DOMAIN	BASELINE PERIOD	PERFORMANCE PERIOD
Safety:	October 1, 2010– June 30, 2012	October 1, 2013– June 30, 2015
CLINICAL CARE:		
Clinical Care: Outcomes	October 1, 2010– June 30, 2012	October 1, 2013– June 30, 2015
Clinical Care: Process	January 1, 2013– December 31, 2013	January 1, 2015– December 31, 2015
Efficiency and Cost Reduction	January 1, 2013– December 31, 2013	January 1, 2015– December 31, 2015
Patient and Caregiver Centered Experience of Care/ Care Coordination	January 1, 2013– December 31, 2013	January 1, 2015– December 31, 2015

FY2018 HVBP Baseline and Performance Periods

FY2018 Value-Based Purchasing Program: Baseline and Performance Periods

DOMAIN	BASELINE PERIOD	PERFORMANCE PERIOD
Safety:	July 1, 2010– June 30, 2012	July 1, 2014– June 30, 2016
CLINICAL CARE:		
Clinical Care: Outcomes	October 1, 2009– June 30, 2012	October 1, 2013– June 30, 2016
Clinical Care: Process	January 1, 2014– December 31, 2014	January 1, 2016– December 31, 2016
Efficiency and Cost Reduction	January 1, 2014– December 31, 2014	January 1, 2016– December 31, 2016
Patient and Caregiver Centered Experience of Care/Care Coordination	January 1, 2014– December 31, 2014	January 1, 2016– December 31, 2016

FY2019 HVBP Baseline and Performance Periods

FY2019 Value-Based Purchasing Program: Baseline and Performance Periods

DOMAIN	BASELINE PERIOD	PERFORMANCE PERIOD
Safety:	July 1, 2010– June 30, 2012	July 1, 2015– June 30, 2017
CLINICAL CARE:		
Clinical Care: Outcomes	July 1, 2009– June 30, 2012	July 1, 2014– June 30, 2017
Clinical Care: Process	January 1, 2015– December 31, 2015	January 1, 2017– December 31, 2017
Efficiency and Cost Reduction	January 1, 2015– December 31, 2015	January 1, 2017– December31, 2017
Patient and Caregiver Centered Experience of Care/Care Coordination	January 1, 2015– December 31, 2015	January 1, 2017– December 31, 2017

2.4.6 Attachment E: FY2014 New Technology Add-On Payments (NTAP)

The following items are listed in the FY2014 Final IPPS Rule as qualifying for NTAP in the fiscal years indicated:

- **FY2013 only: payments for the AutoLITT™**, a laser surgical instrument used to necrotize or coagulate soft tissue through interstitial irradiation (thermal therapy) in general surgery and neurosurgery. Cases involving the AutoLITT™ that are eligible for the NTAP will be identified by assignment to MS-DRGs 25, 26, and 27 with an ICD-9 procedure code of 17.61 (ICD-10-PCS codes D0Y0KZZ and D0Y1KZZ) in combination with one of the following primary ICD-9 diagnosis codes: 191.0, 191.1, 191.2, 191.3, 191.4, 191.5, 191.6, 191.7, 191.8, 191.9 (ICD-10-CM codes C71.0, C71.1, C71.2, C71.3, C71.4, C71.5, C71.6, C71.7, C71.8, and C71.9). The maximum add-on payment for a case involving the AutoLITT™ is $5,300.

- **FY2013–FY2014: DIFICID**, an antibiotic used to treat clostridium difficile-associated diarrhea (CDAD)). Cases involving DIFICID that are eligible for the NTAP will be identified with an ICD-9-CM diagnosis code of 008.45 (the ICD-10-CM diagnosis code is A04.7) in combination with NDC code 52015-0080-01 in data element LIN03 of the 837I. The maximum add-on payment for a case involving DIFICID is $868.

- **FY2013–FY2014: Zenith Fenestrated Graft**, An endovascular graft and adjunctive alignment stent used to treat patients with abdominal aortic aneurysms (AAA). Cases involving the Zenith Fenestrated Graft that are eligible for the NTAP will be identified by ICD-9-CM procedure code 39.78 (the ICD-10-CM procedure codes are: 04U03JZ, supplement abdominal aorta with synthetic substitute, percutaneous approach; 04U04JZ, supplement abdominal aorta with synthetic substitute, percutaneous endoscopic approach; 04V03DZ, restriction of abdominal aorta with intraluminal device, percutaneous approach; or 04V04DZ, restriction of abdominal aorta with intraluminal device, percutaneous endoscopic approach.) The maximum add-on payment for a case involving the Zenith Fenestrated Graft is $8,171.50.

- **FY2013–FY2014: Voraxaze**, an enzyme used to treat patients with toxic levels of methotrexate in their blood due to kidney failure. Cases involving Voraxaze that are eligible for the NTAP will be identified by ICD-9-CM procedure code 00.95 (the ICD-10-CM procedure codes are: 3E033GQ, introduction of glucarpidase into peripheral vein, percutaneous approach or 3E043GQ, introduction of glucarpidase into central vein, percutaneous approach). The maximum add-on payment for a case involving the Voraxaze is $45,000.

- **FY2014–FY2015: Argus**, a retinal prosthetic device designed to help improve blindness due to conditions such as retinitis pigmentosa. Cases involving the Argus® II System are eligible for the NTAP will be identified by ICD-9-CM procedure code 14.81. The maximum add-on payment for a case involving the Argus® II System is $72,028.75 (the ICD-10-CM procedure codes are: 08H005Z, insertion of epiretinal visual prosthesis into right eye, open approach or 08H105Z, insertion of epiretinal visual prosthesis into left eye, open approach).

- **FY2014–FY2015: Kcentra**, a pharmacologic product used for the urgent reversal of acquired coagulation factor deficiency induced by vitamin K antagonist (e.g., warfarin) therapy in adult patients with acute major bleeding. Cases involving Kcentra that are eligible for the NTAP will be identified by ICD-9-CM procedure code 00.96. The maximum add-on payment for a case of Kcentra™ is $1,587.50 (the ICD-10-CM procedure codes are: 30280B1, transfusion of nonautologous 4-factor prothrombin complex concentrate into vein, open approach or 30283B1, transfusion of nonautologous 4-factor prothrombin complex. The ICD-10-CM diagnosis codes are D66, D67, D68.1, D68.2, D68.0, D68.311, D68.312, D68.318, D68.32, and D68.4.)

- **FY2014–FY2015: Zilver® PTX®**, a drug-eluting stent for the superficial femoral artery (SFA), proven to inhibit restenosis and reduce reintervention rates. Cases involving the Zilver® PTX® that are eligible for the NTAP will be identified by ICD-9-CM procedure code 00.60. The maximum add-on payment for a case of the Zilver® PTX® is $1,705.25 (the ICD-10-CM procedure codes are: 047K04Z, dilation of right femoral artery with drug-eluting intraluminal device, open approach; 047K34Z, dilation of right femoral artery with drug-eluting intraluminal device, percutaneous approach; 047K44Z, dilation of right femoral artery with drug-eluting intraluminal device, percutaneous endoscopic approach;

047L04Z, dilation of left femoral artery with drug-eluting intraluminal device, open approach; 047L34Z, dilation of left femoral artery with drug-eluting intraluminal device, percutaneous approach; or 047L44Z, dilation of left femoral artery with drug-eluting intraluminal device, percutaneous endoscopic approach).

2.4.7 Attachment F: Components of the Wage Adjusted DRG Operating Payment and the Base Operating DRG Rate

The following information was extracted from pages 53382–53384 of the FY2013 Final IPPS Rules published in the Federal Register/Vol. 77, No. 170/Friday, August 31, 2012/Rules and Regulations

- After consideration of the public comments we received, we are finalizing the definition of the term "wage-adjusted DRG operating payment" as:

  o The applicable average standardized amount adjusted for:

    ▪ resource utilization by the applicable MS-DRG relative weight

    ▪ differences in geographic costs by the applicable area WI (and by the applicable COLA for hospitals located in Alaska and Hawaii)

    ▪ an applicable transfer under 42 CFR 412.4(f)

- We are also finalizing the definition of the term "base operating DRG payment amount" as that term applies to most subsection (d) hospitals as:

  o the wage-adjusted DRG operating payment plus any applicable NTAP under 42 CFR 412.4(f).

  o We are finalizing that this amount is determined without regard to any payment adjustments under the HRRP and that it does not include any additional payments for:

- indirect medical education under $412.105

- the treatment of a disproportionate share of low-income patients

- outliers

- low-volume of discharges under $412.101

- We are codifying these definitions in our regulations at 42 CFR 412.160.

2.4.8 Attachment G: A Step-by-Step Guide to Calculating the Patient Experience of Care (HCAHPS) Domain Score

FY2014 Actual Percentage Payment Summary Report

This guide summarizes in step-by-step fashion the process by which the CMS and its HCAHPS Project Team calculate the Patient Experience of Care Domain Score for the FY2014 HVBP program. By following these steps, a hospital can approximate its Patient Experience of Care Domain Score.

Step 1: A hospital or its HCAHPS survey vendor submits HCAHPS survey data to the HCAHPS data warehouse for the Hospital Inpatient Quality Reporting program.

- The HVBP Patient Experience of Care (HCAHPS) baseline and performance reporting periods for FY2014–FY2016 are as follows:

HVBP PROGRAM YEAR	BASELINE REPORTING PERIOD	PERFORMANCE REPORTING PERIOD
FY2014	April 1, 2010–December 31, 2010	April 1, 2012–December 31, 2012
FY2015	January 1, 2011–December 31, 2011	January 1, 2013–December 31, 2013
FY2016	January 1, 2012–December 31, 2012	January 1, 2014–December 31, 2014

- HCAHPS data submitted for the hospital IQR program are used in the HVBP program.

- In order to participate in the HVBP program, hospitals must meet the following criteria:
    - be part of the IPPS program
    - be open during the HVBP performance period
    - be located in the fifty states or Washington, DC
    - passed the annual payment update requirements for the performance period
    - have at least 100 completed surveys during the performance period (see Step 7)

Step 2: CMS cleans the submitted HCAHPS data by removing incomplete surveys, surveys from ineligible patients, etc.

"Completed survey" is defined in the HCAHPS Quality Assurance Guidelines.

Step 3: CMS calculates the "top-box" raw score for the nine HCAHPS measures that are used in the HVBP Patient Experience of Care Domain.

- The top-box raw score—which is the percentage of a hospital's patients who chose the most positive, or "top-box," response to HCAHPS survey items—is used in the Patient Experience of Care Domain:
    - See the HCAHPS Summary Analyses page for more information on the HCAHPS top-box: http://www.hcahpsonline.org/SummaryAnalyses.aspx

- Nine measures from HCAHPS are used in HVBP: six composite measures (Communication with Nurses, Communication with Doctors, Staff Responsiveness, Pain Management, Communication about Medicines, and Discharge Information); two individual measures (Cleanliness of Hospital Environment and Quietness of Hospital Environment); and one global measure (Overall Rating of Hospital):
    - CMS combines the Cleanliness and Quietness measures to form a new composite for HVBP, Cleanliness and Quietness of Hospital Environment (see Step 6).

o The HCAHPS global measure Recommend the Hospital is not used in the Patient Experience of Care Domain.

Step 4: CMS applies the patient-mix adjustment for each of the nine HCAHPS measures used in the HVBP program to obtain Patient-Mix Adjusted Scores:

- Information on HCAHPS patient-mix adjustment can be found on the Mode and Patient-mix Adjustment page on the HCAHPS website: http://www.hcahpsonline.org/modeadjustment.aspx

- A detailed description of the HCAHPS patient-mix adjustment process can be found at: http://www.hcahpsonline.org/files/December_2012_PMA_Web_Document_09-12-12.pdf

- The patient-mix adjustment coefficients applicable specifically to the baseline and performance periods for the HVBP program will be made available on the HCAHPS website: www.hcahpsonline.org

Step 5: CMS applies a "survey mode effect adjustment" for each of the nine HCAHPS measures used in the HVBP program. The survey mode adjustment is applied to account for the differences in respondent input based on the method (mode) of survey administration. (i.e., face to face, telephonic, online, etc.):

- Information on HCAHPS survey mode adjustment can be found in the Mode and Patient-mix Adjustment page on the HCAHPS website: http://www.hcahpsonline.org/modeadjustment.aspx

Step 6: CMS combines the Cleanliness of Hospital Environment and Quietness of Hospital Environment measures to create the Cleanliness and Quietness of Hospital Environment dimension for the HVBP program (after having applied the patient-mix and mode adjustments to the Cleanliness of Hospital Environment and Quietness of Hospital Environment measures):

- CMS uses the simple arithmetic average of the Cleanliness and Quietness top-box scores to obtain the Cleanliness and Quietness of Hospital Environment dimension.

- Thus, there are eight HCAHPS measures (called "dimensions") in the HVBP program.

Step 7: CMS performs Steps 1 to 6 separately on each of the quarters of the performance period.

> *Note: If a hospital has fewer than 100 completed surveys in the fiscal year performance period, it will not receive a Patient Experience of Care Domain Score.*

Step 8: CMS calculates the three-quarter average for each of the eight Patient Experience of Care Domain dimensions for each hospital.

- For each hospital, each quarter is weighted according to the number of eligible discharges.

   o Learn more about the weighting of quarters.

Step 9: CMS calculates achievement points and improvement points for each dimension for each hospital:

- Using a hospital's performance rate and the achievement threshold (50th percentile) and benchmark (mean of the top decile) for the fiscal year baseline period, CMS calculates achievement points for each dimension.

- Using a hospital's baseline rate and the achievement threshold (50th percentile) and benchmark (mean of the top decile) for the fiscal year baseline period, CMS calculates improvement points for each dimension:

   o Each eligible hospital received the fiscal year baseline period baseline rate for each dimension in its fiscal year Estimated Payment Report.

   o The Fiscal Year Estimated Report also included the achievement threshold and benchmark for each dimension.

   o The achievement thresholds and benchmarks for the fiscal year baseline period are published in the Hospital Inpatient Value-Based Purchasing Program Final Rule.

- The formula for achievement points is found in the Hospital Inpatient Value-Based Purchasing Program Final Rule (Federal Register/Vol. 76, No. 88/Friday, May 6, 2011/Rules and Regulations, pp. 26517–26520).

- The formula for improvement points is found in the Hospital Inpatient Value-Based Purchasing Program Final Rule (Federal Register/Vol. 76, No. 88/Friday, May 6, 2011/Rules and Regulations, pp. 26517–26520.

Step 10: CMS calculates the HCAHPS Base Score for each hospital:

For each dimension, the greater of achievement points or improvement points is designated the Dimension Score:

- The HCAHPS Base Score is the sum of the eight Dimension Scores.

- The HCAHPS Base Score ranges from 0 to 80 points.

Step 11: CMS calculates the Consistency Score for each hospital.

Using a hospital's performance rate and the floor and achievement threshold for each dimension in the baseline period, CMS determines the lowest dimension score. The formula for determining the lowest dimension score is found in the Hospital Inpatient Value-Based Purchasing Program Final Rule (Federal Register/Vol. 76, No. 88/Friday, May 6, 2011/Rules and Regulations, p. 26519).

- The floors and achievement thresholds for the FY2013 baseline period were published in the Hospital Inpatient Value-Based Purchasing Program Final Rule (Federal Register/Vol. 76, No. 88/Friday, May 6, 2011/Rules and Regulations, p. 26519), http://www.gpo.gov/fdsys/pkg/FR-2011-05-06/pdf/2011-10568.pdf

- The floor and achievement threshold for each dimension are also provided in the Fiscal Year Estimated Report.

  o Having determined the lowest dimension score, CMS calculates the Consistency Score using the formula found in the Hospital Inpatient Value-Based Purchasing Program Final Rule (Federal Register/Vol. 76, No. 88/Friday, May 6, 2011/Rules and Regulations, p. 26519). The Consistency Score ranges from 0 to 20.

Step 12: CMS calculates the Unweighted Patient Experience of Care Domain Score for each hospital by summing the hospital's HCAHPS Base Score (0–80) and HCAHPS Consistency Score (0–20).

- The Patient Experience of Care Domain Score ranges from 0 to 100 points.

- CMS calculates the Weighted Patient Experience of Care Domain Score for each hospital by multiplying the Unweighted Patient Experience of Care Domain Score by 0.30.

- The FY2013 Actual Percentage Payment Summary Report contains the baseline rate, performance rate, achievement points, improvement points, and dimension score for each dimension.

- The report also provides the HCAHPS Base Score, Consistency Score, lowest dimension, number of completed HCAHPS surveys in the performance period, and the Unweighted and Weighted Patient Experience of Care Domain Score. A detailed example of how the Patient Experience of Care Domain Score is calculated can be found in slides 35–61 at Presentation - Special Open Door Forum on Hospital VBP (7-27-11) [PDF, 7MB].

CHAPTER 3

The Hospital Readmissions Reduction Program (HRRP)

Section 3.1: Flash Read!

Hospital readmission rates are an important indicator of quality of care. According to the Centers for Medicare & Medicaid Services (CMS), about 20 percent of Medicare patients discharged from a hospital have historically been readmitted within thirty days. CMS predicts that three-quarters of those readmissions were potentially preventable—and this represents potential savings of $12 billion for Medicare. The Hospital Readmissions Reduction Program (HRRP), created by the Affordable Care Act (ACA), imposes financial penalties for hospitals that have higher-than-expected readmissions within thirty days of discharge for certain conditions.

- The HRRP is a "penalty-only" program. CMS will penalize hospitals that have excessive readmissions (within thirty days of discharge) for specified conditions. The penalties are applied in the form of reduced reimbursements for all Medicare patients admitted to affected hospitals for a given fiscal year.

- For patients with conditions included in the HRRP, readmission is defined as an admission to any acute care hospital within thirty days of a discharge from the same or another acute care hospital, for any cause (with the exception of certain planned readmissions).

- Penalties are calculated based on three years of performance data for Medicare patients over age sixty-five (Medicare Advantage plan data not included). Penalties were first imposed in FY2013, and the maximum penalty will increase by one percent each year through FY2015.

- The following four-step process is used to determine the Payment Adjustment Factor (PAF):

    1. Collect data (extracted from Inpatient Quality Reporting (IQR)).

PROGRAM YEAR (YEAR IN WHICH PENALTY IS APPLIED)	DISCHARGE DATA PERIOD	DATE OF DATA "SNAPSHOT"
FY2013	07/01/08–06/30/11	09/30/11
FY2014	07/01/09–06/30/12	09/30/12
FY2015	07/01/10–06/30/13	09/30/13
FY2016	07/01/11–06/30/14	09/30/14

    2. Calculate the excess readmission ratio for each measure.
    3. Determine the applicable Readmission Adjustment Factor (RAF).
    4. Determine the Payment Adjustment Factor (PAF).

- Penalties will apply for a broader group of conditions as the program is fully phased in.

Implementation Timeline

IMPLEMENTATION YEAR	MAXIMUM PENALTY	APPLICABLE CONDITIONS
FY2013	1 percent	acute myocardial infarction (AMI); heart failure (HF); pneumonia (PN)
FY2014	2 percent	acute myocardial infarction (AMI); heart failure (HF); pneumonia (PN)
FY2015	3 percent	acute myocardial infarction (AMI); heart failure (HF); pneumonia (PN); total knee arthroplasty (TKA); total hip arthroplasty (THA); acute exacerbation of chronic obstructive pulmonary disease (AE COPD)
FY2016 and Beyond	to be determined through future rule-making	

- Excessive readmissions are defined by comparing an individual hospital's excess readmission ratio for each measured condition to the national average for the set of patients with the applicable condition. These are risk-adjusted for clinically relevant factors such as patient demographics, comorbidities, and patient frailty.

- Penalty payment adjustments are applied to the wage-adjusted base operating (WABO) DRG reimbursements for each Medicare discharge in a given program year. They do not include adjustments or add-on payments for indirect medical education, disproportionate share hospitals, outliers, low-volume hospitals or the Hospital Value-Based Purchasing Program (HVBP).

- CMS has established a twenty-five-case-per-condition minimum requirement for evaluation.

- Certain readmissions are excluded, including planned readmissions or transfers to other applicable hospitals.

- Most hospitals are being penalized, but very few are hitting the maximum penalty, and the program is showing promise at reducing readmissions. Still, the penalties have a large fiscal impact:

o For FY2013, the CMS collected a total of $280 million in HRRP penalties. The average per-hospital penalty was a .42 percent reduction in each hospital's base operating DRG rate for each Medicare discharge in that year.

o For FY2014, the CMS estimates $227 million in HRRP penalties, and an average per-hospital penalty of .38 percent.

Estimated HRRP Penalties for FY2014

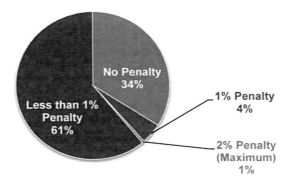

HRRP Penalties for FY2013

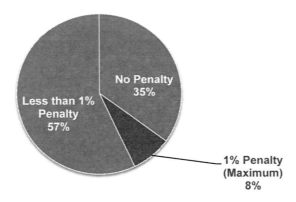

Section 3.2:
Provider Perspectives

The Hospital Readmissions Reduction Program (HRRP) has been one of the most visible of the patient-care improvement initiatives contained in the ACA. Based on early returns, and the level of discussion and investment in the hospital sector, it seems to hold promise for delivering significant results.

3.2.1 Rationale

Unnecessary hospital readmissions can cause undue suffering for patients and families, and may lead to higher spending on health care. High rates of hospital readmission within thirty days of discharge may be attributed to factors such as:

- inadequate treatment

- inadequate care coordination and follow-up care in the community

- complications from treatments received during a hospital stay

- unexpected worsening of disease after discharge from the hospital

For these reasons, hospital readmissions within a short time after discharge have come to be seen as an important indicator of quality of care. Experts believe that by improving communication with patients after discharge, coordinating care, and raising the standard of care on the index admission, many readmissions could be prevented. Yet "Medicare does not reward these efforts," the Medicare Payment Advisory Commission (MedPAC) wrote to Congress in June 2007, in its initial report advising that the status quo was no longer acceptable.

For patients, additional hospital admissions affect their health, their finances, and their state of mind—and many providers feel woefully underprepared to prevent readmissions. "We never learned in medical schools about the risks that patients face soon after leaving the hospital," said Harlan M. Krumholz, MD, a cardiologist and professor of public health at Yale. "Our textbooks lack chapters on this topic.

Most of us learned about inpatient and outpatient care—but somehow the transition from inpatient to outpatient was lost."[107]

Altogether, 17.6 percent of all Medicare admissions led to a second admission within thirty days of discharge in 2005, before the HRRP started. For Medicare, the cost of those readmissions was $15 billion. MedPAC estimated that 76 percent of all discharges within thirty days were potentially avoidable. This represents approximately $12 billion in potential savings for Medicare.[108]

MedPAC recommended that Medicare take the lead in driving change. It said that hospitals should publicly report readmission rates and that their payment should be tied to performance.

Of course, one person's cost is another person's revenue. Hospitals by and large objected to these initiatives. They typically received another payment from Medicare if the patient needed to come back. Why fix something that wasn't broken? Richard J. Baron, MD, president and CEO of the American Board of Internal Medicine, explained how the calculation worked in the real world:

> "You're a doctor working in a hospital and you think that some readmissions to the hospital happen because when patients get home, they confuse their meds, and don't reliably follow up on tests they're supposed to get," Baron said. "You say to the hospital, 'I've had three people in the last three months who have come back. I think that's a quality problem. I think if we had a nurse care manager who called them and went over to their house and reviewed what they are doing, that would make these people healthier. We'd be less likely to have those people readmitted.'

> "You make that case to the hospital CEO and he says, 'That person is going to cost me $100,000 a year. The effect will be great on the quality side. But those three admissions she prevented, I lost revenue because I was being paid for those admissions. I completely agree it would be better for the patients we take care of [and] it would achieve the reason we're in business. But you're

---

[107] Harlan M. Krumholz, MD, *The Incidental Economist*, blog interview, February 5, 2013. http://theincidentaleconomist.com/wordpress/harlan-krumholz-on-hospital-readmissions/

[108] www.medpac.gov/chapters/jun07_ch05.pdf

asking me to pay $100,000 so that I can reduce my revenue by three admissions. That's not a business deal I am interested in.'"[109]

In some parts of the country, readmission rates were going up even during the period when this was being highlighted as a quality issue. Pennsylvania, one of the states that published readmission rates in the mid-2000s, reported that readmission rates rose to 19.1 percent in 2006, up from 18.7 percent in 2004.[110]

Under the fee-for-service system that prevails in US health care, hospitals have never had a strong reason to discourage readmissions as long as the readmissions produced more revenue. Those who tried to do something about it often met with strong opposition. Gene Diamond, Northern Indiana Regional CEO for the Sisters of St. Francis Health Services in Hammond, Ind., said that even though his hospital made money off readmissions, his system has opened clinics to reduce complications and improve care for diabetics, heart patients, and asthmatics.

"I get a lot of resistance from my finance people and cardiologists, who tell me we can't afford to do this," Diamond told *Hospitals and Health Networks* magazine in 2008. "But we have to do what's right for the patient. I want patients here because they need to be here, not because we profit from that. I want us to have complete transparency. We know that Medicare is looking into this and we don't want to be perceived as churning patients."[111]

It wasn't until the Centers for Medicare & Medicaid Services (CMS) decided to change the terms of engagement—by penalizing hospitals for excessive readmissions within thirty days of discharge—that trimming rates of rehospitalization became a business deal that hospitals were interested in, Baron said.

---

[109] *Richard J. Baron, MD, telephone interview, October 1, 2013.*

[110] *Mark Taylor, "The Billion Dollar U-Turn," Hospitals and Health Networks, May 2008. http://www.hhnmag.com/hhnmag/jsp/articledisplay.jsp?dcrpath=HHNMAG/Article/data/05MAY20 08/0805HHN_FEA_CoverStory&domain=HHNMAG*

[111] *Taylor, "The Billion Dollar U-Turn." http://www.hhnmag.com/hhnmag/jsp/articledisplay.jsp?dcrpath=HHNMAG/Article/data/05MAY20 08/0805HHN_FEA_CoverStory&domain=HHNMAG*

The readmissions rate, however, is not anybody's favorite candidate for quality modeling. Many variables can influence the reasons a patient might come back, only some of which can be directly attributed to the hospital.

Many chronically ill or elderly patients face multiple illnesses simultaneously, such as diabetes, obesity, hypertension, asthma, inability to breathe, or heart failure. At the time of discharge, the patient may not be ready to hear and understand complicated changes to medication or diet. The patient may also not be able to act on rehabilitation instructions or even make a follow-up appointment with a personal physician, assuming he or she has one. They may not have anybody to explain their treatment plan.

Krumholz has described this state as "post-hospital syndrome—an acquired, transient condition of generalized risk." At the time of discharge, he said, "physiological systems are impaired, reserves are depleted, and the body cannot effectively defend against health threats."[112] Attending only to the reasons for the admission and treatment may lead caregivers to miss other factors in the patient's condition arising from the hospitalization itself, such as sleep deprivation, reduced nutritional intake, loss of strength, or mood disturbances, which may have little in common with the original diagnosis. These may have greater bearing on the likelihood of readmission.

Even if most readmissions are necessary and inevitable, every hospital in America has patients whose readmissions could be prevented. "If you don't create a reason for the hospital to think of that readmission as something other than a revenue stream," Baron said, the hospital probably won't. By vowing to hurt hospitals' bottom lines for high readmission rates, Medicare has thus turned the customary thinking on its head.

CMS has undertaken a variety of innovations to motivate hospitals to reduce their readmissions rates. These include adding the payment penalties in the HRRP, codified in the ACA, as well as publishing hospital readmission rates on the Hospital Compare website, funding the Partnership for Patients program with the American Hospital Association, and introducing some shared savings initiatives.

---

[112] *Harlan M. Krumholz, MD. "Post-Hospital Syndrome—An Acquired, Transient Condition of Generalized Risk," N Eng J Med 2013; 368:100–102, January 10, 2013. http://www.nejm.org/doi/full/10.1056/NEJMp1212324*

3.2.2 Summary

Under the law, CMS must use three risk-adjusted measures endorsed by the National Quality Forum: acute myocardial infarction (AMI), heart failure, and pneumonia. Hospitals whose rates of readmission within thirty days of discharge exceed certain expected ratios are required to pay what is in effect a fine against their entire annual Medicare reimbursement. For FY2013, the fine could be as high as 1 percent. For FY2014, the maximum fine was raised to 2 percent of Medicare reimbursement, and starting in FY2015, the maximum rises to 3 percent. Hospitals have no possibility for gains as a result of a good readmissions rate. Each fiscal year fine is based on a data period of three years. For example, the base reporting period ran from July 1, 2008, through June 30, 2011 for penalties that went into effect October 1, 2012.[113]

In the first year, 2,217 hospitals (or 71 percent) were assessed penalties, of which 307 received the maximum 1 percent deduction from their Medicare billings in FY2013. Penalties totaled about $280 million.[114]

In response, many, if not most, hospitals have embraced some organized program to focus institutional intent around avoiding readmissions. Two of the most prominent are Boston University Medical Center's Project Re-Engineered Discharge, known as Project RED, and the University of Colorado School of Medicine's Care Transitions Program.

- Project RED is a research group that develops and tests strategies to improve the hospital discharge process in a way that promotes patient safety and reduces readmission rates. The re-engineered discharge has "12 discrete, mutually reinforcing components and has been proven to reduce readmissions and yields high rates of patient satisfaction," according to the university's website.[115]

---

[113]Jordan Rau, "Medicare To Penalize 2,217 Hospitals For Excess Readmissions," KaiserHealthNews.org, August 13, 2012.
http://www.kaiserhealthnews.org/stories/2012/august/13/medicare-hospitals-readmissions-penalties.aspx

[114]Jordan Rau, "Medicare To Penalize 2,217 Hospitals For Excess Readmissions," KaiserHealthNews.org, August 13, 2012.
http://www.kaiserhealthnews.org/stories/2012/august/13/medicare-hospitals-readmissions-penalties

[115] Project RED (Re-Engineered Discharge), Boston University School of Medicine.
http://www.bu.edu/fammed/projectred/

- The widely cited Colorado program, masterminded by Eric A. Coleman, MD, is a comprehensive approach toward smoothing the transitions between care settings; for instance, hospital to nursing home. It includes tools for patients, families, physicians, nurses, and others likely to come in contact with the patient as he or she moves through the care continuum.[116]

The CMS-led Partnership for Patients program, begun in 2011, has promulgated grass-roots education and information exchange throughout the hospital community in support of these goals. Nearly 3,500 hospitals participate, accounting for 75 percent of the index admissions of Medicare fee-for-service patients. The partnership aims to reduce the hospital readmission rate by 20 percent by December 31, 2013, by improving care transitions.

Through an alliance with the American Hospital Association (AHA), much of this work is being done in collaboration with state hospital associations. Via the ACA, the CMS Innovation Center allocated $218 million over two years to create the Hospital Engagement Network (HEN), starting in December 2011, as part of the program. The aim is to test new methods to develop scalable quality improvements in hospitals, targeting such clinical topics as falls, pressure ulcers, surgical site infections, adverse drug events, and preventable readmissions. The funding has been given to twenty-six state, regional, and national hospital organizations, of which the largest is the Health Research & Educational Trust, an affiliate of the AHA. The HRET-HEN includes thirty-one state hospital associations, representing about 1,600 hospitals, many of them small. The goal is to reduce preventable harm by 40 percent and reduce preventable readmissions by 20 percent.[117]

"We are trying to keep it simple and manageable for hospitals, to get the most bang for your buck," said Donna Meador, who leads the HEN in Kentucky on behalf of the state's hospital association. Her hospitals are using the teach-back method to make sure patients understand their medications at discharge or what to do if they've gained three pounds since the day before. They are also making the follow-up appointments for patients.

---

[116] http://www.caretransitions.org/

[117] http://partnershipforpatients.cms.gov/

"Five or six years ago, you never made those appointments," Meador said. "It hasn't traditionally been part of the hospital's role. On a busy med-surg unit, for somebody to stop and call, it's a fairly new thing to do."[118]

The Kentucky hospitals are also trying to communicate better with caregivers across the continuum of care. They're meeting monthly with home health, skilled nursing providers, and pharmacists to make sure nobody is dropping the ball on the patient's needs. For the first time, hospitals are also sharing information with each other. At the monthly coaching call, members of the readmissions collaborative describe what has been successful in reducing readmissions at their hospital.

By September 2013, fifty-seven hospitals in Kentucky were submitting data to the HEN on readmissions. They showed a 13 percent improvement in thirty-day all-cause readmissions and a 14 percent improvement on the heart failure readmission rate—not quite the decline they had desired. "We'd like to be a little farther than three-quarters to our goal," Meador said. They'll keep trying. Congress may or may not extend the HEN program to a third year after the December 2013 cutoff of funding.

The Partnership for Patients has been mostly successful. "Readmission rates at hospitals participating in the program have been, on average, consistently lower than the rates at nonparticipating hospitals," *Medicare & Medicaid Research Review* found.[119] In 73 hospital referral regions, rates fell by more than 5 percent, and in 166 referral regions, readmissions declined between 1 percent and 5 percent. Rates rose by more than 1 percent in just 30 HRRs. The paper's authors admit, however, that the reasons behind the reduction "are not yet clear and merit further investigation."

3.2.3 Current State

Even if the policy researchers don't want to get out ahead of their data, it seems clear that the dial is moving. The analysis by *Medicare & Medicaid Research*

---

[118] *Donna Meador, Kentucky Hospital Association, telephone interview, September 30, 2013.*

[119] *Geoffrey Gerhardt, et al, "Medicare Readmission Rates Showed Meaningful Decline in 2012," Medicare & Medicare Research Review, 2013: Vol. 3, No. 2. http://www.cms.gov/mmrr/Briefs/B2013/mmrr-2013-003-02-b01.html*

Review, published by CMS, showed that the all-cause readmission rate for Medicare averaged 19 percent from 2007 to 2011. In 2012, the rate dropped to 18.4 percent. That is not insubstantial for such a complicated problem in so short a time. A chart in the article shows the trend lines for index admissions and readmissions running in tandem for the years 2007 to 2011. In early 2012, the lines start to diverge as the readmissions rate drops more quickly than that for index admissions.

One possible explanation for the observed rate reduction in 2012 is that "payment reforms and other initiatives aimed at reducing avoidable readmissions are starting to have a measurable impact on provider behavior and are resulting in improved care."[120] But the analysis wasn't designed to determine what caused the rate change, only to find out whether a change had occurred.

Indeed, the CMS-ordained reimbursement penalties for the second year of the thirty-day readmissions reduction program (which measures performance from July 1, 2009–June 30, 2012) are consistent with this finding. CMS announced in mid-2013 that the average fine dropped from .42 percent in the first year of the program to .38 percent in the second year. About two-thirds of eligible hospitals were penalized. Starting October 1, 2013, 2,225 hospitals received lower payments, totaling $227 million withheld over the fiscal year, some $53 million less than the total withhold the preceding year. The maximum penalty of 2 percent was levied against 18 hospitals, and a further 154 institutions lost 1 percent or more of their total inpatient reimbursements. Nationwide, 1,371 hospitals received a lower fine, and 1,074 hospitals a higher one, in the second year, according to an analysis by Kaiser Health News.[121]

The downward trend in readmissions that started in 2012 continued in the first eight months of 2013, according to the CMS blog. Early claims data show the readmission rate was less than 18 percent for the period, resulting in an estimated 130,000 fewer hospital readmissions between January 2012 and August 2013. In 232 of 306 regional hospital markets, readmission rates

[120] *Gerhardt, MMRR, p. E9*

[121] *Jordan Rau, "Armed With Bigger Fines, Medicare To Punish 2,225 Hospitals For Excess Readmissions," Kaiser Health News, August 2, 2013.*
http://www.kaiserhealthnews.org/stories/2013/august/02/readmission-penalties-medicare-hospitals-year-two

averaged at least half a percent less than they did for the period from 2007 to 2011. The trend was widespread across the country.

"I do think we are seeing significant movement and energy in 30-day readmissions," said Craig E. Samitt, MD, executive vice president of DaVita HealthCare Partners Inc. in Denver, and a member of MedPAC. Hospitals and physicians are finally working in tandem to address this concern. "This is one of the earlier quality-improvement cost-reducing strategies that we are seeing bearing a significant amount of fruit. Hospitals have this as a high priority. The fix goes beyond hospitals—physicians are partnering with hospitals post-discharge."[122]

Predictive analytics, a subcomponent of the "big data" approach to population health, helps hospital administrators understand which patients may be most likely to rebound to the Emergency Department, Samitt said. Managers can gather data streams from claims, from the hospital's own electronic health record system, and from historical patterns to intervene earlier in high-risk patients' care. Traditionally, the silo effect in health care has meant that neither hospitals, nor physicians, nor skilled-nursing facilities have had access to the full picture of the patient's case and likely trajectory, Samitt said.

"It's a science that is in development," he added. "It is promising to date."

Hospitals and physician groups—even insurers—that have achieved some success pushing down readmissions have been eager to announce their results. Newspapers around the country have published stories explaining how their local institutions did it. Some examples:

- In Colorado, a collaboration between the state hospital association and UnitedHealthcare at nineteen hospitals avoided 312 potential readmissions, saving $2.9 million in health spending. The readmission rate for same-cause diagnoses declined from 9.8 percent to just over 5 percent in a year.[123]

- Mount Sinai Hospital in New York received a five-year grant from the federal government to hire twenty social workers to support Medicare beneficiaries. They identified more than 600 high-risk patients who were

---

[122] Craig E. Samitt, MD, telephone interview, October 1, 2013.

[123] Michael Booth, "Effort to reduce Colorado hospital readmissions shows results," The Denver Post, August 21, 2013. http://www.denverpost.com/news/ci_23904523/effort-reduce-colorado-hospital-readmissions-shows-results

frequent visitors to the emergency department and who had multiple admissions. Hospital leaders score their high-risk patients each day according to how likely they are to be readmitted. During a pilot from September 2010 to May 2012, the program cut ED visits by 54 percent and trimmed admissions by 43 percent, saving $1.6 million in expenses over six months, the hospital said.[124]

- Western Maryland Health Systems in Cumberland moved readmissions from 16 percent in 2011 to 9 percent in 2013. The hospital is one of a handful in the state, which has regulated hospital reimbursement rates, to receive a fixed budget to include all care required in the community. If hospitals achieve cost savings through admitting or readmitting fewer patients or shifting the locus of care to a doctor's practice, they can make money.[125]

- Cox Medical Center South in Springfield, Mo., which expects to lose $130,000 in revenue from its HRRP penalty in FY2014, evaluates patients on admission to determine whether they have a high, moderate, or low risk of coming back. High-risk patients get a visit with a pharmacist to discuss medications and a meeting with a nutritionist.[126]

In 2011, Barnes-Jewish Hospital in St. Louis suffered a public relations disaster when an enterprising writer splashed across the pages of the *St. Louis Post-Dispatch* that the hospital's readmission rates for the three Medicare target diagnoses well exceeded national averages. She found the numbers she wanted on the newly opened CMS Hospital Compare website (www.HospitalCompare.hhs.gov).

- Heart Failure: US national thirty-day rate:
  24.8 percent; Barnes-Jewish: 28.4 percent

---

[124] Shannon Pettypiece, "Obamacare Incentives Slow Hospitals' Revolving Door," *Bloomberg News*, September 25, 2013. http://www.bloomberg.com/news/2013-09-25/obamacare-keeps-patients-at-home-slowing-hospital-use.html

[125] Julie Appleby, "Hospital effort could reduce readmissions," *The Washington Post* (via KaiserHealthNews.org), December 10, 2010, p. B4. http://www.washingtonpost.com/wp-dyn/content/article/2010/12/06/AR2010120607108.html; Eduardo Porter, "Lessons in Maryland for Costs at Hospitals," *The New York Times*, August 27, 2013. http://www.nytimes.com/2013/08/28/business/economy/lessons-in-maryland-for-costs-at-hospitals.html

[126] "Hospitals trying to reduce patient return rates," *Associated Press*, September 16, 2013.

- Heart Attack: US national thirty-day rate:
  19.8 percent; Barnes-Jewish: 22.4 percent

- Pneumonia: US national thirty-day rate:
  18.4 percent; Barnes-Jewish: 22.9 percent

With 1,259 beds, Barnes-Jewish is the largest hospital in St. Louis and the anchor of the sprawling BJC Health System. It is considered the premier academic medical center in town and is affiliated with the prestigious Washington University School of Medicine.

John Lynch, MD, chief medical officer for Barnes-Jewish, explained the readmission statistics by stating, "If you believe, and we do, that there are significant social and economic factors driving the root causes of readmission, Medicare's strategy to penalize providers who deal with those populations could potentially be flawed." He pointed out that the hospital treats a significant underserved patient cohort. St. Louis closed its public hospital more than twelve years ago, and now Barnes-Jewish fills that role for many patients.

Later, after the newspaper article ran, Barnes-Jewish President Rich Liekweg said the hospital would address the issues raised by the readmission data by creating a post-discharge clinic and by trying to make sure that high-risk patients see a primary care physician within seven days after discharge, at no cost if necessary. He said the problem is rooted in social and economic causes, including lack of access to primary care, absence of a medical home for risky patients, lack of transportation, low health literacy, and poverty.[127]

Barnes-Jewish did suffer a penalty of .98 percent in the first year of the CMS program. In the second year, its fine dropped to .60 percent, indicating progress.[128]

The Barnes-Jewish situation highlights one of the unintended consequences of the government's readmission penalty policy: Teaching hospitals and hospitals that serve large minority and/or low-income populations are more likely to have

---

[127] Duncan Moore, "Barnes-Jewish in Quality Crosshairs," Payer & Providers Midwest Edition, September 8, 2011.

[128] Jordan Rau, "Armed with Bigger Fines, Medicare To Punish 2,225 Hospitals for Excess Readmissions," Kaiser Health News, August 2, 2013.
http://www.kaiserhealthnews.org/stories/2013/august/02/readmission-penalties-medicare-hospitals-year-two

poor scores, and to be penalized. Among safety-net hospitals serving the poor, 77 percent were penalized. Among hospitals that don't serve as many poor patients, about 36 percent saw their reimbursements trimmed, according to the Kaiser analysis.

"It's widely agreed, outside Washington, that the penalty unfairly harms hospitals serving lots of lower-income people by imagining they have more control over readmissions than they really do," said Alan Sager, a professor of health policy at the Boston University School of Public Health. "Lots of income, housing, social, and behavioral factors affect readmissions (as they do admissions themselves)."[129]

Krumholz, who helped devise the CMS policy, is not in favor of including race or socioeconomic status (SES) as a mitigating factor in the formula. "To adjust for that factor would be to hide differences in our population—and I think it is best to confront the differences and then determine the best policy response to reduce or eliminate the disparity."[130] In any case, he does not believe that social determinants of health have a strong bearing on an individual hospital's readmission rates.

3.2.4 The Road Ahead

For all the attention that the hospital readmissions reduction program has received, it's not a perfect measure of quality. Rather, it's fundamentally a proxy for broader concerns about inadequate coordination across the continuum of health care and social services.[131] A study by The Commonwealth Fund and the Institute for Healthcare Improvement called for "a new paradigm... that is relevant to patients, useful for improvement, and fair for accountability." Some of the goals of a revised readmissions program would include:

- Developing a suite of measures that more broadly reflects patients' experiences. Patients and the community should be engaged in the development of measures, as they have the most insight into what matters to them and what barriers they face.

---

[129] Alan Sager, email correspondence, September 27, 2013.

[130] Krumholz, The Incidental Economist.

[131] http://theincidentaleconomist.com/wordpress/harlan-krumholz-on-hospital-readmissions/

- Balancing measures such as mortality, length of stay, and use of observation status—to help ensure health systems aren't eliminating necessary hospital care.

- Creating holistic measures to reflect how instrumental care coordination and community interventions are in relation to outcomes, such as a community's "capacity not to hospitalize."

- Matching measures to the needs of users for improvement and accountability. Improvement measures analyze local performance over time and they indicate whether interventions are producing their intended outcomes. Accountability measures focus on risk adjustment, tend to be outcome-focused, and are collected retrospectively over long periods.

There is little disagreement about the justification for Medicare to use reimbursement penalties as a lever to encourage greater care coordination and risk mitigation. "That the initial policy has flaws is an argument not for abandoning the effort, but for redoubling efforts to improve the measures as well as the incentive system." [132] Readmissions should be considered in balance with other measures, such as mortality, length of stay, and use of observation status, to make sure that providers are not artificially suppressing readmission rates, the study commented.

In June 2013, MedPAC pointed to four issues in the current policy that need refinement, and proposed some technical modifications to address each concern:[133]

- When national readmission rates decline, aggregate penalties remain constant.

- Single-condition readmission rates have significant random variation because of small numbers of observations.

---

[132] *Clifford Marks, Saranya Loehrer, MD, and Douglas McCarthy, "Hospital Readmissions: Measuring for Improvement, Accountability, and Patients," The Commonwealth Fund and The Institute for Healthcare Improvement, September 2013.*
http://www.commonwealthfund.org/Publications/Issue-Briefs/2013/Sep/Measuring-Readmissions.aspx

[133] *http://www.commonwealthfund.org/Publications/Issue-Briefs/2013/Sep/Measuring-Readmissions.aspx*

- Heart failure readmission rates are inversely related to heart failure mortality rates.

- Hospitals that serve many low-income patients have higher readmissions rates and penalties.

In early August 2013, CMS released a rule for the second phase of the readmission penalty program. It made some adjustments to the methodology to account for planned readmissions. However, it declined to adopt an adjustment for patients' socioeconomic status. The rationale given by CMS is that "we do not want to hold hospitals to different standards of patient care simply because they treat a large number of low SES patients."[134]

Hospitals should expect to see a continued evolution of the technical measures, and a further elaboration on the penalty calculations, as more data become available over the next few years.

The end goal, MedPAC wrote, is to see "a decline in readmissions, a decline in the penalties hospitals pay, and a decline in Medicare spending on readmissions."[135] Or, as Krumholz expressed, "From the patient perspective the entire episode of the illness is important and they depend on us to work together on solutions, not debate who is responsible. We are all responsible. And the hospital is the logical actor to pull everyone together."[136]

---

[134] http://www.medpac.gov/chapters/Jun13_Ch04.pdf p. 107.

[135] CMS Federal Register report in 2012, quoted in http://www.medpac.gov/chapters/Jun13_Ch04.pdf p. 107.

[136] Krumholz, The Incidental Economist. http://theincidentaleconomist.com/wordpress/harlan-krumholz-on-hospital-readmissions/

Section 3.3: Technical Appendix: Hospital Readmission Reduction Program (HRRP)

3.3.1 Regulatory Background

With the introduction of the ACA, the Secretary of Health and Human Services (HHS) was charged with the responsibility of creating a National Quality Strategy (NQS) that coordinates health care initiatives throughout the United States, with aims to: (appendix Attachment A)

- improve health care quality

- improve the health of the US population

- reduce the costs of health care

In concert with the establishment of the NQS, a more formalized readmissions reduction program for Medicare patients was mandated under Title III Improving the Quality and Efficiency of Health Care. Section 3025 of the ACA and section 1886(q) of the Social Security Act outline requirements of the HRRP and "requires CMS to reduce payments to Inpatient Prospective Payment System (IPPS) hospitals with excess readmissions, effective for discharges beginning on October 1, 2012." The regulations that implement this provision are in subpart I of 42 CFR part 412 (§412.150 through §412.154).

The basis for the HRRP initiative was established in a set of recommendations made by MedPAC in its June 2007 Report to Congress. In this report, MedPAC presented the results of an FY2005 analysis of hospital admissions and readmissions utilizing a software product by 3M. MedPAC concluded that "in addition to adversely affecting beneficiaries' health and peace of mind," the failure to adequately attend to the care transition at discharge from hospitals resulted in additional Medicare spending. Reported findings by MedPAC indicated that for FY2005:

- 17.6 percent of admissions resulted in readmissions within thirty days of discharge, accounting for $15 billion in spending.

- 76 percent of thirty-day readmissions were flagged as "potentially preventable."

- CMS could potentially save an estimated $12 billion by eliminating such readmissions.[137]

MedPAC analyzed the financial impact of seven clinical conditions that made up almost 30 percent of all Medicare hospital spending:

Hospital readmissions for seven conditions make up almost 30 percent of spending on readmissions.

CONDITION	TYPE OF HOSPITAL ADMISSION	NUMBER OF ADMISSIONS WITH READMISSIONS	READMISSION RATE	AVERAGE MEDICARE PAYMENT FOR READMISSION	TOTAL SPENDING ON READMISSION
Heart Failure	Medical	90,273	12.5%	6,531	590,000,000
COPD	Medical	52,327	10.7%	6,587	345,000,000
Pneumonia	Medical	744,419	9.5%	7,165	533,000,000
AMI	Medical	20,866	13.4%	6,535	136,000,000
CABG	Surgical	18,554	13.5%	8,136	151,000,000
PTCA	Surgical	44,293	10.0%	8,109	359,000,000
Other Vascular	Surgical	18,029	11.7%	10,091	182,000,000
Total for 7 conditions		318,760			2,296,000,000
Total DRG		1,134,483			$7,980,000,000
% of total		28.1%			28.8%

Note: COPD (chronic obstructive pulmonary disease), AMI (acute myocardial infarction), CABG (coronary artery bypass graft), PTCA (percutaneous transluminal coronary angioplasty), DRG (diagnosis related group). Analysis is for readmissions within 15 days of discharge from the initial inpatient stay. Readmissions are identified using 3M's software that defines potentially preventable readmissions.

Source: 3M analysis of 2005 Medicare discharge claims data.

---

[137] Page 103 www.medpac.gov/documents/jun07_entirereport.pdf

Based on this information, Congress elected to focus initial efforts to reduce readmissions on the clinical conditions of acute myocardial infarction, heart failure, and pneumonia. To advance these efforts, two MedPAC recommendations were adopted:

- **Require public reporting of hospital-specific readmission rates for a subset of conditions.**

  - Beginning in 2007, CMS added readmissions measures for acute myocardial infarction, heart failure, and pneumonia to IQR requirements.

  - After collecting data on these measures in 2007 and 2008, CMS included performance reporting on the Hospital Compare website in 2009.

- **Adjust the underlying payment method to financially encourage lower readmission rates.**

  - MedPAC discounted the value of a positive financial incentive payment adjustment saying, "We recognize the importance of pay-for-performance (P4P) measures to improve quality, but find that the underlying payment method may undercut the behavior P4P is trying to encourage. When this is true, other policies may be needed to create stronger incentives to reduce readmissions."[138]

  - Adoption of these recommendations and the resulting actions taken by CMS since 2007 set the stage for the implementation of the HRRP as outlined in section 3015 of the ACA.

3.3.2 The HRRP: Program Overview

Section 3025 of the ACA (P.L. 111–148) required the Secretary of Health and Human Services (HHS) to establish a HRRP to reduce Inpatient Prospective Payment System (IPPS) payments to applicable hospitals with excess

---

[138] www.medpac.gov/documents/jun07_entirereport.pdf

readmissions for applicable conditions, over a specified time period, effective for discharges beginning on October 1, 2012.[139]

The ACA further directed the HHS Secretary to adopt the three NQF-endorsed, 30-day Risk Standardized Readmission measures developed for acute myocardial infarction, heart failure, and pneumonia for HRRP FY2013 and FY2014.

Beginning with program year FY2015, the HHS Secretary was directed "to the extent practicable, expand the applicable conditions beyond the 3 conditions for which measures have been endorsed … to the additional 4 conditions that have been identified by the Medicare Payment Advisory Commission in its report to Congress in June 2007 and to other conditions and procedures as determined appropriate by the Secretary." Section 3025(5)(B).

HHS was charged with developing a methodology to identify excess readmission rates and reduce payment amounts that would otherwise be made by an amount equal to the product of the base operating DRG and a developed adjustment factor.

As currently configured, the HRRP is a "penalty-only" program with payment adjustments made to the wage-adjusted base operating DRG amounts for each Medicare fee-for-service discharge occurring during a program year for "applicable" hospitals determined to have "excessive" readmissions.

3.3.3 Specifications and Standards

Applicable Hospitals

- A hospital in any of the fifty states and the District of Columbia that is classified as a "Medicare Subsection (d) Hospital"—generally defined as hospitals paid under the federal Inpatient Prospective Payment System (IPPS). (defined at section 1886(d)(1)(B) of the Act)[140]

    Note: IPPS-reimbursed hospitals that participate in Accountable Care Organizations (ACOs)—either through the Pioneer ACO initiative or ACOs formed as part of the

[139] Section 3025 http://www.gpo.gov/fdsys/pkg/PLAW-111publ148/pdf/PLAW-111publ148.pdf
[140] Section 1886 (d) (1) (b) http://www.ssa.gov/OP_Home/ssact/title18/1886.htm

Medicare Shared Savings program—are <u>NOT</u> excluded from the HRRP and will be evaluated.[141]

- In addition, for the purpose of determining discharge accountability for the HRRP initiative, the "applicable hospital" is the hospital responsible for discharging the patient to community-based care. In the event of a transfer from one hospital to another, the applicable hospital is the one that receives a patient and subsequently discharges that patient.

- HRRP Excluded Hospitals:

  - Hospitals in the state of Maryland are excluded by a waiver granted by CMS for a state-run initiative to reduce readmissions.

  - All hospitals in US territories and Puerto Rico are excluded.

  - All hospitals and hospital units that are excluded from the IPPS, such as: Long-Term Care Hospitals (LTCHs); cancer hospitals; children's hospitals; Inpatient Rehabilitation Facilities (IRFs); Inpatient Psychiatric Hospitals (IPHs); and Veteran's Administration Hospitals.[142]

Specified Time Period

- Section 3025 of the ACA requires that the HHS Secretary establish a post-discharge time frame for evaluation of readmissions related to "applicable conditions." Currently, the period of time established by the HHS Secretary is thirty days from the date of discharge from an "index admission."

Applicable Conditions

- Conditions that are selected by the HHS Secretary for inclusion must meet the following criteria:

  - Readmissions are high-volume or high expenditure.

  - Measures of such conditions have been endorsed by a contracted, consensus-based entity such as the NQF and such measures

---

[141] Page 53398: http://www.gpo.gov/fdsys/pkg/FR-2012-08-31/pdf/2012-19079.pdf

[142] Page 53397: http://www.gpo.gov/fdsys/pkg/FR-2012-08-31/pdf/2012-19079.pdf

contain exclusions for planned readmissions or transfers to another applicable hospital.

- **FY2013 and FY2014**: For the first two years of the HRRP, the ACA directed HHS to utilize NQF-endorsed readmission measures reported under the IQR program for three of the seven conditions identified in the MedPAC June 2007 Report to Congress. These are: acute myocardial infarction (AMI), heart failure (HF), and pneumonia (PN). Applicable admissions are identified through specific ICD-9 codes for each condition. **(Appendix–Table 1)**

- **FY2015**: Beginning with program year FY2015, the ACA directed HHS to expand the HRRP beyond AMI, HF, and PN. CMS decided to include three additional conditions in the HRRP program. They include:[143]

  o acute exacerbations of chronic obstructive pulmonary disease (AECOPD)

  o total hip arthroplasty (THA)

  o total knee arthroplasty (TKA)

- **Beyond FY2015**: Medicare is currently evaluating the feasibility of an all-condition readmission measure with two models under consideration:

  o **3M Model**: Utilizes a methodology that evaluates readmissions for all clinical conditions that are "clinically related" to the discharge condition. Currently, two states utilize this model for Medicaid readmissions reduction programs (New York and Maryland).

  o **The Yale All-Conditions Model**: This NQF-endorsed model was developed by the Yale New Haven Health Services Corporation—Center for Outcomes Research and Evaluation (YNHHSC/CORE).[144]

    ▪ This model evaluates all conditions and all readmissions, regardless of cause (exclusive of planned readmissions), to

---

[143] *Section 3025 (5) (B) 3025 http://www.gpo.gov/fdsys/pkg/PLAW-111publ148/pdf/PLAW-111publ148.pdf*

[144] *http://www.cms.gov/Medicare/Quality-Initiatives-Patient-Assessment-Instruments/MMS/downloads/MMSHospital-WideAll-ConditionReadmissionRate.pdf*

provide a hospital with one aggregate number for evaluation and assessment of financial incentives/penalties.

- As a precursor to future implementation, this model has received requisite endorsement by the NQF and a new measure for hospital-wide readmissions was added to the hospital IQR for FY2013.

- Per CMS rules, no new IQR measure can be implemented as a program measure until it has been posted on the Hospital Compare website for at least one year.

Index Admission

- An Index Admission is defined as the initial admission for a specified applicable condition. Readmission measures determine whether a patient experiences at least one readmission within thirty days of discharge from this condition-specific "index admission."

- Table 1 of the Appendix lists the ICD-9-CM codes used to identify each applicable condition to calculate excess readmissions for the FY2013– FY2014 HRRP.

- This assessment is a yes/no event, rather than a count of the total number of readmissions that occur in the thirty-day period following an index admission.

- For a given patient, only one readmission during the thirty-day period following a discharge for an index admission will be counted in the calculation under the HRRP.

- If a patient is readmitted within thirty days for another measured condition, the readmission could count as a readmission for the initial index admission *and* an index admission for the second measured condition. **Example:** A patient discharged with an index admission for heart failure returns to the hospital with pneumonia in fifteen days—the readmission would count against the initial index admission of heart failure *and* as a new index admission for pneumonia. Any additional readmissions within thirty days of discharge for pneumonia would count as a pneumonia readmission.[145]

- The measures include CMS fee-for-service beneficiaries with an index admission to an applicable hospital if they have been enrolled in Part A and Part B Medicare for the twelve months prior to the date of admission, and were enrolled in Part A during the index admission. This ensures a full year of administrative data for risk adjustment.

Readmissions

- Readmissions are defined as "occurring when a patient is discharged from the applicable hospital and then is admitted to the same or another acute care hospital within a specified time period (thirty days) from the time of discharge from the index hospitalization."

- Regardless of which hospital the patient is readmitted to, the discharging hospital is held responsible for the readmission.

- The HRRP counts unplanned readmissions for *any* cause, whether or not it is related to the clinical condition responsible for the index admission. In its FY2013 Final IPPS Rule, CMS stated two reasons for this:

  o "First, from the patient perspective, a readmission for any reason is likely to be an undesirable outcome of care after an acute hospitalization."

  o "Second, readmissions not directly related to the index condition may still be a result of care received during the index hospitalization."

- For patients who are transferred between two or more applicable hospitals and readmitted in the thirty days following the final hospitalization, the readmission is attributed to the final hospital that discharged them to a non-acute care setting.

---

[145] Page 53382: http://www.gpo.gov/fdsys/pkg/FR-2012-08-31/pdf/2012-19079.pdf

Readmission Exclusions

CMS *does not* include readmissions for the following:

- for discharges against medical advice as reported in MedPAR

- for admissions where patient died, as reflected in MedPAR discharge info

- for Medicare beneficiaries under the age of sixty-five

- for Medicare Advantage patients

- for admissions for AMI when patient was discharged on the same day

- hospitalizations for patients without at least thirty days post-discharge enrollment in Medicare fee-for-service

- multiple readmissions within thirty days of an index admission (Only the first readmission for an index admission is counted.)

- readmissions to non-applicable hospitals (i.e., VA Hospitals)

Planned Readmissions

- A "planned" readmission is one approved in advance to provide additional treatment not appropriate/available during an index admission and is generally not considered an indication of quality of care. As such, CMS has included provisions for the exclusion of legitimate planned readmissions as part of the HRRP program.

- For the FY2013 program, CMS identified two revascularization procedures (coronary artery bypass graft surgery (CABG) and percutaneous coronary intervention (PCI) as allowed planned readmissions for AMI. However, *no* planned readmissions were identified for the other HRRP clinical conditions of HF or PN.

- Given the limited scope of allowed planned readmissions and the continued expansion of measured HRRP conditions, CMS consulted with experts in the medical community as well as other stakeholders to identify appropriate planned readmissions for procedures and treatments for exclusion from HRRP evaluation, beginning in FY2014.

FY2014 Changes to Assessment of Planned Readmissions

Planned Readmission Algorithm Version 2.1:[146]

- Beginning in FY2014, CMS will utilize a "planned readmission algorithm" developed by Yale New Haven Health Services Corporation—Center for Outcomes Research and Evaluation (YNHHSC/CORE), to be used in more appropriately identifying planned readmissions across its readmission measures.

- The algorithm is a set of criteria for classifying readmissions as planned or unplanned using Medicare claims. The algorithm identifies admissions that are typically planned and may occur within thirty days of discharge from the hospital.

- The algorithm is based on three guiding principles:

  o A few specific, limited types of care are always considered planned (obstetrical delivery, transplant surgery, maintenance chemotherapy, rehabilitation).

  o Otherwise, a planned readmission is defined as a non-acute readmission for a scheduled procedure.

  o Admissions for acute illness or for complications of care are never planned.

- The Planned Readmission Algorithm uses a flowchart and four tables of procedures and conditions to implement these principles and to classify readmissions as planned or unplanned. (The flowchart and tables are available in a report, *CMS Planned Readmission Algorithm Version 2.1*, which is available on the CMS website.

---

[146] *Page 50540 http://www.cms.gov/Medicare/Medicare-Fee-for-Service-Payment/AcuteInpatientPPS/FY2014-IPPS-Final-Rule-Home-Page.html*

Counting of Readmissions following "Planned Readmissions":

- In concert with utilization of the Planned Readmission Algorithm in FY2014, CMS clarified in its FY2014 Final IPPS Rules how readmissions following a planned readmission will be counted:

  - "If the first readmission is planned, it will not count as a readmission, nor will any subsequent unplanned readmission within 30 days of the index readmission. In other words, unplanned readmissions that occur after a planned readmission and fall within the 30-day post discharge timeframe would no longer be counted as readmissions for the index admission."

Estimated Impact of FY2014 Planned Readmission Changes:

- Implementation of the Planned Readmission Algorithm Version 2.1 and associated revisions to the method of counting readmissions following a planned readmission will significantly reduce the number of countable readmissions.

- In comparison to data collected for the FY2013 HRRP program for the period of July 2008–June 2011 for 3,025 hospitals, the application of the FY2014 changes would result in an overall increase in the number of readmissions considered planned (and not counted as a readmission) as follows:[147]

  - AMI: Increase of 4,942

  - HF: Increase of 17,512

  - PN: Increase of 7,084

  Note: For FY2013, only two procedures were considered for planned readmissions for AMI and none for HF and PN.

---

[147] Page 50656 http://www.cms.gov/Medicare/Medicare-Fee-for-Service-Payment/AcuteInpatientPPS/FY2014-IPPS-Final-Rule-Home-Page.html

Risk-Standardized Measures

- Based on the patient population of each hospital, a method of risk assessment is utilized to "level the playing field" among hospitals with regards to patient clinical complexity and chances for readmission.

- To determine a risk-standardization factor, CMS uses Part A and Part B claims (inpatient, outpatient, and physician services) for each patient for the twelve months prior to the index hospitalization as well as the index hospitalization.

- Risk standardization adjusts for key factors that are clinically relevant and have strong relationships with the outcome (for example, patient demographic factors, patient coexisting medical conditions, and indicators of patient frailty).

- Comparisons are made between individual hospital patient data and national measures of risk data to determine relative risk levels.

- The risk adjustment variables that will be used to calculate readmission rates can be found in the readmission measure methodology reports found on the website. (See Resources/Fiscal Year Measure Methodology Report)

3.3.4 Methodology for Payment Adjustments

The process for determining payment adjustments under the HRRP utilizes a fairly straightforward mathematical calculation. However, some components of such calculations are beyond the ability of an individual facility to determine, as they may involve nationally derived data, unavailable to a hospital. It is important to understand the elements that contribute to payment adjustment determinations for the development and implementation of interventional strategies.

The established methodology involves four steps:[148]

- Collect data.
- Calculate the excess readmission ratio for each measure.
- Determine the applicable RAF.
- Determine the PAF.

Step 1: Data Collection Process

- For each HRRP program fiscal year, data on admissions/ readmissions for specified conditions is extracted from the IQR process over a three-year period.

- For FY2013–FY2017, data collection periods are as follows:[149]

PROGRAM YEAR	DISCHARGE DATA PERIOD	DATE OF DATA "SNAPSHOT"*
FY2013	July 1, 2008–June 30, 2011	September 30, 2011
FY2014	July 1, 2009–June 30, 2012	September 30, 2012
FY2015	July 1, 2010–June 30, 2013	September 30, 2013
FY2016	July 1, 2011–June 30, 2014	September 30, 2014
FY2017	July 1, 2012–June 30, 2015	September 30, 2015

*Data "Snapshot" date is ninety days after last discharge in the discharge data period to allow for filing of claims. Although current CMS policy allows for up to one year for file discharge claims, only those filed by the snapshot date are included in the HRRP program year. Such information is extracted from the CMS Common Working File (CWF).

- For FY2013 and FY2014, HRRP-applicable conditions are limited to AMI, HF, and PN. Beginning in FY2015, AECOPD, THA, and TKA will be added.

- Data are collected only for Medicare fee-for-service beneficiaries over the age of sixty-five. Data for patients enrolled in Medicare Advantage plans are not included. This is the same universe of claims used for calculating the NQF-endorsed measures for the purposes of the Hospital IQR Program.

---

[148] http://www.hfma.org/Content.aspx?id=1278

[149] http://www.cms.gov/Medicare/Medicare-Fee-for-Service-Payment/AcuteInpatientPPS/Readmissions-Reduction-Program.html

- A three-year data collection period is utilized to help ensure that each measure meets a minimum of twenty-five cases per measure. In the event that a hospital does not report at least twenty-five cases per measure, results for that measure will not be made.

- Hospitals will receive confidential reports and accompanying discharge-level information from CMS through their QualityNet account once such information has been processed. Once reports are received, hospitals will have thirty days to review and file any corrections.

Note: Information contained in confidential reports for discharge/ readmissions may not match data reported on Hospital Compare. The HRRP program only collects data for subsection (d) hospitals. Data presented on Hospital Compare includes non-subsection data to establish national averages. As a result, relative performance may differ between Hospital Compare and HRRP reports.

Step 2: Calculation of the Excess Readmission Ratio for each Clinical Measure

- An excess readmission ratio is calculated for each NQF-endorsed clinical measure. The methodology used sums the probability of readmission numbers for all patients at an average hospital. The calculation process adjusts for the variation in readmission risk of a hospital's patients, based on how sick they are when admitted, and the variation in the number of patients that a hospital treats in total.

- The excess readmission ratio compares the total adjusted actual readmissions (numerator) at the hospital to the number of expected readmissions (denominator) if the hospital's patients were treated at an average hospital with similar patients.[150]

  o **Actual Adjusted (or predicted) Number of Readmissions**: (numerator) Based on illness and history, an estimate is made of the probability of readmission for each patient. Then, all the patients' probability numbers are summed to produce an actual predicted readmission rate for the hospital.

---

[150] http://www.gpo.gov/fdsys/pkg/FR-2012-08-31/pdf/2012-19079.pdf

- o **Expected Number of Readmissions**: (denominator) This denominator is the sum of all patients' probability of readmissions if they were being treated at an average hospital.

- Dividing the *actual adjusted number* by the *expected number* yields the ratio:

  - o Hospitals with more adjusted actual readmissions than expected readmissions will have a risk-standardized ratio (excess readmission ratio) greater than 1.00.

  - o Hospitals with fewer adjusted actual admissions than expected readmissions will have a ratio less than 1.00.

  - o Such ratios are calculated for each of the clinical measures. Because the HRRP is a penalty-only program, ratios for each measure must be *less* than one to avoid penalty.

- In short, the Excess Admissions Ratio is the sum of all patients' expected probabilities of readmission for a given clinical measure, given their risk factors and the risk of readmission at an average hospital.

Step 3: Determining the "Applicable" Readmission Adjustment Factor (RAF)

- Hospital performance under the HRRP is evaluated against two RAFs:[151]

  - o The first RAF is an annually established national "floor" factor. CMS has established this floor as a numerical factor that determines the maximum HRRP penalty for a given year. The national floor factors for the HRRP are as follows:

    - FY2013   .9900

    - FY2014   .9800

    - FY2015 and beyond   .9700

---

[151] http://www.cms.gov/Medicare/Medicare-Fee-for-Service-Payment/AcuteInpatientPPS/Readmissions-Reduction-Program.html

o The second RAF is an individual hospital's calculated ratio, combining the excess readmission ratios (calculated in Step 2) for each clinical measure with associated base operating DRG amounts.

o The "applicable" RAF utilized to calculate a hospital's payment modifier is selected as the higher of these two RAFs. As described below, higher RAFs are associated with lower penalties.

- The formula used to calculate the RAF is:[152]

  o **Aggregate payments for excess readmissions** = [sum of base operating DRG payments for AMI x (excess readmission ratio for AMI-1)] + [sum of base operating DRG payments for HF x (excess readmission ratio for HF-1)] +[sum of base operating DRG payments for PN x (excess readmission ratio for PN-1)]

  o **Aggregate payments for all discharges** = sum of base operating DRG payments for all discharges

  o **Ratio** = 1-(aggregate payments for excess readmissions/ aggregate payments for all discharges). This ratio is expressed out to the fourth digit and is the RAF ratio.

  o The higher of the RAF ratio or the established annual floor factor will be used to calculate payment modifier.

Step 4: Calculation of the Payment Modifier (PM)

- Payment modifiers are percentage reductions in the wage-adjusted base operating DRG rates for each discharge occurring in a program year.

- The payment modifier is calculated by subtracting the RAF from 1.0000 and expressing the result as a negative percentage modifier applied to the

---

[152]

https://www.qualitynet.org/dcs/ContentServer?c=Page&pagename=QnetPublic%2FPage%2FQne tTier2&cid=1228772412458

base operating DRG rate for each Medicare fee-for-service discharge in a given year.[153]

Note: Since this is a "penalty-only" program, all modifiers are negative numbers.

- o For hospitals that have a RAF *greater* than the annual floor factor, the actual calculated RAF is utilized to determine the payment modifier:

  - For ratios equal to 1.0000, no penalties will be applied (1-1=0).

  - For ratios between .9901 and .9999, the calculated RAF is subtracted from 1 and expressed as a negative percentage payment modifier to be applied to the per-discharge base operating DRG amount.

  - **Example:** RAF=.9950 Modifier=1-.9950 = .005 x100 = -.50% reduction in the per-discharge base operating DRG rate. (In this example, the reported HRRP modifier posted by CMS would be **-.50.**)

- o For hospitals that have a RAF *less* than the floor factor, the established floor factor will be utilized to calculate the payment modifier:

  - The annual floor rate will be subtracted from 1.00 and expressed as a negative percentage.

YEAR	FLOOR	PER-DISCHARGE REDUCTION TO BASE OPERATING DRG RATES
FY2013	.9900	.01 or -1%
FY2014	.9800	.02 or -2%
FY2015	.9700	.03 or -3%

Note: These amounts represent the maximum penalty for each program year.

153

https://www.qualitynet.org/dcs/ContentServer?c=Page&pagename=QnetPublic%2FPage%2FQnetTier2&cid=1228772412458

3.3.5 Estimating the Annual Fiscal Impact of Reimbursement Reductions

- Because HRRP penalties are communicated as a percentage payment modification amount to be applied to a specific portion of per-discharge reimbursement, the resulting financial consequences may be overlooked or minimized. Therefore, it is useful for hospitals to have the ability to develop at least a conservative estimate of revenue loss for a given program year.

- CMS provides modifier reports to hospitals through the hospitals' QualityNet accounts and posts all hospital modifiers on the CMS website.

- Modifiers are expressed as a negative percent reduction to be applied to the wage-adjusted base operating DRG rates for each Medicare discharge only. Modifiers are not universally applied to all Part A charges.

- Penalties are assessed prospectively for a fiscal year. For the FY2013 program, modifiers were applied beginning with all discharges from October 1, 2012 through September 30, 2013.

Wage-Adjusted Base Operating DRG Rate

- In the determination of payment penalties, HHS was directed to develop a methodology to create a modifier that would be applied to a standard reimbursement for each discharge, regardless of case severity. It was agreed that modifiers would be applied to the per-discharge "wage-adjusted base operating Diagnosis Related Group (DRG) payment amount."

  o Hospitals are reimbursed for costs associated with inpatient stays by classifying provided care into defined DRGs. See Attachment A: **Acute Care Inpatient Prospective Payment System (IPPS)** for more information on DRGs.

  o Under the HRRP, *the base operating DRG amounts are utilized to calculate aggregate payments for all discharges and excess discharges. These amounts are then utilized to determine the RAF as described in the methodology section above.*

200

- CMS defines "base operating DRG payment amount" under the HRRP as: "The wage-adjusted DRG operating payment plus any applicable new technology add-on payments."

- Although final reimbursement under the DRG system includes a number of other factors, for the purpose of applying the HRRP penalty amount, the following components are excluded:

  - payments for discharges exceeding base DRG costs (adjustments for condition severity)

  - add-on payments for Indirect Medical Education (IME): the costs associated with a teaching institution

  - payments to hospitals serving low-income populations: Disproportionate Share Hospitals (DSH)

  - "outlier" payments: additional payments made for the most expensive 1 percent of hospital stays

  - additional payments made to low-volume hospitals[154]

Estimating the Wage-Adjusted Base Operating DRG Amount for a Given Hospital

The following information allows hospitals to estimate the current fiscal year impact of the HRRP and to model future changes based on changing patient discharge volumes.

- Each year, CMS establishes a new base DRG rate:

  - FY2013 base DRG rate = $5,348.76

  - FY2014 base DRG rate = $5,370.28[155]

- The base DRG rate is calculated based on annual adjustments made to a "labor-related share" and a "non-labor-related share." The percentage

---

[154] Page 50667 http://www.cms.gov/Medicare/Medicare-Fee-for-Service-Payment/AcuteInpatientPPS/FY2014-IPPS-Final-Rule-Home-Page.html

[155] http://www.cms.gov/Medicare/Medicare-Fee-for-Service-Payment/AcuteInpatientPPS/FY2014-IPPS-Final-Rule-Home-Page.html Final Rules Data tables FY2014 FR Rate table 1A-1E

that each component contributes to the total base DRG can vary, based on the relative wage levels present for a given geographic area. CMS calculates a "wage index" (WI) for specific geographical areas to reflect differences between "high-wage" and "low-wage" areas. High-wage areas are associated with a WI of greater than 1.0 and low-wage areas are indicated by a WI equal to or less than 1.0.[156]

- Hospitals are first grouped according to their location in a high-wage or low-wage area. Based on this designation, the amount of the assigned labor-related share portion of the base DRG is different, as shown below:

For FY2014: base DRG rate = $5,370.28[157]

- High-wage area: (WI>1.00)
  - labor-related share = $3,737.71 or 69.6% of base DRG
  - non-labor-related Share = $1,632.57 or 30.4% of base DRG
  - Total $5,370.28
- Low-wage area: (WI<=1.00)
  - labor-related share = $3,329.57 or 62% of base DRG
  - non-labor-related share = $2,040.71 or 38% of base DRG
  - Total $5,370.28

These labor-related shares are further modified by the application of a hospital-specific WI to determine a *labor-adjusted* base operating DRG rate (before adding in any average adjustments for new technology add-on payments). The impact of the application of the WI can be seen in the following examples:

Low-wage Area Hospital:

- Hospital A is located in Mobile, Alabama with a WI of .8106 (less than 1.0 indicating low-wage area DRG composition).

---

[156] *Page 27498 http://www.cms.gov/Medicare/Medicare-Fee-for-Service-Payment/AcuteInpatientPPS/FY-2014-IPPS-Proposed-Rule-Home-Page-Items/FY-2014-IPPS-Proposed-Rule-CMS-1599-P-Regulations.html*

[157] *http://www.cms.gov/Medicare/Medicare-Fee-for-Service-Payment/AcuteInpatientPPS/FY2014-IPPS-Final-Rule-Home-Page.html Final Rules Data tables FY2014 FR Rate table 1A-1E*

- (WI x labor-related share for *low-wage area*) + non-labor-related share for low-wage area = WABO (Wage-Adjusted Base-Operating DRG)

- (.8106 x $3,329) + $2040.71 = $4,739.20

High-wage Area Hospital:

- Hospital B is located in San Francisco with a WI of 1.6269 (> than 1.0 indicating high-wage area DRG composition).

- (WI x labor-related share for *high-wage area*) + non-labor-related share for high-wage area = WABO DRG

- (1.6269 x $3,737.71) + $1,632.57 = $7,713.45

- View the FY2014 assigned WI table for individual hospitals.

New Technology Add-On Payments (NTAP)[158]

- To account for the NTAP amounts, CMS will assign an additional amount to the labor-adjusted DRG rate based on annual utilization of approved new technology. The aggregate amount reimbursed for new technology will be equally split over total Medicare discharges during a program year.

- DRG rates are recalculated annually, utilizing two years of data. As a result, any newly introduced technology will not be reimbursed for at least two years.

- To address this lag, in 2001 CMS introduced NTAP to allow reimbursement for technologies that met three criteria:

  1. They are considered new (purchased within two to three years of FDA approval).

  2. The average cost of a patient case using the technology is inadequately paid under the current DRG system.

---

[158] http://www.cms.gov/Outreach-and-Education/Medicare-Learning-Network-MLN/MLNMattersArticles/downloads/MM8421.pdf

3. The new technology represents a "substantial clinical improvement" over the existing standard of care.

- CMS has authorized additional payments for specific procedures or drugs that are approved as "new technology" and the WABO DRG rate for a hospital is modified by the application of an average per-discharge adjustment to account for the volume of use of such technology.

The following are designated as qualifying for NTAP:

- **FY2013 only: payments for the AutoLITT™:** A laser surgical instrument used to necrotize or coagulate soft tissue through interstitial irradiation (thermal therapy) in general surgery and neurosurgery. Cases involving the AutoLITT™ that are eligible for the new technology add-on payment will be identified by assignment to MS-DRGs 25, 26, and 27 with an ICD-9 procedure code of 17.61 (ICD-10-PCS codes D0Y0KZZ and D0Y1KZZ) in combination with one of the following primary ICD-9 diagnosis codes: 191.0, 191.1, 191.2, 191.3, 191.4, 191.5, 191.6, 191.7, 191.8, 191.9 (ICD-10-CM codes C71.0, C71.1, C71.2, C71.3, C71.4, C71.5, C71.6, C71.7, C71.8, and C71.9). The maximum add-on payment for a case involving the AutoLITT™ is $5,300.

- **FY2013–FY2014: DIFICID:** An antibiotic utilized to treat clostridium difficile-associated diarrhea (CDAD). Cases involving the treatment of CDAD with DIFICID are eligible for the new technology add-on payment and will be identified with an ICD-9-CM diagnosis code of 008.45 (the ICD-10-CM diagnosis code is A04.7) in combination with NDC code 52015-0080-01 in data element LIN03 of the 837I. The maximum add-on payment for a case involving DIFICID is $868.

- **FY2013–FY2014: Zenith Fenestrated Graft:** An endovascular graft and adjunctive alignment stent utilized to treat patients with abdominal aortic aneurysms (AAA). Cases involving the Zenith Fenestrated Graft that are eligible for the new technology add-on payment will be identified by ICD-9-CM procedure code 39.78. (The ICD-10-CM procedure codes are: 04U03JZ: supplement abdominal aorta with synthetic substitute, percutaneous approach; 04U04JZ: supplement abdominal aorta with synthetic substitute, percutaneous endoscopic approach; 04V03DZ: restriction of abdominal aorta with intraluminal device, percutaneous approach; or 04V04DZ: restriction of abdominal aorta with intraluminal device, percutaneous endoscopic approach.) The maximum add-on payment for a case involving the Zenith Fenestrated Graft is $8,171.50.

- **FY2013–FY2014: Voraxaze:** An enzyme used to treat patients with toxic levels of methotrexate in their blood due to kidney failure. Cases involving Voraxaze that are eligible for the new technology add-on payment will be identified by ICD-9-CM procedure code 00.95. (The ICD-10-CM procedure codes are: 3E033GQ: introduction of Glucarpidase into peripheral vein, percutaneous approach or 3E043GQ: introduction of Glucarpidase into central vein, percutaneous approach.) The maximum add-on payment for a case involving the Voraxaze is $45,000.

- **FY2014–FY2015: Argus:** A retinal prosthetic device designed to help improve blindness due to conditions such as retinitis pigmentosa. Cases involving the Argus® II System that are eligible for new technology add-on payments will be identified by ICD-9-CM procedure code 14.81. (The ICD-10-CM procedure codes are: 08H005Z: insertion of epiretinal visual prosthesis into right eye, open approach or 08H105Z: insertion of epiretinal visual prosthesis into left eye, open approach.) The maximum add-on payment for a case involving the Argus® II System is $72,028.75.

- **FY2014–FY2015: Kcentra:** A pharmacologic product used for the urgent reversal of acquired coagulation factor deficiency induced by vitamin K antagonist (e.g., warfarin) therapy in adult patients with acute major bleeding. Cases involving Kcentra that are eligible for new technology add-on payments will be identified by ICD-9-CM procedure code 00.96. The add-on payment will not be made if any of the following diagnosis codes are on the claim: 286.0, 286.1, 286.2, 286.3, 286.4, 286.5, 286.7, 286.52, 286.53, 286.59. (The ICD-10-CM procedure codes are: 30280B1: transfusion of nonautologous 4-factor prothrombin complex concentrate into vein, open approach or 30283B1: transfusion of nonautologous 4-factor Prothrombin Complex and the ICD-10-CM diagnosis codes are: D66, D67, D68.1, D68.2, D68.0, D68.311, D68.312, D68.318, D68.32, D68.4.) The maximum add-on payment for a case of Kcentra™ is $1,587.50.

- **FY2014–FY2015: Zilver:** Zilver PTX is a drug-eluting stent for the superficial femoral artery (SFA), proven to inhibit restenosis and reduce reintervention rates. Cases involving the Zilver® PTX® that are eligible for new technology add-on payments will be identified by ICD-9-CM procedure code 00.60. (The ICD-10-CM procedure codes are: 047K04Z: dilation of right femoral artery with drug-eluting intraluminal device, open approach; 047K34Z: dilation of right femoral artery with drug-eluting intraluminal device, percutaneous approach; 047K44Z: dilation of right femoral artery with drug-eluting intraluminal device, percutaneous endoscopic approach; 047L04Z: dilation of left femoral artery with drug-eluting intraluminal device, open approach; 047L34Z: dilation of left femoral artery with drug-eluting intraluminal device, percutaneous approach; or 047L44Z: dilation of left femoral artery with drug-eluting intraluminal device, percutaneous endoscopic approach.) The maximum add-on payment for a case of the Zilver® PTX® is $1,705.25.

- Estimates of the average NTAP may be determined by dividing all NTAP by the number of anticipated Medicare discharges. This amount can be added to the WABO DRG to assist in estimating total revenue reductions for a given year.

Estimating Annual Revenue Loss

An estimate of the potential loss of revenue can be made by:

(Labor adjusted base operating DRG rate x payment modifier) x total annual Medicare discharges

Example:

- Hospital B is in a high-wage market and has calculated that average NTAP reimbursements will add $8.00 to each discharge.

- It has received an HRRP payment modifier of -.50 percent.

- It anticipates at least 11,000 Medicare discharges in FY2013.

Labor Adjusted DRG = $7,713.45 + $8 (NTAP Average) = $7,721.45

($7,721.45* x -.005) x 11,000 = $424,679.75 reduction to FY2013 payments

*See above discussion on Base Operating DRG Rates

Note: Modifiers are reported as a negative percentage. To calculate estimated reimbursement reductions, the modifier must be expressed in decimal form. Example: -.50 percent modifier is expressed as -.005.

The example above indicates that reimbursements for each discharge will be decreased by -.50 percent of the WABO DRG standard rate. In the example, each discharge would have approximately $38.61 deducted from each CMS reimbursement.

3.3.6 HRRP Results

FY2013

- Medicare began applying payment modifiers to all Medicare discharges beginning on October 1, 2012, and estimated that the FY2013 penalties would save $280 million.

- FY2013 average reimbursement reduction per hospital was estimated at $125,000, with a range of $0 to over $1 million.

- Based on the FY2013 Payment Modifier Report:

  o 35 percent of hospitals have a factor of 1.0 and will see no change in IPPS payment.

  o 8 percent of hospitals have a factor of 0.9900 and will be subject to the maximum penalty of 1.0 percent. (Original CMS modeling predicted that 14 percent would receive maximum penalties.)[159]

  o The remaining 57 percent of hospitals have factors between 0.9900 and 1.0.

  o Penalties represented .24 percent of all hospital payments for FY2013.

- The data collection period for the FY2014 program ended on June 30, 2012, and modifiers were applied beginning with discharges after October 1, 2012.

---

[159] http://www.advisory.com/Daily-Briefing/2012/08/13/Medicare-will-penalize-2211-hospitals-for-readmissions

FY2014[160]

- The CMS estimate of total penalties for FY2014 indicates a significant decrease over FY2013 (from $300m to $227m), and the average hospital penalty has decreased from -.42 percent in FY2013 to -.38 percent for FY2014.

- Of 3,379 hospitals included in the FY2014 HRRP, 2,225 have received penalties and 1,154 have not.

- 18 hospitals have received the maximum FY2014 penalty of -2.0 percent and 154 have been assessed a -1.0 percent penalty. (In FY2013, 307 hospitals received a -1.0 percent penalty.)

- Based on the FY2014 Payment Modifier Report:

  o average penalty: -.38 percent

  o 34 percent received a payment adjustment factor of 1.0: no penalty

  o 4.5 percent received a payment adjustment factor of 0.9900: -1 percent penalty

  o .5 percent received a payment adjustment factor of 0.9800: maximum penalty of -2 percent

  o 61 percent received a payment adjustment factor between 0.9900 and 1.0

3.3.7 Future Direction

- CMS is continuing to evaluate ways to ensure greater alignment of the HRRP with its goal to reduce preventable readmissions. In a September 2012 MedPAC presentation on Refining the Hospital Readmission Reduction Program, the following goals were identified as "Principles for Refinement":

---

[160] http://www.kaiserhealthnews.org/Stories/2013/August/02/readmission-penalties-medicare-hospitals-year-two.aspx

- o Maintain or increase average hospitals' incentives to reduce readmissions.

- o Increase the share of hospitals that have an incentive to reduce readmissions.

- o Make penalties a consistent multiple of the cost of readmissions.

- o Be at least budget-neutral to current policy, with a preference for lower readmission rates rather than higher penalties.[161]

- A number of issues with HRRP methodology have been voiced by providers and alternatives for future modification are being evaluated.

  - o The method of including national readmission data into the calculation of penalties is such that, as national readmission rates decline, assessed average penalties could increase. In addition, different penalties are calculated for each condition. Possible alternatives to the current penalty methodology being evaluated are:

    - Use readmission information for all conditions.

    - Use a fixed multiplier.

    - Eliminate the use of a multiplier entirely and set a lower target rate for readmissions to maintain budget neutrality.

  - o Because of the small number of cases for many hospitals, it is difficult to distinguish between random occurrence and true performance. Alternatives include:

    - Use all conditions to increase the number of observations.

    - Include more years in the data-collection period.

    - Allow hospital systems to aggregate individual facility data for penalty purposes, but continue to publicly report individual performance.

  - o In contrast to the requirement to include all readmissions regardless of cause, some readmissions are not preventable and are totally unrelated to inpatient care. In addition, the current

---

[161] http://medpac.gov/transcripts/readmissions%20Sept%2012%20presentation.pdf

process recognizes few reasons for planned readmissions. Possible solutions include shifting to an all-conditions measures model that includes planned readmissions and excludes readmissions unrelated to care.

o The current process for risk assessment does not take socioeconomic status (SES) into consideration. In evaluating the impact of SES on the measure of heart failure for the FY2013 program, it was determined that higher rates of HRRP-qualified beneficiaries receiving Social Security Income (SSI) were associated with higher HRRP penalties. Possible remedies include:

- Add SES information to the risk-assessment formula.

- Evaluate the impact on the current incentive program as a means to close the gap between high and low concentrations of lower-income beneficiaries.

- Compare hospitals to similar hospitals to compute penalties.

- Provide financial assistance to hospitals with high levels of low-income beneficiaries.

3.3.8 Conclusion

In summary, although the penalty phase of the HRRP first started with discharges occurring on October 1, 2012 (FY2013), CMS feels that the program is already having the desired effect on hospital readmission rates.

In testimony to the Senate Finance Committee on February 28, 2013, Medicare Director Jonathan Blum concluded that the threat of penalty commencement has already produced results among those hospitals with high rates of readmissions. Blum reported that thirty-day readmissions rates decreased to 17.8 percent in the fourth quarter of 2012, down from between 18.5 percent and 19.5 percent during the past five years.

"This decrease is an early sign that our payment and delivery reforms are having an impact," Blum said in his prepared testimony.[162]

As a cornerstone initiative launched by CME to more closely link payments with quality outcomes and promote value-based care, the HRRP will continue to evolve as a method to hold health care providers more accountable for both cost and quality of care.

---

[162] Statement of Jonathan Blum, Acting Principal Deputy Administrator and Director, Center for Medicare, Centers for Medicare and Medicare Services on: Delivery System Reform: Progress Report From CMS, Before the US Senate Finance Committee, February 28, 2013.

Section 3.4: Appendix

3.4.1 Acronym Guide

3M ....3M Health Information System

ACA............................Affordable Care Act
(Patient Protection and Affordable Care Act of 2010)

ACO ....Accountable Care Organization

AE COPD.................Acute Exacerbation of Chronic Obstructive Pulmonary Disease

AHA...........................American Hospital Association

AHRQ........................Agency for Healthcare Research and Quality

CABG........................Coronary Artery Bypass Graft

CDAD........................Clostridium Difficile-Associated Disease

CMS ....Centers for Medicare & Medicaid Services

COPD........................Chronic Obstructive Pulmonary Disease

CY ....Calendar Year

DRA ....Deficit Reduction Act of 2005, Public Law 109–171

DRG ....Diagnosis-Related Group

DSH ....Disproportionate Share Hospital

FY..............................Fiscal Year

GME.......................... Graduate Medical Education

HCAHPS ....Hospital Consumer Assessment of Healthcare Providers and Systems

HHS .... Health and Human Services

HRRP....................... Hospital Readmission Reduction Program

HVBP .... Hospital Value-Based Purchasing Program

ICD-9-CM.................International Classification of Diseases, Ninth Revision,
Clinical Modification

ICD-10-CM...............International Classification of Diseases, Tenth Revision,
Clinical Modification

ICD-10-PCS..............International Classification of Diseases, Tenth Revision,
Procedure Coding System

IME........................... Indirect Medical Education

IOM .... Institute of Medicine

IPF............................ Inpatient Psychiatric Facility

IPH .... Inpatient Psychiatric Hospital

IPPS .... [Acute care hospital] Inpatient Prospective Payment System

IRF .... Inpatient Rehabilitation Facility

IQR............................ Inpatient Quality Reporting

LTCH .... Long-Term Care Hospital

MA .... Medicare Advantage

MedPAC .... Medicare Payment Advisory Commission

MedPAR .... Medicare Provider Analysis and Review File

MIPPA...................... Medicare Improvements for Patients and Providers Act of 2008, Public Law 110–275

MMA .... Medicare Prescription Drug, Improvement, and Modernization Act of 2003

MRSA........................ Methicillin-Resistant Staphylococcus Aureus

MS-DRG .... Medicare Severity Diagnosis-Related Group

NCQA .... National Committee for Quality Assurance

NQF .... National Quality Forum

NQS .... National Quality Strategy

NTAP .... New Technology Add-on Payment

NVHRI...................... National Voluntary Hospital Reporting Initiative

OMB......................... Executive Office of Management and Budget

PAF .... Payment Adjustment Factor

PCH .... PPS-Exempt Cancer Hospital

PPS.......................... Prospective Payment System

PRA 2.1.................... Planned Readmissions Algorithm Version 2.1

PTCA .... Percutaneous Transluminal Coronary Angioplasty

PVBP .... Physicians Value-Based Purchasing Program

QIG .... Quality Improvement Group, CMS

QIO .... Quality Improvement Organization

RHQDAPU .... Reporting Hospital Quality Data for Annual Payment Update (Now Known as IQR)

RAF.......................... Readmission Adjustment Factor

THA.......................... Total Hip Arthroplasty

TKA .... Total Knee Arthroplasty

VAH.......................... Veterans Administration Hospital

SNF ....Skilled Nursing Facility

WABO DRG..............Wage-Adjusted Base Operating Diagnosis-Related Group

YNHHSC/CORE.......Yale New Haven Health Services Corporation/Center for Outcomes Research and Evaluation

3.4.2 Table 1: Individual Measure ICD-9 Codes, FY2013–FY2014 HRRP

The tables below list the ICD-9-CM codes used to identify each applicable condition to calculate the aggregate payments for excess readmissions for the FY2013–FY2014 HRRP. These codes will also be used to identify the applicable conditions to calculate the excess readmission ratios. Revisions to these tables will be made upon implementation of ICD-10.

ICD-9 Codes to Identify Acute Myocardial Infarction Cases

ICD-9 CODE	DESCRIPTION OF CODE
410.00	AMI (anterolateral wall)-episode of care unspecified
410.01	AMI (anterolateral wall)-initial episode of care
410.10	AMI (other anterior wall)-episode of care unspecified
410.11	AMI (other anterior wall)-initial episode of care
410.20	AMI (inferolateral wall)-episode of care unspecified
410.21	AMI (inferolateral wall)-initial episode of care
410.30	AMI (inferoposterior wall)-episode of care unspecified
410.31	AMI (inferoposterior wall)-initial episode of care
410.40	AMI (other inferior wall)-episode of care unspecified
410.41	AMI (other inferior wall)-initial episode of care
410.50	AMI (other lateral wall)-episode of care unspecified
410.51	AMI (other lateral wall)-initial episode of care
410.60	AMI (true posterior wall)-episode of care unspecified
410.61	AMI (true posterior wall)-initial episode of care
410.70	AMI (subendocardial)-episode of care unspecified
410.71	AMI subendocardial)-initial episode of care
410.80	AMI (other specified site)-episode of care unspecified
410.81	AMI (other specified site)-initial episode of care

| 410.90 | AMI (unspecified site)-episode of care unspecified |
| 410.91 | AMI (unspecified site)-initial episode of care |

ICD-9 Codes to Identify Heart Failure Cases

ICD-9 Code	Description of Code
402.01	Hypertensive heart disease, malignant with heart failure
402.11	Hypertensive heart disease, benign, with heart failure
402.91	Hypertensive heart disease, unspecified, with heart failure
404.01	Hypertensive heart and chronic kidney disease, malignant with heart failure and chronic kidney disease stage I–IV, or unspecified
404.03	Hypertensive heart and chronic kidney disease, malignant with heart failure and with chronic kidney disease stage V or end stage renal disease
404.11	Hypertensive heart and chronic kidney disease, benign, with heart failure and with chronic kidney disease stage I–IV, or unspecified
404.13	Hypertensive heart and chronic kidney disease, benign with heart failure and chronic kidney disease stage I–IV, or unspecified failure and chronic kidney disease stage V or end stage renal disease
404.91	Hypertensive heart and chronic kidney disease, unspecified with heart failure and chronic kidney disease stage V, or end stage renal disease heart failure and with chronic kidney disease stage I–IV or unspecified.
404.93	Hypertensive heart and chronic kidney disease, unspecified with heart failure and chronic kidney disease stage V, or end stage renal disease.

ICD-9 Codes to Identify Pneumonia Cases

ICD-9 CODE	DESCRIPTION OF CODE
480.00	Pneumonia due to adenovirus
480.10	Pneumonia due to respiratory syncytial virus
482.20	Pneumonia due to parainfluenza virus
482.30	Pneumonia due to SARS-associated coronavirus
480.80	Viral pneumonia: pneumonia due to other virus not elsewhere classified
480.90	Viral pneumonia unspecified
481.00	Pneumococcal pneumonia (streptococcus pneumoniae pneumonia)
482.00	Pneumonia due to klebsiella
482.10	Pneumonia due to pseudomonas
482.20	Pneumonia due to hemophilus influenza (h. influenza)
482.30	Pneumonia due to streptococcus unspecified
482.31	Pneumonia due to streptococcus group a.
482.32	Pneumonia due to streptococcus group b.
482.39	Pneumonia due to other streptococcus
482.40	Pneumonia due to staphylococcus unspecified
482.41	Pneumonia due to staphylococcus aureus
482.42	Methicillin resistant pneumonia due to Staphylococcus Aureus
482.49	Other Staphylococcus pneumonia
482.81	Pneumonia due to anaerobes
482.82	Pneumonia due to escherichia coli (e. coli)
482.83	Pneumonia due to other gram-negative bacteria
482.84	Pneumonia due to legionnaire's disease
482.89	Pneumonia due to other specified bacteria
482.90	Bacterial pneumonia unspecified
483.00	Pneumonia due to mycoplasma pneumonia
483.10	Pneumonia due to chlamydia
483.80	Pneumonia due to other specified organism
485.00	Bronchopneumonia organism unspecified
486.00	Pneumonia organism unspecified
487.00	Influenza with pneumonia
488.11	Influenza due to identified novel H1N1 influenza virus with pneumonia

3.4.3 Attachment A:
The National Quality Strategy

With a central aim to "increase access to high-quality, affordable health care for all Americans," the ACA required the Secretary of the Department of Health and Human Services (HHS) to establish a National Strategy for Quality Improvement in Health Care. (ACA, Public Law 111–148 and Public Law 111–152). Designated as the National Quality Strategy (NQS), this effort was tasked with setting priorities and developing a strategic plan to improve:

- the delivery of health care services

- patient health outcomes

- population health

In its initial report to Congress on March 21, 2011, the NQS defined its overarching purpose to: "promote quality health care in which the needs of patients, families, and communities guide the actions of all those who deliver and pay for care."

The proposed strategy was to incorporate the evidence-based results of the latest research and scientific advances in clinical medicine, public health, and health care delivery. The desired end result was the creation of a delivery system that would enhance the quality of patient care and work better for clinicians and provider organizations—reducing the administrative burdens and enhancing collaborative efforts to improve care.

The NQS developed three broad aims with input from across the health care system, including federal and state agencies, local communities, provider organizations, clinicians, patients, businesses, employers, and payers. These aims are used to guide and assess local, state, and national efforts to improve health care quality:

- Better Care: Improve overall quality by making health care more patient-centered, reliable, assessable, and safe.

- Healthy People/Healthy Populations: Improve population health by supporting proven interventions to address behavioral, social, and environmental determinants of health, in addition to delivering higher-quality care.

- Affordable Care: Reduce the cost of quality health care for individuals, families, employers, and government.

As part of its 2011 implementation plan, the NQS identified six specific priorities for the development of quantitative goals and measures. Each of these priorities was identified as having the potential for rapidly improving health outcomes and increasing care for all populations:

- making care safer by reducing harm caused in the delivery of care
- ensuring that all patients and their families are engaged as partners in care
- promoting effective communication and coordination of care
- promoting the most effective prevention and treatment practices for the leading causes of mortality, starting with cardiovascular disease
- working with communities to promote wide use of best practices to enable healthy living
- making quality care more affordable for individuals, families, employers, and governments by developing and spreading new health care delivery models

As a coordinating initiative designed to work across supporting federal agencies, the NQS incorporates HHS agency-specific plans, goals, benchmarks, and standardized metrics where available. In addition, the NQS relies on the additional collaboration and participation of private-sector consultants. The Agency for Healthcare Research and Quality (AHRQ) is tasked with supporting and coordinating implementation planning and strategy updates.

3.4.4 Attachment B: Acute Care Inpatient Prospective Payment System (IPPS)

The Inpatient Prospective Payment System (IPPS) is the method by which facilities are reimbursed for inpatient care of Medicare patients. Facilities

218

contract with Medicare to furnish acute hospital inpatient care and agree to accept predetermined acute rates as payment-in-full under IPPS guidelines.

The inpatient hospital benefit covers beneficiaries for ninety days of care per episode of illness with an additional sixty-day lifetime reserve. Illness episodes begin when beneficiaries are admitted and end after they have been out of the hospital or Skilled Nursing Facility (SNF) for sixty consecutive days.

Basis for IPPS

Generally, hospitals receive Medicare IPPS payment on a per-discharge or per-case basis for Medicare beneficiaries with inpatient stays. All outpatient diagnostic services and admission-related outpatient nondiagnostic services provided by the admitting hospital or an entity that is wholly owned or operated by the admitting hospital on the date of a beneficiary's inpatient admission or within three days immediately preceding the date of a beneficiary's inpatient admission must be included on the claim for the beneficiary's inpatient stay and must not be separately billed to Medicare Part B.

Discharges are assigned to diagnosis-related groups (DRG), a classification system that groups similar clinical conditions (diagnoses) and the procedures furnished by the hospital during the stay. The beneficiary's principal diagnosis and up to twenty-four secondary diagnoses that indicate comorbidities and complications will determine the DRG assignment. Similarly, DRG assignment can be affected by up to twenty-five procedures furnished during the stay. The Centers for Medicare & Medicaid Services (CMS) reviews the DRG definitions annually to ensure that each group continues to include cases with clinically similar conditions that require comparable amounts of inpatient resources. When the review shows that subsets of clinically similar cases within a DRG consume significantly different amounts of resources, CMS may assign them to a different DRG with comparable resource use or create a new DRG.

For discharges occurring on or after October 1, 2007, CMS uses a DRG system called Medicare Severity (MS)-DRG to better account for severity of illness and resource consumption for Medicare beneficiaries. Use of MS-DRGs was transitioned during a two-year period. For the period from October 1, 2007, through September 30, 2008, payment was based on a 50/50 blend of MS-DRGs and the previous DRG system. Beginning October 1, 2008 (FY2009) and after, payment is based solely on the MS-DRGs. Three levels of severity exist in the MS-DRGs based on secondary diagnosis codes:

1. major complication/comorbidity, which reflects the highest level of severity

2. complication/comorbidity, which is the next level of severity

3. non-complication/comorbidity, which does not significantly affect severity of illness and resource use

Payment Rates

The IPPS per-discharge payment is based on two national base payment rates or "standardized amounts": one that provides for operating expenses and another that provides for capital expenses. These payment rates are adjusted to account for:

- the costs associated with the beneficiary's clinical condition and related treatment relative to the costs of the average Medicare case (i.e., the DRG relative weight, as described in the "How Payment Rates Are Set" section below)

- market conditions in the facility's location relative to national conditions (i.e., the wage index, as described in the "How Payment Rates Are Set" section below)

In addition to these adjusted per-discharge base payment rates, hospitals can qualify for outlier payments for cases that are extremely costly. Hospitals that train residents in approved Graduate Medical Education (GME) programs also receive a payment separate from the IPPS for the direct costs of training residents. The operating and capital payment rates for these teaching hospitals are increased to reflect the higher indirect patient care costs of teaching hospitals relative to nonteaching hospitals or indirect costs of graduate medical education (Indirect Medical Education: IME).

Operating and capital payment rates are also increased for facilities that treat a disproportionate share of low-income patients. In addition, hospitals may be paid an additional amount for treating patients with certain approved technologies that are new and costly and offer a substantial clinical improvement over existing treatments available to Medicare beneficiaries. Finally, in some cases, payment is reduced when a beneficiary has a short length of stay (LOS) and is transferred to another acute care hospital or, in some circumstances, to a post-acute care setting.

The steps for determining an IPPS payment are as follows:

1. The hospital submits a bill to the Medicare Administrative Contractor (MAC) for each Medicare patient it treats. Based on the information on the bill, the MAC categorizes the case into a DRG.

2. The base payment rate, or standardized amount (a dollar figure), includes a labor-related and Non-labor-related share. The labor-related share is adjusted by a WI to reflect area differences in the cost of labor. If the area WI is greater than 1.0000, the labor share equals 68.8 percent (indicating a "high-wage" area average). The law requires the labor share to equal 62 percent if the area WI is less than or equal to 1.0000 (indicating a "low-wage" market). The non-labor-related share is adjusted by a cost-of-living adjustment (COLA) factor, which equals 1.0000 for all states except Alaska and Hawaii.

3. The wage-adjusted standardized amount is multiplied by a relative weight for the DRG. The relative weight is specific to each of 751 DRGs (for FY2012) and represents the relative average costs associated with one DRG.

4. If applicable, additional amounts will be added to the IPPS payment as follows:

   o payments to hospitals engaged in teaching medical residents to reflect the higher indirect patient care costs of teaching hospitals relative to non-teaching hospitals

   o disproportionate share payments if a hospital treats a disproportionate share of low-income patients

   o additional payment for cases that involve certain approved new technologies

   o additional reimbursement for high-cost outlier cases

CHAPTER 4

Hospital-Acquired Conditions (HAC) Reduction Initiatives

Section 4.1: Flash Read!

Each month, one in seven Medicare patients is injured as a result of the medical care they receive, according to a November 2010 study by the US Department of Health and Human Services (HHS). Hospital-acquired conditions (HACs) not only pose an enormous threat to patient safety, but are also very expensive. Treating the consequences of medical errors cost Medicare $324 million in October 2008 alone, according to the HHS study, accounting for 3.5 percent of all Medicare expenditures for inpatient care. The Affordable Care Act (ACA) legislates new measures that aim to reduce the incidence of these dangerous and costly events.

- To improve patient care quality and reduce costs, the Centers for Medicare & Medicaid Services (CMS) has undertaken initiatives aimed at reducing the occurrence and severity of HACs—conditions or complications a patient develops during a hospital stay that were not present at admission. CMS began addressing the challenge of HACs in

2008 through a payment modification policy. With the passage of the ACA in 2010, CMS was mandated to implement a more aggressive HAC Reduction Program, with penalties being levied on hospitals beginning in FY2015.

- **The safety and financial impact of HACs is significant:**
  - As many as 98,000 Americans die each year as a result of medical errors, with an associated total national cost of up to $29 billion.
  - A 2007 study found that 1.7 million Hospital-Acquired Infections (HAI) were associated with 99,000 deaths in 2002.
  - Annual deaths from HAC categories involving infections alone are twice as high as those from HIV/AIDS and breast cancer combined.
  - Patients suffering from selected HACs are more likely to incur additional expenses due to increased requirements for post-acute care and a more frequent rate of thirty-day readmissions.

- **The ACA's HAC Reduction Program: Overview**
  - Mandated by the ACA, the program uses an evaluation methodology to identify the 25 percent of hospitals with the highest rates (lowest-performing) of specific HACs occurring during a reporting period.
  - The program imposes a 1 percent payment adjustment on all hospital Medicare reimbursements for the 25 percent of hospitals with the highest rates of specific HACS occurring during a reporting period.
  - **Regardless of how few HACs occur during a given reporting year, the lowest-performing 25 percent will continue to receive a 1 percent penalty on all Medicare reimbursements.**
  - Utilizing data from an initial reporting period of July 1, 2011–December 31, 2013, the 1 percent penalty will apply to all Medicare discharges for the lowest-performing 25 percent, beginning on October 1, 2014 (FY2015).

- **HAC Program Scoring Methodology:**
  - Hospitals will be evaluated on HACs divided into two domains. For FY2015, those are:

    Domain 1: 35 percent weighting (reporting period: July 1, 2011– June 30, 2013) comprises the Agency for Healthcare Research and Quality (AHRQ) Patient Safety Indicator Composite (PSI #90):

    - pressure ulcer rate
    - Iatrogenic pneumothorax rate
    - central venous catheter-related bloodstream infection rate
    - postoperative hip fracture rate
    - postoperative pulmonary embolism (PE) or deep vein thrombosis rate (DVT)
    - postoperative sepsis rate
    - wound dehiscence rate
    - accidental puncture and laceration rate

    Domain 2: 65 percent weighting (reporting period: January 1, 2011–December 31, 2013) comprises health care associated infection measures developed by the Centers for Disease Control and Prevention's (CDC) National Health Safety Network (NHSN):

    - central line-associated bloodstream infection (CLABSI)
    - catheter-associated urinary tract infection (CAUTI)

  - CMS will collect data during the twenty-four-month reporting period assigned for each domain.
  - Each metric of a domain will be individually scored to determine a total domain score.
  - This score will be multiplied by the assigned weighting for the domain.
  - The two weighted domain scores will be summed to determine a total HAC Score.
  - Scores for participating hospitals will be ranked by total HAC Scores, from lowest (best) scores to highest (worst) scores.

- o The 25 percent of hospitals with the highest HAC scores will receive a 1 percent reduction in reimbursements for all Medicare discharges for the program fiscal year.

- Commenters on the 2014 Final IPPS Rule expressed concern about certain elements of the initiative they feel unfairly penalize providers:

  - o The potential exists for "double jeopardy" concerning measures contained in multiple value-based initiatives. For example, Central Line-Associated Bloodstream Infections (CLABSI) and Catheter-Associated UTIs (CAUTI), which are included in the HAC Reduction Program as well as the VBP program.

  - o Regardless of how low the incidence of HACs is in an individual hospital and in the aggregate, the program is built on a bell curve, meaning 25 percent of hospitals will always be penalized.

- Unlike the Inpatient Quality Reporting (IQR) program, which imposes a percentage penalty on the Market Basket portion of the annual payment update for a hospital or the Hospital Value-Based Purchasing (HVBP) and the Hospital Readmissions Reduction (HRRP) programs, which apply penalties in the form of a per-discharge adjustment to the base-operating Diagnosis-Related Group (DRG) rate, the HAC Reduction Program's 1 percent penalty is applied to all of an affected hospital's Inpatient Prospective Payment System (IPPS) payments and represents the largest value-based penalty imposed…so far.

- **The HAC Payment Modification Policy:**

  - o The ACA's HAC Reduction Program is not the CMS's first effort to reduce the occurrence of HACs. Beginning in 2008, hospitals paid under the IPPS no longer received a separate "add-on" payment for costs associated with specific HACs, and CMS identified three "never events" for which no reimbursements would be made.

  - o The fiscal impact of CMS's initial efforts to reduce HAC's has been minimal:

    - ▪ Of the total FY2011 discharges of 8.9 million, only .22 percent (19,839) was identified as discharges involving HACs and only .03 percent (3,006) of total discharges resulted in financial consequences for the hospital. **The average penalty was $5,200 per hospital**.

- The program will continue as before, running concurrently with the ACA's HAC Reduction Program. CMS estimates that this program will generate savings of $26 million in FY2014, increasing to $36 million by FY2018.

Section 4.2: Provider Perspectives

Hospitals are in the business of providing health care services and support for those who cannot be treated on an outpatient basis. From surgery to intensive care, hospitals and the health care providers who work in them do their best to improve the health of their patients and work toward positive outcomes. However, during a hospital stay, patients often are exposed to the threat of HACs, unintended injuries, or illnesses that arise during a hospital stay. During the past twenty years, policy makers and agency officials have become much more cognizant of the threat that HACs pose to patient safety and the nation's health care budget. Any number of problems that can slow recovery, prolong a hospital stay, increase costs, or harm patients—including medication errors, falls, pressure sores, infections, wrong-site surgeries, fires, and unsafe practices—are the focus of renewed attention in the ACA. The law includes specific penalties to ensure that providers remain vigilant and do their best to eliminate or reduce the incidence of some of the most common and dangerous HACs.

4.2.1 Rationale

The landmark Institute of Medicine report issued in 1999, "To Err Is Human: Building a Safer Health System," is often credited with precipitating the health care quality movement that exists today. That publication contained the astonishing suggestion that as many as 98,000 Americans died every year from preventable medical errors.[163]

In reality, today's quality movement has its roots in a March 1995 *Boston Globe* exposé that detailed a catastrophic medical error at the prestigious Dana-Farber Cancer Institute. The newspaper's health columnist, Betsy Lehman, who was being treated at the clinic for breast cancer, was given four times the

---

[163] *http://www.iom.edu/Reports/1999/to-err-is-human-building-a-safer-health-system.aspx*

228

proper dose of a chemotherapy drug. She died as a result. The hospital only caught the dosage error months later.

"The reaction within medicine was: If such a preventable error can happen at an institution like Dana-Farber, it can happen anywhere," said Martin J. Hatlie, president of the Partnership for Patient Safety, in *Medical Economics* magazine. "Celebrated failures often spark change, and this, coupled with the wrong-leg amputation case in Florida a few months later, became patient safety's Chernobyl. The Lehman case helped lead to the recognition that medical errors are most often caused by system-wide failures rather than by an individual who goofs."[164]

Numerous hospitals and health care organizations initiated patient safety improvement efforts in the years that followed. The Institute for Healthcare Improvement, the National Patient Safety Foundation, and other groups offered training sessions for managers, hospital executives, and frontline workers. A cottage industry of quality improvement experts took shape, disseminating strategies that worked to diminish errors in hospitals across the United States and abroad. The term "never event" was invented to describe things that absolutely should not happen within a health care setting, with the goal of analyzing and correcting the systemic failures that allowed them to take place.

A significant share of these errors falls under the category of HACs. Infections from hospitalizations added almost $5 billion to US health care costs, the Center for Disease Control and Prevention (CDC) CDC estimated in 2000. In 2009, Medicare issued an estimated $170 million in extra payments to hospitals because of eight specific HACs.

Yet 14 years after the IOM report, patients in US health care facilities run the risk, albeit low, of being harmed though poor practices, errors and over-treatment. Doctors and nurses still do not always comply with the most basic patient safety protocols, such as washing their hands. Though rare, wrong-site surgeries continue to occur. Fires still break out in operating rooms and, in

---

[164] http://medicaleconomics.modernmedicine.com/medical-economics/news/who-caused-tragic-medication-mistake

some situations, doctors are reluctant to adopt best practice protocol checklists.[165]

"The US Congress, government regulators, accreditation agencies, and the public are growing impatient with our lack of overall progress on safety," said James L. Reinertsen, MD. "We haven't done enough, fast enough, in our industry, and we can expect that the payers and regulators are going to turn up the heat."[166]

In 2008, Congress began to take a more aggressive approach to harm-reduction in hospitals by curbing added payments that resulted from HACs. A few years later, it upped the ante by imposing an across-the-board financial penalty against the worst offenders.

By halting payments for preventable harm to patients, Congress intended to eliminate a perverse incentive built into Medicare's fee-for-service reimbursement system: hospitals could bill to treat nosocomial infections. That is, they gained revenue each time a patient had to be treated for a condition that developed as a result of hospitalization. The new payment structures were based on the principle that hospitals would work harder to avoid losses than they would to gain additional revenues.

4.2.2 Summary

The federal government's effort to reduce HACs comprises two laws: In the Deficit Reduction Act of 2005, Congress instructed CMS not to pay additional costs associated with a condition that the patient acquired during the initial hospitalization. Further, CMS would not pay for costs associated with "never events." Called the HAC Payment Modification Policy, these changes were implemented in FY2009 and were taken up by many private insurers.

As part of the 2010 ACA, Congress enacted a more stringent HAC Reduction Program, which goes into effect in FY2015. In short, CMS will identify the worst

---

[165] See Mark R. Chassin, MD, for a roundup of reasons why quality hasn't improved more than it has. "Improving The Quality of Health Care: What's Taking So Long?" Health Affairs, October 2013 32:10. 1761–1765. http://content.healthaffairs.org/content/32/10/1761.full?sid=11b2a8cc-c2f0-4953-9986-0cb910187999

[166] An interview with James L. Reinertsen, MD, The Joint Commission Journal on Quality and Patient Safety, May 2011, Vol. 37, No. 5

quartile of hospitals for HACs and deduct 1 percent from their total Medicare reimbursements. Data are submitted through the IQR Program. The twenty-four-month data collection period for the initial 2015 penalty year ended on December 31, 2013.

The government established the baseline rate of frequency for HACs at 145 per thousand admissions. The goal was set at a 40 percent reduction in preventable HACs by the end of FY2014, which was estimated to avoid 1.8 million patient injuries and 60,000 deaths. Reducing the number of hospital-related infections—the most frequently encountered HACs—is the No. 1 priority.

4.2.3 Current State

Predictions that the savings from the Payment Modification Policy would be minimal have been borne out. In FY2011, Medicare saved $19.4 million, mostly from two categories: falls and trauma, and PE and DVT after orthopedic surgery. Savings from FY2014 through FY2018 are estimated to fall between $26 million and $36 million per year.

Medicare administrators believe the program has been worthwhile insofar as it has focused the attention of providers on changing behaviors and policies within the hospital. "Our efforts in using payment adjustments and our measurement authority will encourage hospitals to eliminate the incidence of HACs that could be reasonably prevented by applying evidence-based guidelines," CMS wrote in the FY2014 IPPS Final Rule.[167]

Certain organizations that have made a priority of harm reduction have shown that it can be done. Cincinnati Children's Hospital, for example, reduced its infection rate by 80 percent in three years, and is now heading toward zero. Dignity Health, a Catholic system in California, achieved a 52 percent reduction in surgical site infections, a 53 percent reduction in ventilator-associated pneumonia (VAP), and a 70 percent reduction in CLABSI.[168]

---

[167] CMS IPPS Final Rule Home Page, http://www.cms.gov/Medicare/Medicare-Fee-for-Service-Payment/AcuteInpatientPPS/FY2014-IPPS-Final-Rule-Home-Page.html

[168] Agency for Healthcare Research and Quality, 2013 Annual Progress Report to Congress, National Strategy for Quality Improvement in Health Care. www.ahrq.gov/workingforquality/reports.htm

WellStar, a five-hospital system in Atlanta, achieved a 78 percent reduction in safety events. It nearly eliminated Clostridium Difficile (CDI) infections, CLABSI, and VAP. It pushed overall mortality down 23 percent.[169] A project conducted in ICUs in Michigan reduced the median infection rate per thousand catheter-days from 2.7 percent at baseline to zero after interventions that included washing hands, using full-barrier precautions with central-line placement, cleaning the skin with chlorhexidine, avoiding the femoral site if possible, and removing unnecessary catheters.[170]

Yet a comprehensive national study of the effect of the first CMS initiative found "no evidence" that the 2008 policy reducing payments for CLABSI and catheter-associated urinary tract infections (CAUTI) "had any measurable effect on infection rates in US hospitals." The paper's authors commented that the lack of effect may have resulted from the changes in billing practices (the data were derived from billing codes) or the "very small financial incentives at stake"—less than 1 percent of Medicare revenue for the average hospital. The authors went on to cast a skeptical eye on the entire notion of pay-for-performance programs: "The evidence that they improve patient outcomes, either in primary care settings or hospital settings, is mixed... The empirical evidence that financial disincentives improve the quality of care is also limited."[171]

Hospitals attempting to take on these challenges face two main difficulties, said Eric Fontana, practice manager of the data and analytics group at The Advisory Board in Washington, DC. First, there is the culture of the organization and the need for "strong leadership to map out a well-delineated plan for the vision of their organization and how they're going to get there."

Second, hospitals need to adopt and enforce more evidence-based guidelines in practice. Peter Pronovost, MD, and colleagues have shown that if physicians and nurses use a checklist and "do the same thing every time to a predefined

---

[169] An interview with James L. Reinertsen, MD, The Joint Commission Journal on Quality and Patient Safety, May 2011, Vol. 37, No. 5

[170] Peter Pronovost, MD, Dale Needham, MD, et al., "An Intervention to Decrease Catheter-Related Bloodstream Infections in the ICU," New England Journal of Medicine 2006; 355:2725–2732. December 28, 2006. http://www.nejm.org/doi/full/10.1056/NEJMoa061115

[171] Grace M. Lee, MD, Ken Kleinman, et al., "Effect of Nonpayment for Preventable Infections in US Hospitals," New England Journal of Medicine 2012; 367:15 October 11, 2012. www.nejm.org/doi/full/10.1056/NEJMsa1202419

standard—hands are washed, drapes and alcohol used appropriately," central line infections can be avoided, Fontana said.

"Continual vigilance has to be applied to maintain high standards with infections. Each hospital will have [its] own particular challenges," he added. "Hospitals that don't do a lot of surgeries won't have problems with perioperative infections, but they might have trouble with falls and pressure ulcers. I think that's why CMS has written a broad array of measures that apply to many organizations."[172]

There is, of course, much debate, even within the health care quality community, about the direction CMS has taken and the likelihood that the goals will be met. Reinertsen, who has worked for many years with hospital boards and executives to orient organizational culture toward patient safety, is skeptical of the government's approach to value-based purchasing, another arm of the pay-for-performance regimen. Once the whole industry has raised its game, he suggested, the comparative basis of the rankings will be less and less useful for driving further improvement. With HACs, on the other hand, "Anybody can see themselves in that particular effort," he said. "The goal is zero. It has much more clinical meaningfulness than comparing yourself in decile rankings to any other hospital."

Many hospitals get tangled up in how well they compare to their rivals or peer group. It's not always a productive endeavor, Reinertsen argued. "Let's just cut the harm events in half year after year, until they approach zero. Then that hospital would blow past the rest of the field."[173]

Where HACs are concerned, hospitals are sometimes victims of their own low expectations. They don't think they can successfully reduce or eliminate them. Increasingly, that is proving to be wrong. "For years people assumed that if you went into an ICU and got a breathing tube, you had a 10 percent to 15 percent chance of getting ventilator-associated pneumonia. And you did," Reinertsen said. "Now, I know hospitals that have gone four or five years without getting one."

Progress is being held back by two fundamentally wrong approaches, he thinks. First, including quality assurance goals in executive compensation contracts virtually guarantees that the goals will be "some namby-pamby

---

[172] Eric Fontana, telephone interview, November 27, 2013

[173] James L. Reinertsen, MD, telephone interview, November 23, 2013

amount"—in other words, nothing that would threaten the payout of the executive bonus if not met. This just dilutes the organization's willpower to address the issue.

Second, boards of directors have not asserted ownership of the problem. Often they are given clouded versions of the quality statistics in their institutions or meaningless comparisons with neighboring hospitals, which effectively cover up the real number of patients harmed in the most recent reporting period. "They get lulled into this, 'Well, we must be good, because our numbers are good compared to others. We're in the 70th percentile of the database.' Instead they should be asking 'How much harm did we have in our system last year?'" Reinertsen argued.

4.2.4 The Road Ahead

For the HAC Reduction Program that goes into effect in FY2015, CMS will compute HAC scores in two domains. The first domain is an AHRQ patient safety indicator composite (PSI-90) of eight different measures. The second domain consists of selected HACs. In the first year, these will be CLABSI and CAUTI. In FY2016, surgical site infections (SSI) for colon surgery and abdominal hysterectomy will be added. In FY2017, the list will expand to include methicillin-resistant staphylococcus aureus (MRSA) and CDI infections.

The HAC Payment Modification Policy continues as before. Even though the impact of this program is very small, both for CMS and for hospitals, more than revenue is at stake; there is also the added cost of care. A hospital-acquired infection can add anywhere from $30,000 to $150,000 in cost to the case.

It's hard to say whether these programs will be successful, either from the standpoint of the individual hospitals or Medicare, according to Fontana. "We don't have much data," he said. If one looks at the thirty-day readmission penalty program, it's clear that readmissions are starting to come down. Whether that can be attributed to the CMS penalty program is another question. When the first HAC Payment Modification Policy was rolled out "we thought it was going to be dramatic," Fontana said. "In the end it was negligible overall."

Where the Medicare HAC initiatives are going to be felt most strongly are among safety-net hospitals—those with disproportionately higher shares of indigent or minority or uninsured patients, known as Disproportionate Share Hospitals (DSH). CMS has presented some data indicating that a large portion of those receiving penalties would be DSH hospitals, Fontana said. This aligns with reports that DSH hospitals are paying the highest penalties for excessive readmissions and a prediction that they will do worse on value-based purchasing.[174] The reasons for these discrepancies are not yet fully understood.

It's hard to find hospital executives, quality experts, or practitioners who are enthusiastic supporters of the HAC program as conceived. "If you speak to a lot of physicians, purely anecdotally, a lot of folks agree with the premise but not as much with the methodology," Fontana said. He declined to offer an opinion on whether the measures were realistic or of value to providers and patients. "While it's here and being applied and written into law, it's something we have to deal with as an industry," he answered. "Whether we have to deal with these in the future is unknown. They might refine the approaches to measurement."

Even though many of the pay-for-performance demonstration projects have shown "modest or inconsistent effectiveness in improving quality," financial incentives for quality assurance are not likely to go away, wrote Arnold M. Epstein, MD, of the Harvard School of Public Health, in 2012. Pay for performance still has "enormous face validity and ideological support even if success to date has been modest and the optimal program configuration is unclear."[175]

That doesn't offer much solace for the practitioners in America's clinics and hospitals. As Mark Chassin, MD, CEO of The Joint Commission, wrote: "Health care must and can do better… The critics are right. It's not rocket science. It's much more difficult."[176]

---

[174] Ashish Jha, MD, "An Update on Value-Based Purchasing: Year 2," November 19, 2013, posted at https://blogs.sph.harvard.edu/ashish-jha/an-update-on-value-based-purchasing-year-2/

[175] Arnold M. Epstein, MD, "Will Pay for Performance Improve Quality of Care? The Answer Is in the Details," New England Journal of Medicine, 367:19. November 8, 2012. http://www.nejm.org/doi/full/10.1056/NEJMe1212133

[176] Mark R. Chassin, MD, "Improving The Quality of Health Care: What's Taking So Long?" Health Affairs, October 2013 32:10. 1761–1765. http://content.healthaffairs.org/content/32/10/1761.full?sid=11b2a8cc-c2f0-4953-9986-0cb910187999

Section 4.3: Technical Appendix: Hospital-Acquired Conditions (HAC) Reduction Initiatives

Hospital-Acquired Condition (HAC): A medical condition or complication that a patient develops during a hospital stay, which was not present at admission.

Section 2702(b) of the ACA further defines the term "health care-acquired condition" as "a medical condition for which an individual was diagnosed that could be identified by a secondary diagnostic code described in section 1886(d)(4)(D)(iv) of the Act."

4.3.1 Overview

The incidence and frequency of HACs results in significant morbidity, mortality, and an increased financial burden across the health care system:

- The Institute of Medicine's (IOM) 1999 landmark report on medical errors, "To Err is Human: Building a Safer Health System," found that medical errors, particularly largely preventable HACs, were a leading cause of morbidity and mortality in the United States. The report noted:

  o As many as 98,000 Americans die each year as a result of medical errors.

  o The cost burden of HACs is also high. Total national costs of these errors due to lost productivity, disability, and health care costs were estimated at $17 to $29 billion.[177]

---

[177] Kohn, L. T., Corrigan, J. M., Donaldson, M. S. (Institute of Medicine), "To Err is Human: Building a Safer Health System." Washington, DC: National Academy Press, 2000. http://www.iom.edu/Reports/1999/to-err-is-human-building-a-safer-health-system.aspx

- In 2000, the CDC estimated that hospital-acquired infections (HAIs) alone added nearly $5 billion to US health care costs every year.[178]

- A 2007 study found that, in 2002, 1.7 million HAIs were associated with 99,000 deaths.[179]

- In April 2012, RTI International (a Medicare contractor providing data analytic services) reported that Medicare, in FY2009, paid an estimated additional $170 million in Part A (in-hospital) charges as a result of eight identified HACs.[180]

- The financial impact of HACs is not restricted solely to the admission during which they occur. In its September 2012 report to Medicare (evaluating FY2009 and the first ten months of FY2010), RTI International found that patients incurring selected HACs were more likely to incur additional expenses due to increased requirements for post-acute care and a more frequent rate of thirty-day readmissions.[181]

  o For each of three commonly encountered HACs, (falls and trauma, vascular catheter-associated infections, and pulmonary embolisms/DVT following certain orthopedic procedures), which comprised more than 80 percent of restated Medicare Severity (MS) DRG charges, the likelihood of readmission for patients incurring HACs was greater than the comparison group for patients discharged to post-acute care *and* to home.

  o Significantly more HAC patients were discharged to post-acute care for each of the selected conditions than the comparison group.

  o Medicare costs are higher for patients sustaining HACs in both the inpatient and outpatient setting. In addition, beneficiaries

---

[178] *www.cms.hhs.gov/AcuteInpatientPPS/downloads/CMS-1390-F.pdf*

[179] *Klevens et al. Estimating Health Care-Associated Infections and Deaths in US Hospitals, 2002. Public Health Reports. March–April 2007. Volume 122.*

[180] *April 18, 2012 Analysis Report: Estimating the Incremental Costs of Hospital-Acquired Conditions (HACs) http://www.cms.gov/Medicare/Medicare-Fee-for-Service-Payment/HospitalAcqCond/index.html?redirect=/HospitalAcqCond*

[181] *Readmissions Due to Hospital-Acquired Conditions (HACs): Multivariate Modeling and Under-coding Analyses [PDF, 662KB] http://www.cms.gov/Medicare/Medicare-Fee-for-Service-Payment/HospitalAcqCond/Downloads/Final-Report-Readmissions.pdf*

experiencing HACs face increased costs in the form of additional coinsurance and deductibles.

Relationship between discharge to a post-acute care (PAC) setting and the likelihood of readmission for beneficiaries in the hospital-acquired condition and comparison groups

Hospital-acquired condition	Likelihood of readmission: HAC group	Likelihood of readmission: Comparison group
Falls and trauma		
Discharged to PAC setting	23.7%	19.8%
Not discharged to PAC	19.7%	14.5%
Vascular catheter-associated infection		
Discharged to PAC setting	32.0%	30.0%
Not discharged to PAC	28.0%	16.6%
DVT/PE following certain orthopedic procedures		
Discharged to PAC setting	12.8%	9.8%
Not discharged to PAC	6.8%	5.2%

NOTES: HAC = Hospital-acquired condition; PAC = Post-acute care; DVT/PE = Deep vein thrombosis or pulmonary embolism

**indicates statistically significant difference using negative binomial regression with $p<0.01$.

Source: September 2012 RTI Final Report, Readmissions Due to Hospital-Acquired Conditions (HACs) Multivariate Modeling and Under-coding Analyses

Discharge destination for selected hospital-acquired conditions

Hospital-acquired condition	HAC group	Comparison group	Difference
Falls and trauma			
Discharged to PAC setting	76.9%	57.4%	19.5%**
Discharged home	13.7%	33.7%	-20.0%**
Other	9.4%	8.9%	0.5%
Vascular catheter-associated infection			
Discharged to PAC setting	67.9%	53.2%	14.7%**
Discharged home	25.0%	24.9%	0.1%
Other	7.1%	21.9%	-14.8%**
DVT/PE following certain orthopedic procedures			
Discharged to PAC setting	88.0%	81.8%	6.2%**
Discharge home	8.5%	13.9%	-5.4%**
Other	3.5%	4.3%	-0.8%**

NOTES: HAC = Hospital-acquired condition; PAC = Post-acute care; DVT/PE = Deep vein thrombosis or pulmonary embolism

**indicates statistically significant difference using negative binomial regression with $p<0.01$.

Source: September 2012 RTI Final Report, Readmissions Due to Hospital-Acquired Conditions (HACs) Multivariate Modeling and Under-coding Analyses

238

- A 2012 study by McNair and Luft estimated that Medicare could recoup an additional $103 million in payments if the HAC Payment Modification policy was applied to HAC-related readmissions.[182]

- For beneficiaries, HAC-related incremental liabilities associated with extended hospitalization stays, readmissions, and increased utilization of skilled nursing facilities totaled an estimated $19 million in coinsurance and additional deductible costs.[183]

Overview Summary:

HACs can result in:

- overall increases in patient morbidity and mortality

- increased costs to the hospitals that provide care where such events occur, to third parties who pay for care, and to patients themselves

- subsequent health care encounters that might not have been necessary or might not have been as resource-intensive, if that patient did not incur a HAC

- a greater net burden on quality and efficiency across the health care environment

4.3.2 CMS "Two-Part" Strategy

1. The Hospital-Acquired Conditions Payment Modification Policy
   FY2009–Present

2. The Hospital-Acquired Conditions Reduction Program
   FY2015

To address the dangers and costs associated with HACs, Medicare first implemented a Hospital-Acquired Conditions Payment Modification Policy in

---

[182] *McNair, P. D., & Luft, H. S.: Enhancing Medicare's hospital-acquired conditions policy to encompass readmissions. Medicare Care & Medicaid Res. Rev. 2012; 2(2), E1-E15.*

[183] *Readmissions Due to Hospital-Acquired Conditions (HACs): Multivariate Modeling and Timing of Clinical Presentation Analysis http://www.cms.gov/Medicare/Medicare-Fee-for-Service-Payment/HospitalAcqCond/index.html*

2008. The program, which prohibits Medicare from paying for the additional cost of treating a HAC, was part of an array of Medicare value-based reimbursement initiatives that CMS currently uses to promote increased quality and efficiency of care. This payment modification policy was among the first of such initiatives, through which the Medicare program seeks to tie payment to performance and transform Medicare from a passive payer to an active purchaser of higher-value health services.

In 2015, CMS will further enhance HAC-reduction efforts through the implementation of the Hospital-Acquired Conditions Reductions Program, an initiative mandated by the ACA of 2010. The program imposes a 1 percent payment adjustment on all hospital Medicare reimbursements for the 25 percent of hospitals with the highest rates of specific HACS during a reporting period.

Through the combination of individual discharge payment reductions and the potential for a global Medicare payment penalty, CMS expects to further reduce the incidence of potentially preventable HACs, decrease excess costs, and improve patient care.

4.3.3 Hospital-Acquired Conditions Payment Modification Policy

Background

With the signing of the Deficit Reduction Act (DRA) of 2005 by President Bush on February 8, 2006, CMS was required to implement a hospital payment modification system aimed at reducing the incidence of HACs. The initial effort was contained in DRA Section 5001(c) (QUALITY ADJUSTMENT IN DRG PAYMENTS FOR CERTAIN HOSPITAL-ACQUIRED INFECTIONS). With this measure, CMS sought to improve patient care quality and end a reimbursement policy through which hospitals could actually recoup financial returns as a result of complications.[184]

Under this directive, by October 1, 2007, the secretary of the US Department of Health and Human Services (HHS) was required to select ICD-9 CM

---

[184] DRA 2005 Sec.5001(c) *www.gpo.gov/fdsys/pkg/PLAW-109publ171/.../PLAW-109publ171.htm*

diagnosis codes associated with at least two conditions, each of which met all of the following requirements (as determined by the secretary):

- Cases described by such codes had high cost or high volume, or both.

- The code resulted in the assignment of a case to a DRG that had a higher payment when the code was present as a secondary diagnosis.

- The code described such conditions that could reasonably have been prevented through the application of evidence-based guidelines.

The secretary was given the flexibility to revise (through addition or deletion of codes) the diagnosis codes over time so long as there were diagnosis codes associated with at least two conditions selected for discharges during any fiscal year. In selecting and revising diagnosis codes, the secretary was directed to consult with the CDC and other appropriate entities. An initial listing of eight potentially preventable conditions for FY2008 was developed and has since been revised to include eleven HAC conditions for FY2013.

Section 5001(c) further specified:

- For discharges occurring on or after October 1, 2008, the DRG to be assigned for a discharge shall be a DRG that does *not* result in higher payment based on the presence of a secondary diagnosis code, not included upon admission.

- The discharge includes a condition identified by a diagnosis code selected as a secondary diagnosis for a condition that was not present upon admission.

- Absent provisions of this amendment, the discharge would have been classified as a DRG that results in a *higher* payment based on the presence of a secondary diagnosis code selected.

For the specified HACs, the DRA mandated that for discharges occurring on or after October 1, 2008, the acquisition of one or more of these preventable conditions during a hospital stay could *not* lead to the patient being assigned to a higher-paying DRG. As such, Medicare would no longer reimburse hospitals paid under the IPPS for a separate "add-on" payment that had been previously allowed when such conditions were acquired during the course of a hospital stay.

- This provision will only apply when one or more of the selected conditions are the only secondary diagnosis or diagnoses present on the claim that will lead to higher payment.

- Because Medicare beneficiaries will generally have multiple secondary diagnoses during a hospital stay, beneficiaries having a major complication or comorbidity (MCC) or complication and comorbidity (CC) will frequently have additional conditions that also will generate higher payment.

- Thus, only a small percentage of the cases will have *only* one secondary diagnosis that would lead to a higher payment. Therefore, if at least one nonselected secondary diagnosis that leads to higher payment is on the claim, the case will continue to be assigned to the higher-paying MS-DRG and hospitals will not incur financial penalties.[185]

Inclusion of "Never Events"

In addition to the mandated development of HACs categories, CMS also adopted a limited listing of "never events" for payment modification evaluation:

- Ken Kizer, MD, former CEO of the National Quality Forum (NQF), first introduced the term "never event" in 2001 to describe particularly shocking medical errors that should never occur.[186]

- In 2002, the NQF published "Serious Reportable Events in Healthcare: A Consensus Report," which listed twenty-seven adverse events that were "serious, largely preventable and of concern to both the public and health care providers." These events and subsequent revisions to the list became known as "never events."

- The NQF's "Consensus Standards Maintenance Committee on Serious Reportable Events" maintains and updates the list, which currently contains twenty-nine items.

---

[185] *53734 Federal Register/Vol. 77, No. 170/Friday, August 31, 2012/Rules and Regulations www.gpo.gov/fdsys/pkg/FR-2013-08-30/pdf/FR-2013-08-30.pdf*

[186] *http://psnet.ahrq.gov/primer.aspx?primerID=3*

- This list of "Never Events" includes adverse events that are clearly definable, measureable, serious, and usually preventable. For 2013, the list includes twenty-nine events grouped into seven categories: surgical, product or device; patient protection; care management; environmental; radiologic; and criminal.

- "Never events" rarely occur, as illustrated in a 2006 study by Kwaan et al. that estimated the average hospital might experience one wrong-site surgery every five to ten years.[187]

- However seldom they are, such events are devastating to patients—71 percent of such events reported to the Joint Commission during the past twelve years were fatal.[188]

- In 2008, as part of the HAC Payment Modification initiative introduction, CMS identified three "never events" for which no reimbursements would be made. These conditions are identified by the issuance of three National Coverage Determinations (NCDs), under which CMS does not provide reimbursement for a particular surgical or other invasive procedure to treat a specified medical condition when the practitioner erroneously performs:

  1. a different procedure altogether

  2. the correct procedure but on the wrong body part

  3. the correct procedure but on the wrong patient

  - Medicare also will not cover hospitalizations and other services related to these non-covered procedures.

  - Payment prohibition for services related to these conditions extends to state Medicaid programs, mandated by CMS Final Rule, June 6, 2011.[189]

The full listing of 2013 "never events" may be viewed at: http://psnet.ahrq.gov/primer.aspx?primerID=3

---

[187] Kwaan, M.R., Studdert, D.M., Zinner, M.J., Gawande, A.A. "Incidence, Patterns, and Prevention of Wrong-Site Surgery." Arch Surg. 2006; 141:353–358

[188] http://psnet.ahrq.gov/primer.aspx?primerID=3

[189] Federal Register/Vol. 76, No. 108/Monday, June 6, 2011/Rules and Regulations page 32817 www.copyright.gov/fedreg/2011/76fr32316.pdf

Expansion of HAC Payment Modification Policy to State Medicaid Programs

- The CMS HACs Payment Modification Policy was extended to state Medicaid programs effective in July 2012, with the mandated implementation of Section 2702 of the ACA. This section directed the HHS secretary to issue Medicaid regulations effective as of July 1, 2011, prohibiting federal payments to states under Section 1903 of the Social Security Act for any amounts expended for providing medical assistance for HACs.[190]

  - Provisions of Final Rule, published on June 6, 2011:

    - CMS delayed the Medicaid implementation of the HAC initiative until June 2012.

    - States were given the authority to determine the extent to which they paid for Provider Preventable Conditions (PPCs) through amendments to state Medicaid plans.

    - As specified in the Final Rule: "A State plan must provide that no medical assistance will be paid for 'provider-preventable conditions' as defined in this section; and as applicable for beneficiaries dually eligible for Medicare and Medicaid services." As a minimum, States were directed to adopt Medicare's three NCD "never events" (see below):

      - Provider Preventable Condition (PPC): an "umbrella" term for hospital and nonhospital-acquired conditions identified by the state for nonpayment. PPCs are clearly divided into two separate categories:

        - Health Care-Acquired Conditions (HCACs): conditions identified as Medicare's HACs (with the exception of DVT/PE following total knee replacement or hip replacement in pediatric and obstetric patients) for IPPS purposes, applied broadly to Medicaid inpatient hospitals.

---

[190] *Federal Register/Vol. 76, No. 108/Monday, June 6, 2011/Rules and Regulations www.copyright.gov/fedreg/2011/76fr32316.pdf*

       ○ Other Provider Preventable Conditions (OPPCs): conditions that are applicable in any health care service setting apply as required under the statute. OPPCs would be applicable to other conditions that states identify and have approved through their Medicaid state plans. OPPCs are *minimally* defined as Medicare's three NCD events: surgery on the wrong patient, wrong surgery on a patient, and wrong-site surgery.

Commercial Adoption of Similar HAC Payment Policies:

Many commercial payers—including Aetna, CIGNA health care, Anthem Blue Cross Blue Shield of New Hampshire, Blue Cross and Blue Shield of Massachusetts, United Healthcare, WellPoint, and other private insurers—have adopted similar payment provisions for reasonably preventable health conditions.[191]

FY2013 HAC Categories:

Under the authority given the HHS secretary under provisions of Section 5001(c) of the DRA, the list of HACs may be modified over time. The current FY2013 list contains eleven HAC categories, as follows:[192]

1. foreign object retained after surgery
2. air embolism
3. blood incompatibility
4. Stage III and IV pressure ulcers
5. falls and trauma:
    a. fractures
    b. dislocations

---

[191] http://www.cms.gov/Medicare/Medicare-Fee-for-Service-Payment/HospitalAcqCond/Downloads/HAC-SpilloverEffects.pdf

[192] Federal Register/Vol. 78, No. 160/Monday, August 19, 2013/Rules and Regulations www.gpo.gov/fdsys/pkg/FR-2013-08-19/pdf/2013-18956.pdf

c. intracranial injuries

d. crushing injuries

e. burn

f. other injuries

6. manifestations of poor glycemic control :

   a. diabetic ketoacidosis

   b. nonketotic hyperosmolar coma

   c. hypoglycemic coma

   d. secondary diabetes with ketoacidosis

   e. secondary diabetes with hyperosmolarity

7. catheter-associated urinary tract infection (CAUTI)

8. vascular catheter-associated infection

9. surgical site infections:

   a. mediastinitis, following coronary artery bypass graft (CABG):

   b. surgical site infection following bariatric surgery for obesity

   c. laparoscopic gastric bypass

   d. gastroenterostomy

   e. laparoscopic gastric restrictive surgery

   f. surgical site infection following certain orthopedic procedures:

   - spine

   - neck

   - shoulder

   - elbow

   g. surgical site infection following:

   - cardiac implantable electronic device (CIED)

10. deep vein thrombosis (DVT)/pulmonary embolism (PE) following certain orthopedic procedures:

   a. total knee replacement

   b. hip replacement

11. Iatrogenic pneumothorax with venous catheterization

FY2014 HAC Categories:

In the FY2014 IPPS/LTCH PPS proposed rule (78 FR 27511), CMS did not propose to add or remove categories of HACs and the final FY2013 HAC list will be used to determine payment modifications for FY2014.

Present on Admission (POA) Reporting Requirement:

This companion reporting requirement was implemented along with the Medicare HAC Payment Modification policy to more accurately capture the presence or absence of HACs as part of the hospital admissions process:

- Section 5001(c) of the DRA requires providers paid under the inpatient prospective payment system (IPPS) to code Present on Admission (POA) indicators on all ICD-9-CM diagnoses for all claims submitted, beginning October 1, 2007.

- There are five POA indicator reporting options, as defined by the ICD-9-CM Official Coding Guidelines:

POA	DESCRIPTOR
Y	Indicates that the condition was present on admission.
W	Affirms that the provider has determined, based on data and clinical judgment, that it is not possible to document when the onset of the condition occurred.
N	Indicates that the condition was not present on admission.
U	Indicates that the documentation is insufficient to determine if the condition was present at the time of admission.
1	Signifies exemption from POA reporting. CMS established this code as a workaround to blank reporting on the electronic 4010A1. A list of exempt ICD-9-CM diagnosis codes is available in the ICD-9-CM Official Coding Guidelines.

  - Under HAC policy, CMS treats HACs coded with "Y" and "W" indicators as POA and allows the condition on its own to cause an increased payment.

247

> o HACs coded with "N" and "U" indicators are classified by CMS as NPOA and will not allow the condition on its own to cause an increased payment.

- This requirement provides a method to record the presence of conditions included on the HAC list upon admission to avoid discharge payment modification.

- POA indicator reporting requirement only applies to IPPS-reimbursed hospitals.

- Non-Inpatient Prospective Payment System hospitals are exempt from POA reporting requirements and the HACs Payment Modification policy. This includes:

  - o long-term care hospitals (LTCHs)
  - o Maryland waiver hospitals*
  - o cancer hospitals
  - o children's inpatient facilities
  - o rural health clinics
  - o federally qualified health centers (FQHCs)
  - o religious non-medical health care institutions
  - o inpatient psychiatric hospitals
  - o inpatient rehabilitation facilities (IRFs)
  - o Veterans Administration/Department of Defense hospitals.

*Hospitals in Maryland operating under waivers are not subject to the HAC payment modification provisions (as long as they are not paid under the IPPS). However, in the FY2014 IPPS Final Rule, CMS will require hospitals in Maryland currently paid under section 1814(b)(3) to report the POA indicator on their claims beginning with discharges on October 1, 2013.

HAC Frequency of Occurrence and Financial Impact:

HAC Frequency of Occurrence FY2011:

- In a study involving selected HACs in California conducted by McNair and Luft in 2009, the authors predicted that payment reductions under the HAC Payment Modification program would be "negligible" and "unlikely to promote measurable quality improvements."[193]

- An analysis of the FY2011 Medicare's HAC Payment Modification program by Medicare analytics contractor RTI reveals the following:[194]
  - For FY2011, there were more than 8.9 million Medicare IPPS hospital discharges with an average of ten listed secondary conditions per discharge.

  - Of total secondary conditions, 5.9 million (6.7 percent) were classified as "N" or "U" (HACs not present on admission) and were subject to evaluation for payment modification.

Table 1: POA Code Distribution Across All Secondary Diagnoses

		Number	Percentage
Total Discharges in Final File		8,941,507	
Total Number of Secondary Diagnoses Across Total Discharges		89,252,194	100.00
POA	Indicator Description		
Y	Condition present on admission	69,231,189	77.57
W	Status cannot be clinically determined	21,796	0.02
N	Condition not present on admission	5,748,769	6.44
U	Documentation not adequate to determine if condition was present on admission	207,258	0.23
1	Exempted ICD–9–CM code	14,043,182	15.73

Source: RTI Analysis of MedPAR IPPS Claims, October 2010 through September 2011.

- Of total FY2011 Medicare discharges, 287,993 discharges had a HAC as a secondary diagnosis.

- Of these 287,993 discharges, 19,839 were identified as a HAC and 3,006 MS-DRGs were changed due to HACs.

- Of total FY2011 discharges of 8.9 million, only .22 percent (19,839) was identified as discharges involving HACs and .03 percent (3,006) of total discharges had MS-DRG reimbursement restated.

---

[193] hlthaff.28.5.1485 Health Aff September/October 2009 vol. 28, no. 5, 1485–1493

[194] Federal Register/Vol. 78, No. 160/Monday, August 19, 2013/Rules and Regulations/Pages 53293-53296, www.gpo.gov/fdsys/pkg/FR-2013-08-19/pdf/2013-18956.pdf

- 78 percent of restated MS-DRGs occurred as the result of just two HACs:

  o falls and trauma: 1,259 cases requiring MS-DRG restatement

  o PE and DVT orthopedic: 1,082 cases requiring MS-DRG restatement

- No cases involving crushing injuries or electric shock required MS-DRG restatement and only one case involving blood incompatibility required MS-DRG restatement.

Table 2: FY2011 Discharge Frequencies of Current CMS HACs

CHART C—DISCHARGE FREQUENCIES OF CURRENT CMS HACS OCTOBER 2010 THROUGH SEPTEMBER 2011

Selected HAC category	Discharges with this condition as secondary diagnosis		Discharges Identified as a HAC		Discharges that change MS–DRG due to HAC	
	Number (column A)	Percent[2] (column B)	Number (column C)	Percent[3] (column D)	Number (column E)	Percent[4] (column F)
1. Foreign Object Retained After Surgery	606	0.01	284	46.86	37	13.03
2. Air Embolism	45	0.00	34	75.56	14	41.18
3. Blood Incompatibility	22	0.00	11	50.00	1	9.09
4. Pressure Ulcer Stages III & IV	96,646	1.08	1,770	1.83	286	16.16
5. Falls and Trauma	147,684	1.65	4,596	3.11	1,259	27.39
a. Fracture	128,065	1.43	3,829	2.99	996	26.01
b. Dislocation	1,014	0.01	22	2.17	2	9.09
c. Intracranial Injury	15,478	0.17	694	4.48	258	37.18
d. Crushing Injury	55	0.00	1	1.82	0	0.00
e. Burn	2,147	0.02	42	1.96	3	7.14
f. Electric Shock	925	0.01	8	0.86	0	0.00
Less: Discharges with multiple Falls & Trauma	3,764	0.04	41	1.09	18	43.90
5. Falls & Trauma: Unduplicated Total	143,920	1.61	4,555	3.16	1,241	27.24
6. Catheter-Associated UTI	16,807	0.19	3,918	23.31	160	4.08
7. Vascular Catheter-Associated Infection	11,324	0.13	5,921	52.29	20	0.34
8. Poor Glycemic Control	15,145	0.17	555	3.66	152	27.39
9a. SSI Mediastinitis CABG	58	0.07	50	86.21	5	10.00
9b. SSI Orthopedic	351	0.31	244	69.52	6	2.44
9c. SSI Bariatric	25	0.19	24	96.00	2	8.33
10. Pulmonary Embolism & DVT Orthopedic	3,044	0.76	2,473	81.24	1,082	43.75
Total [1]	287,993	3.22	19,839	6.54	3,006	15.96

[1] Discharges can appear in more than one row. The total figure is not adjusted for the 207 discharges with more than one HAC that appear as secondary diagnoses (15 of these resulted in MS–DRG reassignment).
[2] Percent computed relative to total discharges "at risk" for this HAC. For HACs 1–8, this is 8,941,507. For HAC 9a, this is 77,744. For HAC 9b, this is 112,951. For HAC 9c, this is 13,404. For HAC 10, this is 401,246.
[3] Percent computed relative to discharges with condition as a secondary diagnosis.
[4] Percent computed relative to discharges with this HAC (Column C).
Source: RTI Analysis of MedPAR IPPS Claims, October 2010 through September 2011.

- The DRG category rarely changes either because:

  o the discharge was already grouped to a simple DRG (rather than a DRG "with complications and comorbidities")

  o the HAC was not the only condition or complication converting the discharge from a simple DRG to one "with complications and comorbidities." The 2009 Medicare IPPS Final Rule CMS specified:

- ▪ "However, if any nonselected CC/MCC appears on the claim, the claim will be paid at the higher MS-DRG rate.

- ▪ "To cause a lower MS-DRG payment, all CCs/MCCs (complications, comorbidities/major complications, comorbidities) on the claim must be selected conditions for the HAC payment provision.

- ▪ Given the example above for FY2011, each discharge has an average of ten secondary conditions, any of which may cause a discharge to be reimbursed at a higher rate due to CC/MCC status.

HAC Financial Impact on Medicare and Hospitals:

- An examination of the financial impact to hospitals conducted for Medicare by RTI in FY2011 reveals minimal effect:[195]

  - o Of 19,839 HAC discharges, 3,006 required a reassignment of the MS-DRG.

  - o HAC-caused MS-DRG adjustments summary for FY2011:

average MS-DRG adjustment:	$6,456
largest single HAC-caused MS-DRG adjustment: (SSI mediastinitis CABG)	$12,088
smallest single HAC-caused MS-DRG adjustment: (burns)	$1,528

  - o Two HAC categories resulted in 80 percent of annual HAC-related Medicare savings:

Falls and trauma:	$7,362,538
PE & DVT post-orthopedic surgery:	$8,313,098
Total FY2011 Medicare savings:	**$19,375,777**

---

[195] *http://www.rti.org/reports/cms/*

Table 3: Payment Savings by MS-DRG Reassignment by HAC

Discharge FY2011

SELECTED HAC CATEGORY	Discharges identified w/ this HAC	Discharges w/ reassigned MS-DRG	Changes in IPPS per reassigned discharge	Changes in IPPS, total
1. foreign object retained after surgery	284	37	$4,536	$167,818
2. air embolism	34	14	$8,901	$124,620
3. blood incompatibility	11	1	$7,115	$7,115
4. pressure ulcer Stages III & IV	1,770	286	$6,456	$1,846,449
5. falls and trauma	-	-	-	-
a. fracture	3,829	996	$6,257	$6,232,020
b. dislocation	22	2	$4,538	$9,075
c. intracranial Injury	694	258	$4,738	$1,222,290
d. crushing Injury	1	0	-	$0
e. burn	42	3	$1,528	$4,583
f. electric shock	8	0	-	$0
Less: multiple falls and trauma HACs1	-41	-18	($5,857)	($105,430)
6. unduplicated falls and trauma	4,555	1,241	$5,933	$7,362,538
7. catheter-associated UTI	3,918	160	$3,069	$491,053
8. vascular catheter-associated infection	5,921	20	$4,605	$92,100
9. poor glycemic control	555	152	$6,595	$1,002,378
10a. SSI mediastinitis CABG	50	5	$12,088	$60,438
10b. SSI orthopedic	244	6	$6,917	$41,503
10c. SSI bariatric	24	2	$1,656	$3,312
11. PE & DVT post-orthopedic	2,473	1,082	$7,683	$8,313,098
Total	19,839	3,006	$6,491	$19,512,422
Less: adjustment for discharges with multiple HACs 2	-207	-15	($9,110)	($136,645)
Unduplicated total	**19,632**	**2,991**	**$6,478**	**$19,375,777**

Source: HAC-POA Evaluation, RTI Evaluation of FY2011 Data

HAC Statistical Validity Analysis

The statistical validity of using HACs that occur so infrequently as a valid measurement in determining payment modification and assessing overall care quality has come under increased scrutiny:

- In a November 2011 memorandum to Medicare, Mathematica Inc. (Mathematica Policy Research, a CMS contractor) reported the results of an evaluation of the statistical validity of eight HAC measures to determine their accuracy in reflecting the quality of care on average.[196]

- Data collected was for the seven-month period from March to September 2010 and presented: minimum caseloads required to meet a reliability standard; percentage of hospitals having such caseloads; and achievement of each measure in meeting standards over time.

- The methodological standard for reliability was established at .4, which is considered to be the lower limit of "moderate" reliability.

  Note: The statistical concept of reliability (R) used to determine minimum case size for a particular measure is whether a hospital's ranking on that measure, compared to its performance in other periods or compared to other hospitals, is likely to be the same if repeated samples of the hospital's cases were taken.

- **Results of the analysis:**

  o At twelve, eighteen, and twenty-four months, the median reliability standard exceeded the minimum standard of .4, indicating that aggregated HAC measurement could adequately reflect overall hospital quality of care.

  o At twenty-four months, 66 percent of hospitals would have an adequate caseload for effective HAC evaluation.

  o The falls and trauma measurement failed to achieve 50 percent of the reliability standard of .4, even at twenty-four months. In addition, only 6 percent of hospitals were determined to have a sufficient caseload to make this a valid measure.

  o Because of the rarity of blood incompatibility and air embolism, no standards could be set.

- **Conclusions:**

  o The overall reliability of individual HAC measures varies widely.

---

[196] *www.mathematica-mpr.com/Publications/.../hvbp_measure_reliability.pd... : , Memorandum to Sophia Chan–Reporting Period and Reliability Period and Reliability of AHRQ, CMS 30-Day and HAC Quality Measures–Revised*

  o Significant fluctuations in a hospital's performance classification are possible when unreliable measures are evaluated at different points in time.

  o The more reliable measures and the composite score indicate that a majority of hospitals meet the standard after accumulating twelve to twenty-four months of data experience.

Table 4: Reliability and Time Period of Calculation

HAC Measures

Measure	N at which R=0.4	6 Months		12 Months		18 Months		24 Months	
		Median Reliability*	R≥0.4** (%)	Median Reliability*	R≥0.4** (%)	Median Reliability*	R≥0.4** (%)	Median Reliability*	R≥0.4** (%)
Foreign object retained after surgery	15,417	0.05	0	0.09	1	0.12	4	0.14	7
Air embolism	UNDEF	UNDEF	UNDEF	UNDEF	UNDEF	UNDEF	UNDEF	UNDEF	UNDEF
Blood incompatibility	UNDEF	UNDEF	UNDEF	UNDEF	UNDEF	UNDEF	UNDEF	UNDEF	UNDEF
Pressure ulcer stages III & IV	2,195	0.28	31	0.40	50	0.50	62	0.53	66
Falls and trauma	16,119	0.05	0	0.08	1	0.12	4	0.14	6
Vascular catheter-associated infection	3,498	0.19	15	0.29	34	0.38	48	0.42	52
Catheter-associated UTI	1,070	0.44	55	0.57	70	0.67	80	0.70	83
Manifestations of poor glycemic control	27,888	0.03	0	0.05	0	0.07	0	0.08	1
All HAC	1,950	0.30	35	0.42	53	0.53	65	0.56	69

Note: Estimated over hospitals required to submit POA data, March 2010 to September 2010. Reliability estimate based on 200 largest hospitals. N=3401.

* Reliability of measure of hospital of median case size.
** Proportion of hospitals with case size large enough that R≥0.4.

UNDEF – Undefined because estimated signal variance negative or undefined

Source: *Mathematica Policy Research 11/18/2011 Memorandum: Reporting Period and Reliability of AHRQ, CMS 30-day and HAC Quality Measures – Revised*

Hospital-Acquired Conditions Payment Modification Policy Conclusion:

Although the relative incidence of patients acquiring one of the identified HACs under the HACs Payment Modification initiative is small, CMS expects that increased provider awareness of the incidence and costs of HACs will lead to improved hospital protocols and reductions in the number of reasonably preventable events across all patients. As CMS officials Barry Staube and Jonathan Blum commented in an editorial in response to the 2009 McNair study:

- "Although the projected payment reductions are not large, small payment penalties have been effective in changing human behavior and ultimately in improving the hospital care experience for patients."

- "Medicare's total payment reductions may understate the overall cost savings of preventing hospital-acquired conditions. In addition to a general recognition that performance-sensitive payment methods can contribute to improved quality and efficiency in the health care system, increasing attention is being paid to economic arguments that health care providers are more likely to take action to avoid definite losses than to capture potential gains."[197]

- In the FY2014 Proposed IPPS Rule, CMS estimates savings through HAC Payment Modifications during the next five fiscal years to be:

YEAR	SAVINGS
FY2014	$26 million
FY2015	$28 million
FY2016	$30 million
FY2017	$33 million
FY2018	$36 million

Hoped-for "spillovers" are expected to occur as hospitals create new procedures and adapt behaviors in response to the payment incentives or POA documentation requirements. Each of the new policy responses by other payers or state governments increases the likelihood of desirable spillover effects to the non-Medicare population.

4.3.4 Hospital-Acquired Conditions Reduction Program (FY2015)

Building upon the FY2008 HAC Payment Modification policy, provisions contained in the 2010 ACA mandated that CMS implement a broader incentive program aimed at further reducing the incidence and frequency of HACs.

---

[197] http://content.healthaffairs.org/content/28/5/1494.full

Regulatory Overview

Under Section 3008 of Part I, Subsection A, Title III of the ACA, CMS is directed to implement the Hospital-Acquired Conditions Reduction Program (HAC Program), under which payments to applicable hospitals are adjusted to provide an additional incentive to reduce HACs, effective for discharges beginning on October 1, 2014 (FY2015) "and for subsequent years." CMS is directed to:

- Design the HAC Program with clearly identified metrics, against which all applicable hospitals will be evaluated.

- Develop an evaluation methodology by which CMS is able to identify the 25 percent of applicable hospitals with the highest rates of determined HACs, relative to the national average of conditions acquired during an applicable period.

- Implement a payment adjustment for the identified 25 percent of hospitals with the highest rates of HACs equal to 99 percent of the amount that hospitals would ordinarily receive for discharges. This 1 percent reduction in payments will be applied to all Medicare discharges occurring during FY2015.

- Proposed specifications of the HAC Program were introduced with the May 10, 2013, publication of the FY2014 Proposed IPS Rule. Upon consideration of received public comments, CMS published final modifications of the HAC Program in the FY2014 Final IPPS rule, published on August 19, 2013:

  o Hospitals were provided their first look at domain specifications, to include data collection time periods, for the FY2015 program in August 2013.

  o The final data collection period for assessment of the FY2015 penalty ends on December 31, 2013.

Background

- The HAC Reduction Program is constructed to align with the long-term goals established as part of the National Strategy for Quality

Improvement in Health Care, [National Quality Strategy (NQS)] as outlined in Section 3011 of the ACA.

- In its 2013 Report to Congress on the NQS, HHS reviewed HAC occurrence and outlined NQS HAC reduction goals:[198]

    - The baseline frequency of HAC occurrence used to establish NQS improvement goals was set as 145 HACs per 1,000 admissions. The most recently reported tracking data (contained in the 2013 Report to Congress) was an annual HAC rate of 142 per 1,000 admissions for FY2011.

    - HAC reduction goals are specified under NQS Priority 1: Making Care Safer by Reducing Harm Caused in the Delivery of Care.

        - The HAC reduction goal by the end of FY2014 is to achieve a 40 percent reduction in *preventable* HACs from a baseline rate of 145 HACs per 1,000 admissions.

    - Achieving this goal is estimated to save 60,000 lives and reduce injuries to patients by 1.8 million.

- Although many common HACs can be prevented through the proper application of evidence-based guidelines, surveys have revealed that 87 percent of hospitals fail to follow such guidelines:[199]

    - When established guidelines are stringently adhered to, significant reductions in the occurrence and severity of HACs can be realized. In its 2013 NQS Progress Report to Congress, HHS cited HAC reductions made by Dignity Health as an example of the impact of effective guideline implementation:[200]

---

[198] *2013 Annual Progress Report to Congress National Strategy for Quality Improvement in Health Care: 2013 Annual Progress Report to Congress (PDF, 1.5 MB)* http://www.ahrq.gov/workingforquality/reports.htm

[199] *Federal Register/Vol. 78, No. 160/Monday, August 19, 2013/Rules and Regulations/Page 50708* www.gpo.gov/fdsys/pkg/FR-2013-08-19/pdf/2013-18956.pdf

[200] *2013 Annual Progress Report to Congress National Strategy for Quality Improvement in Health Care: 2013 Annual Progress Report to Congress (PDF, 1.5 MB)* http://www.ahrq.gov/workingforquality/reports.htm

- Founded in 1986 and headquartered in San Francisco, Dignity Health is the fifth largest hospital provider in the nation and the largest hospital system in California.

- Dignity Health is a participating member of the CMS Partnerships for Patients (PfP) initiative. The PfP:

  - is a voluntary portfolio initiative under the direction of the CMS Innovation Center

  - involves twenty-six Hospital Engagement Networks (HENs) representing 4,111 hospitals

  - requires participants to adopt NQS quality improvement goals and share proven practices, such as the use of clinical decision support and quality measures

- Since 2011, Dignity Health has dramatically reduced rates of HAI in four areas representing 80 percent of all health care-associated infections nationwide:

  - 70 percent reduction in CLABSI

  - 53 percent reduction in VAP

  - 52 percent reduction in surgical site infections SSI

  - 24 percent reduction in CAUTI

- HAI are the most frequently encountered HACs and are associated with significant morbidity and mortality. CMS reports that annual deaths from HAC categories involving infections alone are twice as high as those from HIV/AIDS and breast cancer combined.[201]

- In the FY2011 IPPS/LTCH PPS Final Rule (75 FR 50196), CMS adopted eight HAC measures as part of the Hospital IQR Program for the FY2012 payment determination to promote quality of care by reducing HAC occurrence in acute care settings. Hospital performance on these

---

[201] *Federal Register/Vol. 78, No. 160/Monday, August 19, 2013/Rules and Regulations/Page 50708 www.gpo.gov/fdsys/pkg/FR-2013-08-19/pdf/2013-18956.pdf*

measures has been publicly reported on the Hospital Compare website since September 2010.

- In outlining implementation steps for the HAC Program, CMS stated in the FY2014 IPPS Final Rule:

  o "Our goal for the HAC Reduction Program is to heighten the awareness of HACs and reduce the number of incidences that occur through implementing the adjustments required by section 1886(p) of the Act."

  o "We believe that our efforts in using payment adjustments and our measurement authority will encourage hospitals to eliminate the incidence of HACs that could be reasonably prevented by applying evidence-based guidelines."

- These goals reflect the opinions expressed by Medicare Director Jonathan Blum in a 2009 editorial regarding the effectiveness of the (then) newly implemented HAC Payment Modification policy, in which he stated:

  o "Although the projected payment reductions are not large, small payment penalties have been effective in changing human behavior and ultimately in improving the hospital care experience for patients."[202]

Jonathan Blum, Medicare deputy administrator and director of the Center of Medicare at the CMS, is responsible for overseeing the regulation and payment of Medicare fee-for-service providers, privately administered Medicare health plans, and the Medicare prescription drug program.

Key HAC Program Terms

(2014 Final IPPS Rule):

Hospital-Acquired Condition:

A condition identified as part of the current HACs Payment Modification initiative as specified in subsection 1886(d)(4)(D)(iv) of the Social Security Act

---

[202] *http://content.healthaffairs.org/content/28/5/1494.full*

and "*any other condition determined appropriate by the Secretary that an individual acquires during a stay at an applicable hospital, as determined by the Secretary.*" This intentionally broad definition grants exceptional flexibility to the secretary in designing a HAC Program.

Applicable Hospital:

Subsection (d) hospitals (those reimbursed under the IPPS) do not include hospitals and hospital units excluded from IPPS reimbursement, such as:

- long-term care hospitals (LTCHs)
- Maryland waiver hospitals*
- cancer hospitals
- children's inpatient facilities
- rural health clinics
- federally qualified health centers (FQHCs)
- critical access hospitals (CAHs)
- religious non-medical health care institutions
- inpatient psychiatric hospitals (IPFs)
- inpatient rehabilitation facilities (IRFs)
- Veterans Administration/Department of Defense hospitals.
- *In the FY2014 Final Rule, Maryland hospitals may be granted an exemption for application of payment adjustment under the HAC program. However, such hospitals must report HAC measures and these will be included in the national determination of hospital quartiles.

Applicable Period:

The twenty-four-month period (specified by the secretary) from which data are collected in order to calculate a total HAC Score for each applicable hospital participating in the HAC Program. Specific and separate twenty-four-month data collection periods are established for each of two domains of the HAC Program (see HAC domains below).

Domains:

These are sets of measures used to determine payment adjustment under the HAC Program.

4.3.5 HAC Program Methodology

Overview:

- All applicable hospitals will be evaluated against metrics divided into two domains.
- CMS will collect data during the twenty-four-month reporting period assigned for each domain.
- Each metric of a domain will be individually scored to determine a Total Domain Score.
- This score will be multiplied by the assigned weighting for the domain.
- The two weighted domain scores will be summed to determine a total HAC Score.
- Scores for participating hospitals will be ranked by total HAC Scores, from lowest (best) scores to highest (worst) scores.
- The hospitals with the highest 25 percent of HAC scores will receive a 1 percent reduction in all Medicare discharges for the program fiscal year.

HAC Program Domains:

- All measures selected for each of two domains follow criteria established by the Deficit Reduction Act (DRA) of 2005:
  - high volume or high cost
  - preventable through the use of evidence-based guidelines
- All measures recommended for inclusion in the HAC Program have been endorsed by the NQF Measures Application Partnership (MAP), on their own or as part of a composite, or represent one of the twelve HACs identified by the HHS secretary.

- CMS will use the Hospital IQR Program's data submission, review, and correction processes. This process allows for review and correction of data on a continuous basis as data are being submitted quarterly for the Hospital IQR Program

- Two domains have been identified for use in the FY2015 HAC Program with separate associated data-collection periods and relative weightings:

  o **Domain 1:**

FY2015 Domain Data:	AHRQ PSI-90 Composite
FY2015 Data Period:	July 1, 2011–June 30, 2013
FY2015 Domain Weighting:	35 percent

  o **Domain 2:**

Domain Data:	- Select CDC HAI
	- CLABSI (FY2015)
	- CAUTI (FY2015)
	- SSI (FY2016)
	- MRSA (FY2017)
	- Clostridium Difficile (CDI) (FY2017)
FY2015 Data Period:	Jan. 1, 2011–Dec. 31, 2013
FY2015 Domain Weighting:	65 percent

Domain 1: PSI-90 Composite

Note: To address concerns expressed (especially by large and teaching hospitals) that some events included within the PSI-90 were more likely to be seen with increased patient volumes, CMS reduced the proposed weighting of 50 percent for the PSI-90 Composite to 35 percent.

Component Measures and Weighting

- Patient Safety Indicators (PSIs) have been developed by the AHRQ and are sets of collected data that provide information on potential in-hospital complications and adverse events during surgeries and procedures.

- Under the Reporting of Hospital Quality Data for Annual Payment Update (RHQDAPU) program, CMS adopted PSIs as an Inpatient Quality Reporting (IQR) requirement affecting annual hospital reimbursement updates (RHQDAPU is now known as IQR).

- One such adopted indictor is the PSI-90 Composite.[203]

  - The NQF endorsed the PSI-90 as a valid measure of hospital safety in 2009 and began reporting measures on the Hospital Compare website in 2010.

  - The PSI-90 composite is an AHRQ measure in the Outcomes Domain for the FY2014–FY2017 hospital value-based purchasing (HVBP) program.

Individual Measures and Relative Weighting

The PSI-90 for the FY2015 HAC Program consists of eight separate risk-adjusted and weighted measures:

PSI-90 MEASURE	MEASURE'S WEIGHT IN COMPOSITE
PSI 03 – pressure ulcer	0.1357
PSI 06 – Iatrogenic pneumothorax	0.0614
PSI 07 – central venous catheter-related bloodstream infections	0.0831
PSI 08 – post-operative hip fracture	0.0005
PSI 12 – PE/DVT	0.2209
PSI 13 – post-operative sepsis	0.0536
PSI 14 – post-operative wound dehiscence	0.0159
PSI 15 – accidental puncture or laceration	0.4289
Total:	**1.0000**

[203] *"AHRQ Patient Safety Indicators Adopted for the Hospital Inpatient Quality Reporting Program,"* June 2013. www.qualityindicators.ahrq.gov/Downloads/Modules/PSI/V44/Composit...

Calculation and Interpretation of Composite Score

- The AHRQ PSI-90 measures use Medicare FFS *claims* data and are calculated using ICD-9-CM diagnosis and/or procedure codes and, for the secondary diagnoses, the POA value associated with each secondary diagnosis in the claim:

    o PSI-90 measures capture occurrences of adverse events for Medicare FFS discharges only.

    o PSI-90 measure results are risk- and reliability-adjusted based on a twenty-four-month data period.

    o PSI-90 measures identify adverse events occurring across units within a facility.

    o The HAC Domain 1 PSI-90 score is calculated using a data extract taken at the conclusion of the ninety-day period following the last date of discharge used in the applicable period. For example, if the last discharge date in the applicable period for a measure is June 30, 2013, data would be extracted by CMS on September 30, 2013, and that data would be used to calculate the claims-based measures for that applicable period.

        ▪ PSI-90 Composite calculation is made by multiplying the event incidence by the weighting factor and summing the result.

    o Hospitals will receive their Domain 1 Scores in confidential QualityNet reports upon score determination and will be provided 30 days to review and submit corrections.

- Interpretation of a hospital's PSI composite ratio by itself is complex—lower ratios indicate better quality. A ratio of "1" does not indicate that a hospital is performing as expected.

    o The most relevant interpretation of a PSI composite ratio is in a comparison—for example, a hospital with a PSI composite ratio of .5 represents higher quality than the national median (i.e., threshold) of .622879.

- Commenters responding to the proposed inclusion of the PSI-90 for the HAC Domain 1 measure for FY2015 expressed concern about the potential for "double payment adjustments" due to overlapping requirements with the HVBP program. In addition, concern was expressed that a PSI-90 condition potentially overlaps with a HAC Domain 2 measure for CLABSI.

  - CMS responded in the Final FY2014 rule that "we believe that the importance of these measures to patient safety, coupled with the numerous comments asking for measure alignment, justifies the use of PSI-90 in more than one program."

  - In addition, CMS emphasized that the HAC program and the HVBP programs are separate programs with different purposes and goals:

    - HAC program: Penalty program to improve patient safety in hospitals through percentage reductions in global Medicare payments made to the top 25 percent of hospitals reporting HACs.

    - HVBP program: Incentive program that redistributes reductions made to the base operating DRG payment amounts, based on certain performance measures.

    - "The Statute does not prohibit the use of the same measures in both the HAC Reduction Program and the Hospital VBP Program."[204]

Domain 2: CDC Hospital-Acquired Infections (HAI)

Background:

- FY2015 Domain 2 measures consist of two selected HAI measures developed by the CDC National Health Safety Network:

  - CLABSI
  - CAUTI

---

[204] *Federal Register/Vol. 78, No. 160/Monday, August 19, 2013/Rules and Regulations/Page 50716 www.gpo.gov/fdsys/pkg/FR-2013-08-19/pdf/2013-18956.pdf*

- HAI rates show how often patients in a particular hospital contract certain infections during the course of their medical treatment, when compared to like hospitals.

    o To receive payment from CMS, hospitals are required to report data about selected infections to the CDC's National Healthcare Safety Network (NHSN).

    o The NHSN is a free web-based tool hospitals use to input the required information.

    o For many HAI measures, hospitals have the ability to transmit data electronically directly from Electronic Health Record systems (EHRs) or EHR components.

    o Most hospitals that track the incidence of HAIs still rely on infection-control specialists, using chart-abstracted data, to manually identify such infections.

- As opposed to the PSI-90 Composite measures that used claims data, the CDC HAI measures use chart-abstracted data.

- CMS will use the same inclusion criteria as used under the Hospital IQR Program for the Domain 2 measures:

    o CDC HAI measures are reportable for all patients treated in acute care hospitals, including adult, pediatric, neonatal, Medicare, and non-Medicare patients.

    o CDC HAI measures identify adverse events at the *unit* level. For the FY2015 HAC Program, Domain 2 measures of CAUTI and CLABSI will be measured at the Intensive Care Unit (ICU) level *only*, including pediatric and neonatal ICUs.

Note: Beginning in January 2015, the Hospital IQR program will begin collecting non-ICU data for CAUTI and CLABSI measures.

HAI Measurement Utilizing the Standardized Infection Ratio (SIR)

Calculations for the HAI measures adjust for differences in the characteristics of patients at a hospital using a Standardized Infection Ratio (SIR), based on quarterly reporting:[205]

- The SIR is a summary measure accounting for differences in patient types, account location, hospital affiliation with an Academic Medical Center (AMC) and hospital bed counts.

- It compares the actual number of HAIs in a facility or state to a national benchmark based on previous years of reported data and adjusts the data based on several factors.

- CDC SIR Measures are calculated by dividing the total facility number of *observed* HAI events by the total facility number of *predicted* HAI events.

- In order to calculate a Standard Infection Ratio (SIR), a hospital's number of expected HAIs must be >1:

  o A confidence interval with a lower and upper limit is displayed around each SIR to indicate that a high degree of confidence exists that the true value of the SIR lies within that interval.

  o SIRs with a lower limit that is greater than 1.0 mean that more HAIs occurred in a facility or state than were predicted, and a SIR with an upper limit that is less than 1 means that fewer HAIs occurred than were predicted.

  o For hospitals that have an expected number of HAIs < 1, a score of zero (0) would be inserted in order to calculate the domain score.

  o For hospitals that have no ICU and have an active waiver for the Hospital IQR program, HAI quality reporting also would receive zero (0) points.

  o If a hospital is eligible to report HAIs, does not have an active IQR waiver, and fails to report to NHSN, it would receive the maximum

---

[205] http://www.medicare.gov/hospitalcompare/Data/Healthcare-Associated-Infections.html

penalty of 10 points for that measure to calculate the Domain 2 (See "Scoring" below):

4.3.6 FY2015 HAI Measures:

Central Line-Associated Bloodstream Infections (CLABSI)

- CLABSI: a primary laboratory-confirmed bloodstream infection in a patient with a central line at the time of (or within 48 hours prior to) the onset of symptoms and the infection is not related to an infection from another site.

- The CLABSI measure assesses the rate of laboratory-confirmed cases of such infections among ICU patients.

- CLABSI is one of the two Hospital Acquired Infection measures (along with CAUTI) contained in the Outcomes Domain for the FY2016 hospital value-based purchasing program.

  o Commenters responding to the proposed inclusion of CLABSI as a HAC Domain 2 condition for FY2015 expressed concern about the potential for "double payment adjustments" due to overlapping requirements with the HVBP program.

- For additional information regarding CLABSI identification and reporting see: *www.cdc.gov/nhsn/pdfs/pscmanual/4psc_clabscurrent.pdf*

Catheter-Associated Urinary Tract Infections (CAUTI)

- A urinary tract infection (UTI) is an infection involving any part of the urinary system, including urethra, bladder, ureters, and kidney. UTIs are the most common type of HAI reported to the NHSN. Among UTIs acquired in the hospital, approximately 75 percent are associated with a urinary catheter.

4.3.7 HAC Program Scoring Methodology[206]

The adopted scoring methodology for the HAC Reduction Program is similar to that used for the HVBP program in that:

- the HAC program uses multiple domains consisting of individually weighted metrics

- selected measures are assigned performance points

- metric performance within domains is summed to determine a domain score

- each domain has a weighted impact on determining an overall program score

Domain 1: Rules and Scoring of PSI-90 Composite

- Data used to calculate the PSI-90 Composite is claims-extracted by CMS ninety days after the end of the "applicable period." For FY2015, CMS extracted data for Domain 1 calculation on September 30, 2013.

- To be scored for Domain 1, a hospital must have three or more eligible discharges for at least one of the PSI-90 Composite indicators:

  - If a hospital meets the above criteria, for other measures with less than three eligible discharges, the national average rate is substituted for the hospital rate for calculation.

- If the number of eligible discharges for a hospital is fewer than three for *all eight* component indicators comprising the composite, the composite value would *not* be calculated and the HAC score would depend entirely on Domain 2 scoring.

---

[206] *Federal Register/Vol. 78, No. 160/Monday, August 19, 2013/Rules and Regulations/Page 50723 www.gpo.gov/fdsys/pkg/FR-2013-08-19/pdf/2013-18956.pdf*

Domain 1: Scoring:

- Higher scores are associated with lower performance.

- For each PSI-90 measure, applicable discharge rates are multiplied by the measure-weighting factor to determine the individual measure score.

- The Domain 1 composite score is determined by adding all individual measure scores of the PSI -90.

- Based on the distribution of PSI-90 for all hospitals, CMS will divide the results into percentiles in increments of 10, with the lowest percentile ranges meaning better performance:

  o Hospitals with PSI-90 rates within the lowest percentile will receive a point score of 1.

  o Hospitals with PSI-90 rates in the second-lowest percentile (between the 10th and 20th percentile) will receive two points, and so on through the highest percentile.

IF A HOSPITAL'S PSI-90 FALLS WITHIN THESE PERCENTILES:	POINTS ASSIGNED
1st-10th	1
11th-20th	2
21st-30th	3
31st-40th	4
41st-50th	5
51st-60th	6
61st 70th	7
71st-80th	8
81st-90th	9
91st-100th	10

  o The assigned Domain 1 score will then be weighted at 35 percent and added to the Domain 2 score.

Domain 2: Rules and Scoring of CDC HAI (CLABSI/CAUTI):

- Measure results are obtained through data submitted to CDC as part of the Hospital IQR Program.

- Events for the FY2014 HAC program are collected only from ICUs (to include pediatric and neonatal ICUs).

- CMS must be able to calculate a SIR for at least one of the two CDC HAI measures (CLABSI/CAUTI). If at least one SIR cannot be calculated, no Domain 2 score will be included and the Domain 1 score will be used to calculate the total HAC Score.

Domain 2: Scoring

- For each CDC HAI (CLABSI and CAUTI), the SIR is calculated and points will be awarded based on a national percentile ranking as described for Domain 1 scoring (1 point for 0–10th percentile, 2 points for 11th—20th percentile, etc.).

- The points awarded to each CDC HAI will then be averaged and the result multiplied by the weighting factor for Domain 2 of 65 percent.

- Some hospitals participating in IQR reporting do not have ICUs. If such facilities have received a waiver for ICU reporting as a result, CMS will only use Domain 1 scores to determine the total HAC Score.

- If an IQR-reporting hospital has not received an ICU waiver and fails to report data for at least one of the CDC HAI measures, CMS will assign 10 points for that measure.

4.3.8 Total HAC Score Determination:

For each of the descriptions of domain data reporting, the calculation of the total HAC Score is accomplished as indicated:

Example 1:

- Domain 1: at least three discharges for one PSI-90 Composite indicator.
- Domain 2: sufficient cases to calculate a SIR for at least one measure.

- Scoring: Domain 1 score (weight 35 percent) + Domain 2 score (weight 65 percent)

Example 2:
- Domain 1: at least three discharges for one PSI-90 Composite indicator.
- Domain 2: insufficient data to calculate at least 1 SIR for CDC HAI.
- Scoring: Domain 1 score (weight 100 percent)

Example 3:
- Domain 1: less than three discharges for one of the eight PSI-90 Composite indicators.
- Domain 2: sufficient cases to calculate a SIR for at least one measure.
- Scoring: Domain 2 score (weight 100 percent)

Example 4:
- Domain 1: at least three discharges for one PSI-90 Composite indicator.
- Domain 2: hospital participates in IQR reporting, doesn't have an ICU waiver, and does not report CDC HAI.
- Scoring: Domain 1 Score (weight 35 percent) + Domain 2 Score of 10 (weight 65 percent)

Example 5
- Domain 1: less than three discharges for one of the eight PSI-90 Composite indicators.
- Domain 2: insufficient cases to calculate a SIR for at least one measure.
- Scoring: no total HAC Score will be calculated for this hospital.

Data Dissemination, Confidential Reporting, and Public Posting:

- CMS will provide hospitals with confidential reports via QualityNet that include:

- discharge-level information related to claims-based data for PSI measures, the domain score for each domain, and the total HAC Score.

- Hospitals will have a thirty-day period upon receipt of these reports to review/contest results.

- Upon the conclusion of the allowed review period, CMS will review final results to determine the 25 percent of hospitals with the highest total HAC Scores. These hospitals will receive a 1 percent reduction in all Medicare reimbursements for FY2015.

- CMS will post each hospital's scores with respect to each measure, each hospital's domain-specific score, and the hospital's total HAC Score on the Hospital Compare website.

Additional information on the HAC Reduction Program may be found at: www.cms.gov/Medicare/Medicare-Fee-for-Service.../hacfactsheet.pdf

Section 4.4: Acronym Guide

ACA ....Affordable Care Act of 2010

AHRQ ....Agency for Healthcare Research and Quality

AMA ....American Medical Association

ARRA.......................American Recovery and Reinvestment Act of 2009,
Public Law 111–5

ATRA ....American Taxpayer Relief Act of 2012, Public Law 112–240

BBA ....Balanced Budget Act of 1997, Public Law 105–33

CABG ....Coronary Artery Bypass Graft

CAH ....Critical Access Hospitals

CAUTI ....Catheter-Associated Urinary Tract Infection

CC............................Complication or Comorbidity

CCN ....CMS Certification Number

CDAD.......................Clostridium Difficile-Associated Disease
CDC Center for Disease Control and Prevention

CERT ....Comprehensive Error Rate Testing

CDI ....Clostridium Difficile

CLABSI ....Central Line-Associated Bloodstream Infection

CMI ....Case-Mix Index

CMS ....Centers for Medicare & Medicaid Services

CRNA ....Certified Registered Nurse Anesthetist

CY ....Calendar Year

DOD ....Department of Defense

DRA ....Deficit Reduction Act of 2005, Public Law 109–171

DRG ....Diagnosis-Related Group

DSH ....Disproportionate Share Hospital

DVT/PE....................Deep Vein Thrombosis/Pulmonary Embolism

EHR ....Electronic Health Record

EMR.........................Electronic Medical Record

FQHC.......................Federally Qualified Health Centers

FR ....Federal Register

FTE ....Full-Time Equivalent

FY	Fiscal Year
HAC	Hospital-Acquired Condition
HAI	Healthcare-Associated Infection
HCAHPS	Hospital Consumer Assessment of Healthcare Providers and Systems.
HHS	Department of Health and Human Services
HQI	Hospital Quality Initiative
ICD-9-CM	International Classification of Diseases, Ninth Revision, Clinical Modification
ICD-10-CM	International Classification of Diseases, Tenth Revision, Clinical Modification
ICD-10-PCS	International Classification of Diseases, Tenth Revision, Procedure Coding System
ICU	Intensive Care Unit
IOM	Institute of Medicine
IPF	Inpatient Psychiatric Facility
IPPS	[Acute care hospital] Inpatient Prospective Payment System
IRF	Inpatient Rehabilitation Facility
IQR	Inpatient Quality Reporting
LTCH	Long-Term Care Facility
LTCH PPS	Long-Term Care Facility Prospective Payment System
MAP	Measure Application Partnership
MCC	Major Complication or Comorbidity
MedPAC	Medicare Payment Advisory Commission
MedPAR	Medicare Provider Analysis and Review File
MMA	Medicare Prescription Drug, Improvement/ Modernization Act of 2003
MRSA	Methicillin-Resistant Staphylococcus Aureus
MS-DRG	Medicare Severity Diagnosis- Related Group
MS-LTC-DRG	Medicare Severity Long-Term Care Diagnosis-Related Group NAICS North American Industrial Classification System
NCD	National Coverage Determination
NCHS	National Center for Health Statistics
NCQA	National Committee for Quality Assurance
NHSN	National Healthcare Safety Network
NQF	National Quality Forum

NQS .... National Quality Strategy

OPPC........................ Other Provider Preventable Conditions

PCH .... PPS-Exempt Cancer Hospital

PfP .... Partnership for Patients

POA .... Present on Admission

PPC........................... Provider Preventable Conditions

PAC........................... Post-Acute Care

PSI .... Patient Safety Indicators

PQRS........................ Physician Quality Reporting System

QIG .... Quality Improvement Group

RHQDAPU................ Reporting Hospital Quality Data for Annual Payment Update

SIR .... Standardized Infection Ratio

SNF.......................... Skilled Nursing Facility

SSI .... Surgical Site Infections

VA .... Veterans Administration

VAP.......................... Ventilator-Associated Pneumonia

VBP.......................... [Hospital] Value-Based Purchasing [Program]

PART 2

Value-Based Medicare
Reimbursement Programs
Affecting Physicians

PART 2

Value-Based Medicare
Reimbursement Programs
Affecting Physicians

CHAPTER 5

The Physician Quality Reporting System (PQRS)

Section 5.1: Flash Read!

The Physician Quality Reporting System (PQRS) is a federal program designed to increase the transparency of health care quality among physicians. The program has been in place since 2007. From the program's beginning in 2007 through recently, physicians were rewarded financially for voluntary participation. However, participation in PQRS has not reached the level hoped for by the Centers for Medicare & Medicaid Services. The Affordable Care Act aims to change that by converting PQRS to a penalty-only program, meaning those providers who do not successfully participate will suffer financial penalties, and there are no bonus payments for participation.

- The Physician Quality Reporting System (PQRS) is a voluntary program structured to encourage eligible health care providers to report information on various selected quality measures.

- As a result of the Affordable Care Act (ACA), the PQRS program will apply financial penalties starting in 2015 (based on 2013 performance) to those providers who do not satisfy reporting requirements. Financial penalties are a new element of the PQRS program, which has been in existence since 2007. Previously called the Physician Quality Reporting Initiative, the program once used only financial incentives to encourage provider participation.

- For 2014, providers and group practices can report quality information on 284 individual measures and twenty-five measures groups. The measures are developed by provider associations, quality groups, and CMS, and are used to assign a quantity to the quality of care provided. Factors to be considered by providers when choosing which measures to report include clinical conditions usually treated, types of care typically provided, setting where care is usually delivered, quality improvement goals for 2014, and other quality reporting programs in use.

- Measures are selected based on patient clinical demographics, the method of reporting selected, and whether PQRS data is being submitted as an individual provider or as a group practice.

- **Financial incentives and penalties under PQRS will be implemented as follows:**

PERFORMANCE PERIOD	INCENTIVE AMOUNT (assessed on total estimated Medicare Part B PFS allowed charges)	PENALTY AMOUNT (assessed on total estimated Medicare Part B PFS allowed charges)
2013	0.5%	–
2014	0.5%	–
2015	–	-1.5% (based on PQRS participation during the 2013 reporting period)
2016	–	-2.0% (based on PQRS participation during the 2014 reporting period)

Note: 2014 is the final year to earn an additional 0.5 percent payment incentive for participation in the Maintenance of Certification Program (MOC).

- →IMPORTANT! While the PQRS payment adjustment penalty on Medicare Part B reimbursement will be capped at -2.0 percent for the program year of 2016 (2014 reporting) and beyond. Up to 7 percent of Medicare Part B reimbursements are at risk via other value-based reimbursement programs that utilize PQRS as the reporting system. This exacerbates the financial exposure for providers who do not meet PQRS participation requirements, ultimately placing 9 percent of

Medicare Part B revenue at risk by 2018. Other value-based reimbursement programs dependent on PQRS-reported data include:

- o The PQRS MOC Incentive Initiative
- o The Electronic Health Records (EHR) Incentive Program
- o The Physician Value-Based Payment Modifier (VBM) Program
- o The Medicare Shared Savings Program (MSSP)

- For 2014, CMS has provided a broad array of reporting methods to meet the needs of individuals and group practices. The following table represents the success of each option as reported in the most recent data year of 2011:*

2014 Reporting Options and % of Participants Successfully Reporting Using this Option to Earn PQRS Incentive in 2011	Number and % of Participants Using Each Reporting Option in 2011 (Latest Data Year)	2014 Reporting Methods for Individuals or Group Practices and Type of Data Reportable Through Each Option
claims: 77%	229,282 71.5%	**individual eligible professionals**: individual measures only (beginning in 2014)
qualified registry: 90%	50,125 16%	**individuals and groups of 2+:** individual measures and measures groups
electronic heath records (EHR): 90%	560 .15%	**individuals and groups of 2+:** individual measures
GPRO web-based interface: 98%	40,193 12%	**groups of 25+:** individual measures
qualified clinical data registry (QCDR): NA	new for 2014	**individuals:** individual PQRS measures and those determined by the QCDR
CMS-certified survey vendor: NA	new for 2014	**groups of 25+:** individual measures and CG CAHPS results

*Of 320,422 participants listed in the 2011 PQRS Experience Report, published in March 2013 (most recent data available)

Note: Beginning in 2014, group practices of 100+ eligible professionals are required to report Clinician Group (CG) Consumer Assessment of Healthcare Providers and Systems (CAHPS) Survey results. CG-CAHPS is a standardized tool that measures patient perceptions of care provided by a physician in an office setting. In 2014, CMS will fund survey administration for these groups. Groups of 25–99 providers are "encouraged" to participate in CG-CAHPS reporting, but CMS will not fund survey administration or reporting for such groups in 2014.

- With the 2015 implementation of payment adjustments (2013 reporting year) and the use of PQRS data for the upcoming physician value-based payment modifier (VBM), CMS estimates that participation rates in the 2014 PQRS will rise to 40 percent of the more than 1 million eligible professionals. (PQRS incentive payments offered by CMS since 2007 have had little impact on the overall participation rate, which has been around 25 percent.)

- Out of 1 million potential participants for 2014 PQRS, CMS estimates in the CY2014 Final PFS Rule 270,000 eligible professionals will each receive incentive payments averaging $1,059 (total of $286 million to be paid in incentives):

  o 730,000 providers, due to a lack of participation in FY2014, will be penalized 2 percent of their Medicare Part B reimbursements in FY2016

  o Costs for providers to comply with PQRS reporting requirements will be $66.7 million (an estimated $166.73 per individual provider).

  *Potential participants include all CMS-defined "eligible professionals."

Section 5.2:
Provider Perspectives

Quality improvement, like health care reform itself, is nothing if not an iterative process. The Physician Quality Reporting System (PQRS), one of the cornerstones of system quality improvement embedded in Title III of the overarching reform law, is the culmination of many years of thought, experiment, and discovery. In its current form, as mandated by the ACA, it uses a combination of incentive payments and penalties to promote reporting of quality information for services rendered under Medicare Part B fee-for-service.

5.2.1 Rationale

The PQRS, in effect, represents the government's effort to codify all that is known about the full gamut of measures—from process metrics to actual outcomes and mortality/morbidity statistics—and introduce a means to underscore their importance by tying reimbursement to performance and resource consumption.

The quality movement in health care began in the 1990s using process measures, for the most part, as proxies for things that researchers couldn't get at: for example, the rate at which patients experiencing a heart attack are given aspirin and beta-blockers. The Joint Commission, the National Committee on Quality Assurance, and other organizations created measures that they believed would improve compliance with best practices, and lead to better patient outcomes, lower morbidity, and reduced mortality. But the link of process measures to improved patient outcomes turned out to be not as obvious as the innovators had hoped.

The Institute of Medicine reports, "To Err Is Human" and "Crossing the Quality Chasm," attempted to accelerate the quality revolution. They fundamentally changed the understanding of medical errors from a focus on individual culpability to an emphasis on the need for systems thinking and high-reliability processes in organizations.

By 2004, five years after the first IOM report, Donald M. Berwick, MD, then the president of the Institute for Healthcare Improvement (IHI), declared that a more radical effort was required. Arguing that "some is not a number, soon is not a time," he devised the 100,000 Lives Campaign to give a sense of urgency to hospital patient-safety efforts. The IHI and partners promoted a series of rapid response innovations to keep care teams focused on quality.[207]

Around the same time, Robert M. Wachter, MD, a patient-safety expert at the University of California-San Francisco, published an assessment. "There has been progress, but it has been insufficient," he wrote. "Error-reporting systems have had little impact, and scant progress has been made in improving accountability." He blamed, in part, the reimbursement system: "Hospitals and physicians are paid the same regardless of the safety of the care they deliver. The system thus creates no incentive to invest in safety; indeed, in many situations precisely the opposite occurs, as error-prone care leads to higher revenues through more per diem payments or more lucrative diagnosis-related group (DRG) designations." The underinvestment by hospitals and physicians "demonstrates that the business case for safety, although more compelling than it was before 1999, remains inadequate to the size of the task." He then expressed the need to determine what would be the right mix of financial, educational, regulatory, and organizational forces to pull in the investment to make health care safer.[208]

In 2006, Congress took up the gauntlet. It ordered development of the Physician Quality Reporting Initiative (PQRI), a voluntary program that began July 1, 2007. The intent was to collect data on how well doctors cared for Medicare beneficiaries. It was expanded the next year. Gradually, it turned into the Physician Feedback Program, in which doctors received individualized reports depicting their quality of care and risk-adjusted cost metrics.

As a robust technical infrastructure did not yet exist to facilitate these communications, the goals were laid out in hopes that physicians would respond to the power of suggestion and alter their practice patterns. Simultaneously, the government introduced the tools to pull the pieces

---

[207] Donald M. Berwick, MD, et al., "The 100,000 Lives Campaign: Setting a Goal and a Deadline for Improving Health Care Quality," JAMA, 2006; 295(3):324–327, January 18, 2006. http://jama.jamanetwork.com/article.aspx?articleid=202194

[208] Robert M. Wachter, MD, "The End of the Beginning: Patient Safety Five Years After 'To Err Is Human'," Health Affairs, November 30, 2004. http://content.healthaffairs.org/content/early/2004/11/30/hlthaff.w4.534/suppl/DC1

together: financial support for electronic prescribing and electronic health records came on line during this period.

By 2009 and 2010, as what became the ACA was being drafted, the government was prepared to push through the fully developed PQRS.

5.2.2 Summary

With the current evolution of the PQRS, physicians' reimbursements are tied to how well they report on the various quality measures included in the PQRS. The measures form the basis for the value-based modifier payments (described in Chapter 7) and the new and evolving payment systems that reward doctors for quality of care rather than just volume of services. Physicians' reporting in 2013 determines whether they will get reimbursements trimmed by 1.5 percent in 2015; their 2014 reporting performance could lead to a 2 percent subtraction in 2016.

PQRS applies not just to licensed physicians but to a panoply of what are referred to as eligible professionals (EPs) as well; that is, physicians plus physician assistants, nurse practitioners, midwives, clinical psychologists, physical therapists, language therapists, and others.

Eligible health care professionals (EPs) who work with a qualified MOC entity and complete certain other requirements will qualify for a bonus of .5 percent in 2013 and 2014. The 2014 MOC incentive will be paid as a lump sum amount in March 2015, in addition to the 2014 PQRS incentive. Through successful PQRS reporting in 2013 and 2014, participants will avoid the penalty payment adjustments of 2015 and 2016 respectively. As with the CMS programs for electronic prescribing and meaningful use of an electronic health record, the sooner that medical groups enter and qualify for PQRS, the more likely they will end up with a positive cumulative payment over three years, instead of a negative one.

The American Academy of Family Physicians has calculated that a three-physician practice with annual revenue of $1.425 million and a 20 percent Medicare patient mix would have the opportunity to gain as much as $2,850 over three years if it qualified for PQRS at the earliest (in 2013). A practice that didn't qualify until 2014 would gain $1,425 but could lose $4,275 in 2015, while a practice that didn't start on PQRS until 2015 could lose as much as $4,275, with no possibility of offsetting gain.

Additionally, if the practice didn't participate in PQRS, it can't participate in the Value-Based Modifier Program, which carries another 2 percent penalty, or $5,800. If it also didn't participate in EHR or meet meaningful use benchmarks in 2014, it would be penalized another $5,800 (3 percent, or $8,700 next year). Altogether, PQRS is aligned with up to $15,875 in potential penalties for this hypothetical group of family physicians.

To qualify for the 2014 PQRS incentive payment (to be made as a lump sum payment in March 2014), CMS provides a variety of reporting methods for individual eligible professionals and group practices. The number of measures required for reporting, as well as the required percent of patient encounters for data submission, varies depending on the reporting method chosen and whether the reporting is accomplished as an individual professional or as a group practice. For example, individual eligible professionals may choose between claims, electronic health records (EHR), qualified registry or (new for 2014) qualified clinical data registry (QCDR) reporting methods. Group practices may report using a qualified registry, the group practice reporting option (GPRO) web-based interface (for groups of 25+ EPs), EHR or (new for 2014) a CMS-certified survey vendor.

For the 2014 PQRS, there are a total of 284 individual quality measures from which to choose. In addition, there are twenty-five separate measures groups—groupings of at least four clinically related measures—for use primarily by specialists. However, not all of these measures may be reported by each reporting method. For example, only 64 measures may be reported via EHR, 111 by claims, 200 by registry, and 22 for the GPRO web-based interface. To participate in the 2014 PQRS program, individual eligible professionals or groups of 2+ eligible professionals must self-nominate by October 15, 2014, and state their chosen reporting method.[209]

Practices may report on their own or they may use a registry service. Many physicians who have looked at these issues have formed the opinion that registry is the best option for most, as it will save staff time and provider time.

---

[209] AMA, Physician Quality Measure Reporting. http://www.ama-assn.org/ama/pub/physician-resources/clinical-practice-improvement/clinical-quality/physician-quality-reporting-system.page

CMS paid out $261,733,236 in PQRS incentives in program year 2011 to the 27 percent of professionals eligible to participate. That included 26,515 practices with 266,521 eligible professionals. CMS estimated that more than 1 million professionals were eligible to participate. The average amount paid out per EP was $1,059.

5.2.3 Current State

With the publication of the Final PFS Rule in November 2014, CMS outlined revised technical requirements for the 2014 PQRS incentive payment of +.5 percent and reporting specifications to avoid the 2016 PQRS penalty of -2.0 percent. Such revisions to PQRS may impact successful participation in other CMS value-based initiatives which can put up to 7 percent of Medicare Part B reimbursements at risk.

Both skeptics and supporters of the PQRS initiative may wish to regard this piece of the federal government's QI agenda as an evolving work in progress. Most doctors, even those who are on board with the QI program, haven't fully engaged with PQRS and stand to lose a significant amount of annual revenue as a result.

The majority of physicians support the movement toward assuring quality in medical practice. As David M. Shahian, MD, wrote in 2011, "Practitioners should not fear the increasing emphasis on performance measurement—it is impossible to improve what you cannot measure, and we all want the very best for our patients. Quality care is our professional responsibility, and it is a challenge and an opportunity that we must embrace."[210]

That doesn't mean it's easy. "There is so much happening, with exchanges, with value-based modifiers, with PQRS," said Lawrence Kosinski, MD, a gastroenterologist in Elgin, Illinois. "There is a significant slope of knowledge [physicians] have to take on. The government for the first time has access to data that they've never had before, because of the EHR and because of the

---

[210] David M. Shahian, MD, "Clinical Data Registries and the Future of Healthcare Quality" (editorial), Progress in Pediatric Cardiology 32 (2011) 71–74. December 2011. http://www.ppc-journal.com/article/S1058-9813%2811%2900060-9/fulltext

large registries that have been developed. They're starting to flex their muscles on the providers."[211]

Some physicians have serious doubts about whether PQRS is entirely the right methodology to achieve these aims. Many of the metrics are "straw dogs," said Arthur Palamara, MD, a vascular surgeon in Broward County, Florida. An active delegate to the American Medical Association (AMA) from Florida and a former head of the county medical association, Palamara is as plugged into the medical community as any doctor is likely to be. "There's a lot of things that we as organized medicine could have done but never did," he said. "Does government have a role in improving outcomes? Absolutely. There needs to be certain goals built in and ways of documenting whether physicians are supporting them. It's metrics. I'm a big supporter."[212]

Still, he has serious reservations about the direction the Medicare authorities are going. For one thing, too many of the metrics are based on billing codes, which are not sufficient to ascertain a physician's level of care. For a vascular surgeon, he points out, a useful measure of quality might be whether the patient has been discharged on a statin, on Plavix, or on an ACE inhibitor. "The difficulty is, are you going to be able to document whether that has been done or not?" he said. It's not always easy to determine whether the patient has actually filled the prescription—and if she has, whether she is taking the medication as indicated. The concept of pay-for-performance "puts the burden on us. If the patient didn't comply, then we're the person who is criticized for not fulfilling our responsibilities," he observed.

Alicia Cool, MD, an internist in Maryland, described her irritation at the fact that her reimbursement is now tied "to diabetics who eat Twinkies and hypertensives and congestive heart failure patients eating steamed crabs— one of the biggest causes for admission in Baltimore. And people thinking your med list is a suggestion box [such as] the college professor who only takes his insulin sometimes and is a dead ringer for Santa Claus." She is happy to run her practice as a patient-centered medical home, "but you cannot legislate or control human behavior, and all the education in the world doesn't affect their personal habits—at least, not often."[213]

---

[211] *Lawrence Kosinski, MD, telephone interview, September 26, 2013.*

[212] *Arthur Palamara, MD, telephone interview, August 25, 2013.*

[213] *Alicia Cool, MD, email correspondence, August 16, 2013.*

In the view of William L. Rich, III, MD, director of health policy for the American Academy of Ophthalmology, the basic methodology behind the PQRS is flawed. This is in part because the mechanisms for designing and certifying measures are inadequate to the task, according to Rich. Further, he believes the requirement by Congress that the reimbursement reforms be budget-neutral was unwise. At this point, the private sector is more likely to produce meaningful quality measures that should then be adopted by CMS, he added.[214]

Robert A. Berenson, MD, a Medicare policy expert with the Urban Institute, said that CMS's current efforts "require reporting on a raft of measures of varying usefulness and validity." This may divert providers' attention from efforts to make culture and work-process improvements "that could produce larger improvements in outcomes."[215] What is missing is a commitment to invest in the "basic science" of measurement development, he said.

Berenson advocates building an infrastructure to achieve a national consensus on: "what to measure; how to collect the data needed to calculate measures; the accuracy of EHR data for use in performance measurement; how to measure the cost-effectiveness of particular measures; how to reduce the costs of data collection; what thresholds to use to ensure measure accuracy; and how to prioritize which measures to collect." With Harlan M. Krumholz, MD, at Yale, and Peter J. Pronovost, MD, at Johns Hopkins, Berenson drafted a comprehensive report for the Robert Wood Johnson Foundation assessing the state of performance measurement and public reporting.[216]

That work—creating serious, reliable, outcome-centered measures—is actually being done by specialty societies and registry services, Berenson and Rich both said, and the thoracic surgeons have been in the lead.

"We've been pushing for the federal government to use clinical data registries (when available), as opposed to claims data, for performance measurement and reimbursement," said Shahian, vice president for quality and safety at

---

[214] William L. Rich, III, MD, telephone interview, September 17, 2013.

[215] Robert A. Berenson, MD, "Seven Policy Recommendations to Improve Quality Measurement," Health Affairs blog, May 22, 2013. http://healthaffairs.org/blog/2013/05/22/seven-policy-recommendations-to-improve-quality-measurement/

[216] http://www.rwjf.org/en/research-publications/find-rwjf-research/2013/05/achieving-the-potential-of-health-care-performance-measures.html

Massachusetts General Hospital and chair of the Society of Thoracic Surgeons (STS) National Database and its Quality Measurement Task Force.[217]

The problem with claims data is they were not devised for clinical purposes, but rather for billing. They lack the granularity and specificity necessary to support the subtle distinctions that clinicians make in diagnosis and treatment. In many cases the data are entered by billing coders with limited medical knowledge.

By contrast, the clinical data put into professional registries are entered by trained data managers, who understand the minutiae of the clinical specifications (a clinical registry is a database of health information on specific clinical conditions, procedures or populations). It is important, when comparing results across hospitals, that all the important data elements are defined the same at each site. For example, there must be strict criteria for how everyone defines whether or not a patient experienced a stroke after surgery.

"I think you're going to see more and more willingness" on the part of the federal government to work with data registries, Shahian said. "And they are so much better accepted by the provider community."

Clinical data have the further strength of being better at defining homogeneous categories of procedures for the purpose of comparing results among providers. You want to compare apples to apples, Shahian said. A common misclassification issue is lumping together patients who are having a coronary artery bypass operation (isolated CABG) with other patients who are having CABG plus some other procedure (e.g., a valve repair).

"You'd like to base hospital comparisons on diagnoses and procedures that are frequent and well-defined," Shahian said. "For example, big centers like Massachusetts General Hospital do many cases in which coronary artery bypass grafting surgery (CABG) is combined with something else—a combined procedure with higher inherent risk—whereas a smaller hospital might do proportionately more lower-risk, isolated CABG procedures," he explained. It's important to base performance estimates on similar categorizations of procedures at various hospitals. Risk factors used in risk-adjustment are also much more accurate and granular when obtained from clinical as opposed to claims data.

---

[217] David M. Shahian, MD, telephone interview, September 25, 2013.

For 2013, CMS has approved some seventy-one vendors of registries qualified to handle these reporting requirements, including such familiar names as Allscripts, Fresenius, Massachusetts General Physicians Organization, Johns Hopkins Disease Registry, Rush Health, and the National Committee for Quality Assurance. Some support individual measures, others support groups of measures. They charge fees for use of their registries, unless medical groups are already members. Numerous specialty professional societies, such as the American Board of Family Medicine, American Board of Internal Medicine, American College of Cardiology Foundation, American College of Surgeons, and the STS National Database, are also listed as offering registry services.

In July 2013, CMS set forth requirements for a qualified clinical data registry. If physicians practices met the requirements and submitted nine measures from the database (up from three in 2012), they would fulfill the PQRS mandate.

The problem is that the informatics standards that CMS established "were so onerous that few if any clinical registries in the world can meet it in that time frame," Shahian said. Even the STS, which has established a reputation for good measures, will not be able to meet it.

There is no shortage of performance measures in health care. The National Quality Forum, which acts as a gatekeeper and standard-setter for medical quality measures, currently endorses nearly 700 performance measures, and there are many more measures used by individual societies, states, and payers that are not NQF-endorsed.[218]

In that case, how are doctors supposed to know which measures to pick?

"You have to have someone in the practice examine the list of measures and figure out which ones apply," Kosinski said. "If you're a primary care physician, it's easy. For a gastroenterologist, it's a little more difficult. We can't use something for diabetes or congestive heart failure."

Many PQRS measures are also measures for attesting to meaningful use of an EHR, he said, a result of CMS attempting to harmonize the various reporting requirements. That means if you're already compliant with meaningful use, "you can pick up the patient's BMI," Kosinski said. "You can also pick up 'counsel them on smoking.' You can double dip, you can meet both those requirements."

---

[218] David M. Shahian, MD, *Progress in Pediatric Cardiology* editorial.

However, CMS noted in July 2013 that less than 1 percent of the 320,422 eligible professionals participating in PQRS used the EHR-based reporting mechanism in 2011. It estimates that 50,000 EPs would use EHR reporting in 2014.[219]

Kosinski's practice, the Illinois Gastroenterology Group, had "no trouble" coming up with PQRS measures. The challenge, he said, is to arrive at a process for recording these values in the EHR that's within the normal work flow for doctors and office staff, "so people don't have to go out of their way to meet the requirements." It needs to be "built in, part of the normal everyday process of seeing patients. It's invisible."

His practice, with thirty-eight board-certified physicians spanning the Chicago region, has sufficient staff and expertise to push through remedies. "We met all the MU requirements for Stage 1—twice. We were able to do this fairly seamlessly. But if a practice is on paper, or doesn't have staff in-house, that is tough." His group is the largest gastroenterology practice in Illinois and is gearing up to handle population-based medicine for GI services. "But half the docs are in practices under five members," he commented, and their staff knowledge base isn't as large.

For a practice without deep resources, these can be expensive undertakings. Doctors might not have staff members in the office who are savvy enough to handle these new requirements. They might have to send employees to training or call in an expert consultant.

Yet in a rule published in the *Federal Register* on July 19, 2013, CMS estimated that it would cost an eligible professional who is reporting as an individual just $80 to handle the PQRS administrative burden: two hours to review the measures and pick a reporting option and three hours to review the specifications and incorporate reporting into the office work flow. So that is five hours at a $16 hourly wage, making $80. Providers may view other CMS estimates as equally far-fetched:

- Using claims-based reporting, an EP might spend between $9 to $432 to comply.

---

[219] *43508 Federal Register/Vol. 78, No. 139/Friday, July 19, 2013/Proposed Rules*

- For a group practice to submit quality measures for a year it would cost $3,160.

- It would cost a registry $160 to become qualified to submit data.

Another unresolved question is the value of public reporting on individual physicians' quality measures. As a starting point for discussion, take cardiac surgery outcomes. The basic idea is that patients will choose providers with better performance and insurance companies (and possibly Medicare and Medicaid) will steer their clients toward those providers. "Hospitals and surgeons will, in response, be motivated to excel in an effort to attract referrals," Shahian wrote in an essay for the *Journal of Cardiac Surgery*. The problem is that studies of public reporting in several states (Massachusetts, New York, Pennsylvania) "have shown limited, transient, and in some cases negligible impact of public report cards on referral patterns and market share."[220]

Berenson, too, is skeptical about how useful public reporting is as a lever to raise overall quality of medicine. "If I were running my own ACO, I would want to have a measure of the percentage of patients with chronic stable coronary disease who are getting stents." His reasoning is that stents are now regarded as overused in treating coronary disease.

But how well does this work as a publicly reported measure? Can the public grasp the subtleties (i.e., more stents might not be "better" stents)?

"I'm not sure," Berenson answers. Not only do the numbers have to be case-mix adjusted, they have to be explained in terms the public can understand and act on. This is a fundamentally different approach from applying the data for purposes of internal quality improvement. For one thing, Berenson notes, "You can afford to be wrong when data is used for internal improvement, but you can't for public reporting."

Furthermore, there is evidence that the public isn't able to use the comparative reports and prefers this data to be used internally for improvement. Focus groups conducted by David Lansky, president of the Pacific Business Group on Health, showed that patients would rather have their doctors use the comparative data to improve their own care; they don't want to use the

---

[220] David M. Shahian, MD, "Public Reporting of Cardiac Surgery Outcomes—What Do We Know, What Can We Expect?" *Journal of Cardiac Surgery*, 2010; 25:710–712. November 2010. http://onlinelibrary.wiley.com/doi/10.1111/j.1540-8191.2010.01147.x/full

information to locate a new doctor. "They have found a physician," Berenson said. "They want to trust that physician."

5.2.4 The Road Ahead

The question remains whether, even as the measures grow more sophisticated and reliable, the penalties and rewards are too small to drive changes in behavior, particularly since they take time, staff, and money to report. If the penalties were to increase to a higher proportion of a practice's revenues, the practice patterns would be more likely to change.

"Doctors want to do things that will positively impact care of patients," Shahian said. To the extent that government and commercial payers can design the incentive programs to be clinically relevant, doctors will more readily accept them as valuable. When particular measures are not seen as advancing outcomes and clinical care of their patients, then they are going to be viewed as a nuisance, and ultimately detracting from patient care. "It's a zero-sum game," Shahian said. "There are only 24 hours in a day. If you're wasting time and money on measures that don't have clinical relevance, it takes time from things that do."

Berenson doesn't intend to "throw in the towel" on measures. "I just think we should use them more opportunistically and strategically," he said. For instance, there's good literature on the fact that patients die more often on weekends. "That is unacceptable."

For all the resentment of PQRS and related reporting requirements, organized medicine has indicated a willingness to accept it if it leads to the demise of the sustainable growth rate (SGR) formula, imposed by Congress in 1999 as a way to discipline spending on physician services. The SGR, however, has never worked as intended to balance the budget. Instead, every year, Congress passes a fix to stop the SGR from cutting physicians' pay by an amount that grows more unreasonable with each annual postponement of the reckoning day. In 2013, according to the formula, payments should have been cut by almost 25 percent. Clearly, that was never going to happen. Still, despite the fact that the SGR is almost universally viewed as a flawed and outdated formula, it falls to organized medicine to lobby intensively each year to make sure Congress overturns it in time.

"Everybody knows it's a farce," said Michael L. Millenson, a health care quality expert in Highland Park, Illinois, and author of *Demanding Medical Excellence.*[221] That's why medical societies let it be known that they were willing to be paid differently. "If the alternative is, you're going to squeeze my fee-for-service reimbursements so badly and make it a bureaucratic nightmare, then all right, let's talk about another way of doing things." Pay-for-value now looks preferable to the agonizing annual fee adjustment squabble, in Millenson's view.[222]

Berenson is not aware of any groundswell to overturn the misbegotten measures. Organized medicine's No. 1 priority is to get rid of the SGR, and it is reluctant to muddy its message by asking for something else on the side. "It seems like legislators on the House side want more measurement," Berenson said. If that's what they want, "the AMA will hold their tongue. There's reasons you don't say the emperor has no clothes. The way the lobbying works, the groups that want something constrain themselves on items that are not at the top of their list. Don't spend political capital on things that are second order. I think they believe this is second order or they will have more time later to fix it."

In December 2013, a three-month temporary SGR fix averting a 23.7 percent payment cut had been incorporated into the budget bill and had been passed by committees in both houses of Congress with the president promising to sign the bill. The challenge of finding a permanent substitution for the SGR was pushed into 2014. The legislative language in the bill creates a three-month transition period prior to the final sunsetting of the SGR. During this time congressional committees will finalize language to permanently eliminate the SGR formula. Legislative language to replace the SGR won't be finalized until March 2014. However, Congressional committees have discussed replacing the SGR with a ten-year freeze in Medicare reimbursement rates and additional

[221] Michael L. Millenson, *Demanding Medical Excellence: Doctors and Accountability in the Information Age.* University of Chicago Press, 1997.
http://press.uchicago.edu/ucp/books/book/chicago/D/bo3683442.html

[222] David Pittman, "SGR Repeal Bill Gains Broad Support," *MedPage Today,* July 23, 2013.
http://www.medpagetoday.com/PublicHealthPolicy/Medicare/40646

value-based incentives and penalties to improve the quality of patient care and lower costs.[223]

In a sign of further loosening by CMS, the agency also agreed in late 2013 to allow specialty societies to determine the measures that their physicians would report starting in January 2014. Doctors would need to send in data on nine quality measures covering at least three domains established by the National Quality Strategy. At least one measure should deal with patient outcomes. The new rule would create more incentive for specialists to participate in PQRS and give them opportunities to take control of the process, which had until then been directed toward primary care doctors, a physician told Modern Healthcare.[224]

Thus, through this unlikely combination of legislative initiatives, such as the HITECH Act and the ACA, and through sheer economic pressure on the federal budget, as evinced in the SGR, quality measurement and pay-for-value are gaining a degree of traction that had eluded policymakers and health care visionaries for some fifteen years.

Even if the measures and methodologies for improving quality are "still in evolution," Palamara said, overall, "I think we're moving in the right direction."

[223] Jessica Zigmond, "Budget bill with short-germ SGR fix clears Congress, ready for Obama to sign," Modern Healthcare, December 18, 2013.
http://www.modernhealthcare.com/article/20131218/NEWS/312189951

[224] Andis Robeznieks, "Specialists notch victory in new CMS rule on quality reporting," Modern Healthcare, December 4, 2013.
http://www.modernhealthcare.com/article/20131204/NEWS/312049948/specialists-notch-victory-in-new-cms-rule-on-quality-reporting

Section 5.3: Technical Appendix: Physician Quality Reporting System (PQRS)

5.3.1 Background

The Tax Relief and Health Care Act (TRHCA) of 2006 (Public Law 109423) mandated the secretary of Health and Human Services (HHS) implement a program to collect information related to physician-provided care for Medicare beneficiaries. The result was the creation of the Physician Quality Reporting Initiative (PQRI), which began with a trial period from July 1, 2007–December 31, 2007. In 2008, provisions contained under Section 131 of the Medicare Improvement for Patients and Providers Act of 2008 (MIPPA), expanded the PQRI to full implementation. Reflecting expectations for a broader role in CMS's emerging value-based purchasing initiative, MIPPA designated PQRI as the Physician Quality Reporting System (PQRS).

Information from the PQRS was to be used to provide the quality of care component for another MIPPA 2008 directive. HHS was to develop a program to provide confidential feedback to physicians on the resources used to provide care to Medicare beneficiaries. The resulting initiative was the Physician Resource Use Measurement and Reporting Program (Physician Feedback Program or PFP). By providing physicians with individual reports combining risk-adjusted cost and quality of care metrics to illustrate the "value" of services provided, CMS sought to:[225]

- encourage higher-quality beneficiary care

- enhance the efficiency of the medical practice

- create a transparent process to develop meaningful, actionable, and fair physician performance indicators

---

[225] http://www.gao.gov/products/GAO-11-720

- develop physician performance indicators to be used as part of CMS's value-based purchasing initiative

Much of the requisite supporting infrastructure needed to achieve the value-related aims of both the PQRS and PFP was not in place in 2008. As a result, a number of support processes were developed and related initiatives were introduced to encourage relevant physician behaviors. Parallel incentive/payment adjustment programs such as EHR and electronic prescribing (eRx) were introduced to enhance the data collection and reporting process.

With the passage in March 2010 of the ACA, physician value-related initiatives and processes were extended and enhanced under:

Title III: Improving the Quality and Efficiency of Health Care

Subtitle A: Transforming the Health Care Delivery System

- Part I: Linking Payment to Quality Outcomes Under the Medicare Program

  - Section 3002: Improvements to the Physician Quality Reporting System

  - Section 3003: Enhancements to the Physician Feedback Program

  - Section 3007: Value-Based Modifier Under the Physician Fee Schedule

5.3.2 Overview

Section 1848 of the Social Security Act (SSA) established the PQRS under subsections (a), (k), and (m). These provisions were subsequently amended by Sections 3002 and 10327 of the ACA of 2010 and Section 601(b) of the American Taxpayer Relief Act (ATRA) of 2012.

As currently configured, PQRS is a voluntary pay-for-reporting program that is structured to provide incentive payments and payment adjustments to eligible professionals to promote reporting of quality information. PQRS incentive payments will be made through 2014 to eligible professionals who satisfactorily report data on quality measures for covered physician fee schedule (PFS) services furnished to Medicare Part B fee-for-service (FFS) beneficiaries.

Beginning with the PQRS program year of 2015, PQRS becomes a "penalty-only" program with payment adjustments assessed against eligible professionals failing to achieve satisfactory reporting of quality measures related to professional covered services during a specified reporting period. Reporting periods are established as the calendar year (CY) occurring two years prior to the program calendar year. As such, reporting performance occurring during calendar years 2013 and 2014 will determine the final incentive qualification payments *and* payment adjustments for calendar years 2015 and 2016, respectively.

To provide the greatest flexibility in the reporting of quality data, the PQRS has been designed by CMS as a multifaceted system allowing reporting customization based on the unique needs and capabilities of each provider. To account for variations in patient populations and supporting practice infrastructure, many options for reporting quality data have been provided to encourage participation. With each option selected, requisite standards for satisfactory reporting differ, depending on:

- **specifications of selected measures for reporting**: The Medical Characteristics of Patients, Medical Demographics, Required Reporting Frequency, Reporting Method, Reportable Codes, and Selection of Individual Measures or Measures Groups to report

- **selected reporting period**: six months or twelve months

- **submitter status**: Individual Reporting or Group Reporting

- **manner of report submission:** claims, registry, EHR, and (new for 2014 reporting) QCDR

In addition, participation in other quality programs requiring data collection and reporting further complicate the choices facing providers. The eRx initiative and the EHR incentive program require additional levels of technological complexity and add another layer of specifications to required reporting.

5.3.3 PQRS-Related Programs

As configured for 2014 reporting, there are several related quality programs using data collected through PQRS that have the potential to financially impact providers:

	INCENTIVES OFFERED	PENALTIES ASSESSED
1. traditional PQRS reporting	2014	2015 forward
2. maintenance of certification (MOC)	2014	None
3. EHR incentive program	2014–2016	2015 forward
4. eRx	None	2014
5. physician value-based modifier (VBM)	None	2015 forward
6. Medicare Shared Savings Program	Payment adjustments are dependent on program performance.	

In addition, the ACA mandated the creation of a Physician Compare website to allow consumers to search for physicians and other health care professionals who provide Medicare services. CMS will post the first set of PQRS-reported quality measure data on the site in CY2014, reflecting data collected no sooner than program year 2012. These data will include PQRS GPRO measures for group practices and Accountable Care Organizations (ACOs).

Each of these programs will be covered in detail below, to include satisfactory participation requirements and information on how incentives can be earned and penalties/payment adjustments avoided. The following summarizes program-associated projected incentives and penalties:

5.3.4 Table 1: CMS PQRS and Associated Programs: Incentives and Penalties

| Year | eRx | EHR Incentive Program | | PQRS Program | | MOC | Value-Based Modifier | | Annual Penalty/Incentive Range[4] | Annual Net Potential |
	eRx Penalty	EHR Incentive	EHR Penalty	PQRS Incentive	PQRS Penalty	MOC Incentive	VBM Incentive[3]	VBM Penalty		
2014	-2.0%	Fixed Pay	0	+.5%	0	+.5%	+1.0% to +3.0%	0.0% to -2.0%	-4.0% to + 4%	0.00%
2015	0	Fixed Pay	-1% to -2%[1]	0	-1.5%	0	+1.0% to +3.0%	0.0% to -2.0%	-5.5% to +3.0%	-2.5%
2016	0	Fixed pay	-2%	0	-2.0%	0	+1.0% to +3.0%	0.0% to -2.0%	-6.0% to +3.0%	-3.0%
2017	0	0	-3%	0	-2.0%	0	+1.0% to +3.0%	0.0% to -2.0%	-7.0% to +3.0%	-4.0%
2018 On	0	0	-4% to -5%[2]	0	-2.0%	0	+1.0% to +3.0%	0.0% to -2.0%	-9.0% to +3.0%	-6.0%

1. Under HITECH Act Rules, EHR users who fail to achieve meaningful use for 2015 (2013 reporting year) *and* were subject to the eRx penalty in 2014, (2013 reporting year) will receive a -2% EHR penalty in 2015.

2. For 2018 and thereafter, if the Secretary HHS determines that less than 75% of eligible professionals meet EHR meaningful use criteria, penalties can be increased by 1% per year, not to exceed a maximum of 5%.

3. The calculation of the VBM incentive payment involves the application of an annual modifier to ensure budget neutrality. For purposes of the chart, a modifier amount of 1.0% was assumed. The actual modifier amount will be determined after calculation of total penalty dollars is made.

4. Ranges presented represent the consequences of **not meeting any** program requirements (penalty) or **fully meeting** all program requirements (incentive).

5.3.5 Eligible Professionals for PQRS Reporting

Overview

Eligible Professionals (EPs) are individuals who provide covered professional services for Medicare beneficiaries that are paid under the Medicare PFS. EPs are identified on claims by their individual National Provided Identifier (NPI) and Tax Identification Number (TIN). Providers included in this definition are:[226]

- **Medicare Physicians**: Doctor of Medicine; Doctor of Osteopathy; Doctor of Podiatric Medicine; Doctor of Optometry; Doctor of Oral Surgery; Doctor of Dental Medicine; and Doctor of Chiropractic.

- **Practitioners**: Physician Assistant; Nurse Practitioner*; Clinical Nurse Specialist*; Certified Registered Nurse Anesthetist* (and Anesthesiologist Assistant); Certified Nurse Midwife*; Clinical Social Worker; Clinical Psychologist; Registered Dietician; Nutrition Professional; and Audiologists. *This list includes Advanced Practice Registered Nurse (APRN).

---

[226] http://www.cms.gov/Medicare/Quality-Initiatives-Patient-Assessment-Instruments/PQRS/index.html?redirect=/pqrs

- **Therapists**: Physical Therapist; Occupational Therapist; and Qualified Speech-Language Therapist.

  Practitioners and Therapists are excluded from PQRS reporting as part of the EHR incentive program.

- In the 2011 Physician Quality Reporting System and eRx Reporting Experience and Trends Report, published in March of 2013, CMS reported that the overall participation rate for PQRS-eligible providers was 29 percent. Out of 1,101,773 eligible providers, 320,422 participated in PQRS. In the final CY2014 Final PFS Rule, CMS estimated that the overall PQRS participation rate "hovers around 25 percent."

Excluded (Non-Eligible) Professionals

All PFS payments to EPs qualify for PQRS incentive payments and/or payment adjustments. However, services payable under fee schedules or methodologies other than the PFS are not included in PQRS, even if such service is provided by a recognized EP. Non-PQRS eligible services would include those provided by:

- federally qualified health centers
- independent diagnostic testing facilities
- independent laboratories
- hospitals (including method I critical access hospitals)
- rural health clinics
- ambulance providers
- ambulatory surgery center facilities

5.3.6 PQRS Incentives and Penalties

Background

Beginning in 2007, CMS established an incentive system to encourage participation in the PQRS. Incentive payments will continue to be available to reward satisfactory reporting through 2014. However, beginning in 2015, PQRS incentives will no longer be offered. Instead, payment adjustments (penalties) will be assessed against eligible providers who fail to achieve satisfactory reporting under PQRS.

2014 Base PQRS Incentive Payments:

- The final reporting year for qualification to receive the +.5 percent PQRS incentive is CY2014.

- To qualify for incentive payments, participants must achieve:

  - **satisfactory reporting**: This means that measures were reported using the claims, EHR, registry or GPRO methods and standards were achieved.

  OR

  - **satisfactory participation**: This is a new term introduced in the CY2014 Final PFS Rule that applies to the use of a Qualified Clinical Data Registry (QCDR) by an EP to satisfy the PQRS, beginning with 2014 reporting.

- Incentive amounts are paid as a lump sum to EPs who satisfactorily reported PQRS in the year following the reporting period.

- The allowed PQRS incentive is a percentage of the total estimated Medicare Part B allowed fee-for-service (FFS) charges for all covered services furnished by the EP during the reporting period. For participating group practices, this incentive amount is based on the estimated Medicare Part B allowed charges for all covered services furnished by the group.

2014 Enhanced PQRS Incentive for Maintenance of Certification (MOC) Participation

- **MOC 2014 incentive:**

  - An additional +.5 percent incentive payment is available for 2014 only to PQRS EPs who elect to participate in an additional MOC program. MOC participants may use any of the approved reporting mechanisms to meet the data submission requirements of PQRS, but must participate in an extensive specialty recertification program to qualify for incentive payment.

  - MOC program means a continuous assessment program, such as a qualified American Board of Medical Specialties MOC program or an equivalent program that advances quality and the lifelong learning and self-assessment of board-certified specialty physicians by focusing on the six core competencies of patient care, medical knowledge, practice-based learning, interpersonal and communication skills, and professionalism. Such a program must include the following:

    - **licensure and professional standing**: The program requires physicians to maintain a valid unrestricted license in the United States.

    - **lifelong learning and self-assessment**: The program requires physicians to participate in educational and self-assessment programs that require an assessment of what was learned.

    - **cognitive expertise**: The program requires physicians to demonstrate, through a formalized secure examination, that they have the fundamental diagnostic skills, medical knowledge, and clinical judgment to provide quality care in their respective specialties.

    - **practice assessment**: The program requires successful completion of a qualified MOC program practice assessment.

- **MOC recertification process:**[227]

    o Through the MOC program, EPs or group practices must work with a MOC entity that will recertify physicians through the American Board of Medical Specialties (ABMS) MOC process. EPs must participate in, and successfully pass, a MOC recertification program at a "greater frequency required to qualify for, or maintain, board certification." The frequency of review is defined by the qualified MOC program. Currently there are twenty-four participating member boards of the ABMS to conduct the MOC evaluation.

- **MOC reporting requirements:**

    o EPs may participate in a MOC program as an individual physician or as a member of a selected group practice. PQRS data submission may be made by any CMS-approved method to meet the following:

        ▪ EPs must satisfactorily submit data on quality measures under Physician Quality Reporting, using an approved reporting method of choice.

        ▪ Data must be submitted for a twelve-month period.

Note: Although the MOC incentive is available only through 2014, CMS is evaluating the feasibility of incorporating MOC reporting into a "composite of measures" of quality provided under the VBM program for all providers.

PQRS Payment Adjustment Penalties 2015–2021:

- Beginning with the initial reporting year of CY2013, payment adjustment penalties will be applied two years later to any eligible professional who fails to satisfactorily report PQRS.

- Currently, payment adjustments are planned to occur through CY2021 (reporting year CY2019).

---

[227] *http://www.cms.gov/Medicare/Quality-Initiatives-Patient-Assessment-Instruments/PQRS/Maintenance_of_Certification_Program_Incentive.html*

- Program year payment adjustment penalties are levied as a percentage reduction in overall Medicare Part B PFS reimbursements.

- For CY2016 (CY2014 reporting year) and forward, the PQRS penalty is -2.0 percent (providers would be reimbursed at a rate of 98 percent of allowed charges).

5.3.7 PQRS Quality Measures

The core function of the PQRS is the collection and reporting of information related to the provision of health care to patients. As such, a number of quality measures are used for annual reporting by individual providers or group practices. Measures listings are published each year by CMS and reporting may be accomplished by the collection of data for individual measures or established "measures groups."

Overview

Defined by the Agency for Health Care Research and Quality (AHRQ) as "a quantitative tool (e.g., rate, ratio, index, percentage) that provides an indication of performance in relation to a specified process or outcome," PQRS measures fall into one of three broad categories:[228]

- **process measure**: a measure that focuses on a process that leads to a certain outcome, meaning that a scientific basis exists for believing that the process, when executed well, will increase the probability of achieving a desired outcome

- **outcome measure**: a measure that indicates the result of the performance (or nonperformance) of a function(s) or process(es)

- **structure measure**: a measure that assesses whether organizational resources and arrangements are in place to deliver health care, such as the number, type, and distribution of medical personnel, equipment, and facilities

---

[228] *Agency for Health Care Research & Quality (AHRQ) National Quality Measures Clearinghouse Glossary*

To ensure alignment with the three broad aims of the National Quality Strategy (NQS), CMS has aligned each measure with one of six domains for quality measurement.

- **NQS aims**:[229]

    o **patient safety:** better care—improve the overall quality, by making health care more patient-centered, reliable, accessible, and safe.

    o **population/public health:** healthy people and communities—improve the health of the US population by supporting proven interventions to address behavioral, social, and environmental determinants of health in addition to delivering higher-quality care.

    o **improved clinical process/effectiveness**: affordable care—reduce the cost of quality health care for individuals, families, employers, and government.

- **CMS-Adopted Domains for Quality Measurement**:

    o Clinical Care; Care Coordination; Population and Community Health; Efficiency and Cost Reduction; Safety and Person/Caregiver Experiences; and Outcomes.

PQRS Individual Measures

Individual PQRS measures reflect specific aspects of patient health care that represent recognized standards of care. These measures encourage adherence to standards related to various aspects of care, such as prevention, chronic and acute-care management, procedure-related care, resource utilization, and care coordination.

- Measures are developed by the National Committee for Quality Assurance (NCQA) or other organizations that provide consensus-based guidelines for care, such as the American Medical Association (AMA), the American Heart Association (AHA), the Physician Consortium for Performance Improvement® (PCPI), and others.

---

[229] http://www.healthcare-informatics.com/article/aligning-emeasures-national-quality-strategy

Developers ensure that measures are aligned with the National Quality Strategy and the six CMS domains for quality measurement. Upon approval for inclusion in the PQRS, each measure is assigned an individual PQRS identifying number and an accompanying National Quality Forum (NQF) number if the measure is NQF-endorsed.

- For 2014, there are a total of 284 individual measures as listed in Table 52 of the CY2014 Final PFS rule. Each measure is listed and fully described in a PQRS Measures Specifications Manual and has a specific set of reporting instructions and a required method for reporting assigned to it. Participants must ensure that specified information is collected and reported through the appropriate mechanism as described in the 2014 PQRS Specifications Manual.[230]

PQRS Measures Groups

To provide an alternative to the reporting of individual measures, CMS has created a measures groups reporting process. Measures groups are composed of four or more individual PQRS measures that are all related to a specific clinical condition or share a common process/outcome focus. Use of measures groups is particularly useful for EPs who have many patients with the same or similar medical conditions. For 2014, CMS has established twenty-five measures groups as follows:

MEASURES GROUP TITLE	INDIVIDUAL MEASURES	REPORTING OPTIONS*	MEASURES GROUP** G-CODE
diabetes mellitus (DM)	5	registry	G8485
chronic kidney disease (CKD)	4	registry	G8487
preventive care	9	registry	G8486
coronary artery bypass graft (CABG)	10	registry	G8544

[230] Page 839, Table 52, CMS-1600-FC: Centers for Medicare & Medicaid Services Regulation #: CMS-1600-FC; Display Date: 2013-11-27; Publication Date: 2013-12-10; Calendar Year: 2014; Regulation Type: Final Rule with Comment ... http://www.cms.gov/Medicare/Medicare-Fee-for-Service-Payment/PhysicianFeeSched/PFS-Federal-Regulation-Notices-Items/CMS-1600-FC.html

rheumatoid arthritis (RA)	6	registry	G8490
perioperative care	4	registry	GG8492
back pain	4	registry	G8493
hepatitis C	8	registry	G8545
heart failure (HF)	4	registry	G8548
coronary artery disease (CAD)	4	registry	G8489
ischemic vascular disease (IVD)	4	registry	G8547
HIV/AIDS	6	registry	G8491
asthma	4	registry	G8645
chronic obstructive pulmonary disease (COPD	5	registry	G8898
inflammatory bowel disease (IBD)	8	registry	G8899
sleep apnea	4	registry	G8900
dementia	9	registry	G8902
Parkinson's disease	6	registry	G8903
hypertension (HTN)	8	registry	G8904
cardiovascular prevention	6	registry	G8905
cataracts	4	registry	G8906
oncology	8	registry	G8977
total knee replacement (new for 2014)	4	registry	to be published
general surgery (new for 2014)	5	registry	to be published
optimizing patient exposure to ionizing radiation (new for 1024)	6	registry	to be published

*Beginning with 2014 reporting, measures groups may only be reported through the registry reporting option.[231]

**Submission of the measures group G-code serves as indication that an EP is choosing to report on a specific measures group and CMS analysis is initiated.

Note: Tables 55 through 79 (pages 1091–1107) of CMS-1600-FC: Centers for Medicare & Medicaid Services specify the final measures groups that are reportable for the PQRS for 2014 and beyond.

---

[231] Page 1091 52, CMS-1600-FC: Centers for Medicare & Medicaid Services Regulation #: CMS-1600-FC; Display Date: 2013-11-27; Publication Date: 2013-12-10; Calendar Year: 2014; Regulation Type: Final Rule with Comment ... http://www.cms.gov/Medicare/Medicare-Fee-for-Service-Payment/PhysicianFeeSched/PFS-Federal-Regulation-Notices-Items/CMS-1600-FC.html

5.3.8 PQRS Reporting: Considerations for Measures Selection

Overview

- Providers have the choice of PQRS reporting as an individual provider, using their individual National Provider Identifier (NPI) or as a group, reporting under a common Tax Identification Number (TIN).

- In addition, CMS provides options for reporting of selected individual measures or groups of similar measures through several reporting mechanisms. The 2014 PQRS submission of quality data may be accomplished through claims, registry, EHR or through the GPRO. In addition, starting in 2014, PQRS reporting may be accomplished through a QCDR or through the use of a new CMS-certified survey vendor. Regardless of the selected reporting option, the general reporting process is similar.

- Providers select clinical measures from an annually updated list provided by CMS that most closely match the medical characteristics of their Medicare patient population. The selection of measures for reporting can be for individual measures or for measures groups. At a minimum, the following factors should be taken into consideration by PQRS participants when selecting measures:

- clinical conditions usually treated:
  - o measures that do not or seldom apply to their Medicare patients should not be selected for reporting

- election to use measures groups:
  - o This option should only be selected if *all* the measures within the group reflect services provided to Medicare patients.

- types of care typically provided:
  - o preventive, chronic or acute

- settings where care is usually delivered:
  - o in-office, emergency department (ED) or surgical suite

- annual quality improvement goals.

Annual Measures Specifications

- In order to correctly report data, providers research measure (or measures groups) reporting requirements/options found in the applicable PQRS Specification Manual and review clinical recommendations related to each measure.

- Within the Specifications Manual, each measure or measures group description contains specific reporting requirements. Most importantly, information is provided on two major components for reporting, which allows for the calculation of the percentage of a defined population that receives a specific process of care or achieves a particular outcome:

  - a defined denominator component:

    - This is a description of eligible cases for the measure and is identified by specific ICD-9-CM, CPT Category I, and HCPCS codes, patient demographics, and place of service.

  - a defined numerator component:

    - This component identifies the clinical action required by the measure for reporting and performance as listed in the Specification Manual. The measure specification includes reporting instructions for the measure and the applicable quality data codes (QDC) to be used.

Note: The Measures PQRS Specifications Manuals for Individual and Measures Groups may be viewed at:
http://www.cms.gov/Medicare/Quality-Initiatives-Patient-Assessment-Instruments/PQRS/MeasuresCodes.html

General Measures Reporting Guidelines

- To ensure credit for reporting, providers must assign the appropriate identifying QDC (CPT Category II or "G" code) for each measure or measures group to indicate patient care provided. To view 2014 QDC information, consult the 2014 PQRS Measures Groups Specifications, Release Notes to be published on the CMS.gov website.[232]

---

[232] *http://www.cms.gov/Medicare/Quality-Initiatives-Patient-Assessment-Instruments/PQRS/MeasuresCodes.html*

- For submission of measures data, providers must select the reporting mechanism that is appropriate for the selected measure. EPs can choose more than one reporting option (individual measures or measures groups) but can only earn a maximum of one incentive payment.

- All applicable measures within a group must be reported for each patient within the sample that meets the required criteria (such as age or gender).

Note: Annual reporting requirements (and associated incentives/payment adjustments) vary depending on selected reporting mechanism, election of reporting as an individual provider or as a group, and reporting of individual measures versus measures groups.

The Measure Applicability Validation (MAV) Process[233]

- For each PQRS reporting year, CMS uses a process to ensure the validity of individual measures reported. The Measure Applicability Validation (MAV) process is used to determine an appropriate number of reported measures for providers meeting minimum reporting standards.

- For those eligible providers who report fewer than nine measures covering three NQS domains via the registry or claims-based reporting option for the 2014 reporting year, the MAV process will determine whether they should have submitted additional measures through a two-step evaluation process: a "clinical relation" test and a "minimum threshold" test.

- **clinical relation test**: This test is based on:

  o the assumption that if EPs submit data for a measure, then that measure applies to their practice.

  o and the concept that if one measure in a cluster of measures is applicable to an EP's practice, then other closely related measures (measures in that same cluster) may also be applicable.

---

[233] *http://www.cms.gov/Medicare/Quality-Initiatives-Patient-Assessment-Instruments/PQRS/Downloads/2013_PQRS_MeasureApplicabilityValidation_Docs_030413.zip*

- **minimum threshold test**: This test is based on:

  o the concept that during the 2014 reporting year, if an EP treated more than a certain number of Medicare patients with a condition to which a certain measure applied (that is, the EP treated more than a "threshold" number of patients or encounters), then that EP should be accountable for submitting the QDC(s) for that measure.

Note: As reported in the CY2014 Final PFS Rule, the 2014 MAV process for registry-reported measures will "be similar to the "clinical relation" test used in the 2013 claims MAV process.

- Those who fail the validation process will not earn the 2014 PQRS incentive payment and may be subject to the 2016 payment adjustment.

- A description of the current claims MAV process is available at: http://www.cms.gov/Medicare/Quality-Initiatives-Patient-Assessment-Instruments/PQRS/AnalysisAndPayment.html

- CMS will post a guidance document on the 2014 claims MAV process, which will include a list of the measure clusters that are used for the "minimum threshold" test, prior to January 1, 2014 (the start of the 2014 reporting periods).

5.3.9 PQRS Reporting Options

Overview

The selection of a reporting mechanism results from an evaluation of a number of variables:

- the decision to report individual measures or measures groups

- the required reporting option assigned to each measure or measures group in the Specifications Manual

- the type and number of eligible professionals within a practice

- the level of a participant's technological support infrastructure

- participation in available incentive/payment adjustment programs

The available options for PQRS reporting has evolved from a singular "claims-only" choice, provided in 2007, to the current suite of alternative mechanisms. By combining a wider range of reporting options with an established plan of participation incentives and non-participation penalties, CMS seeks to meet the unique needs of each provider and encourage participation.

Reporting Mechanisms:

Satisfactory PQRS reporting to qualify for the 2014 +.5 percent incentive payments or to avoid the CY2016 payment adjustment may be accomplished through several mechanisms which are specific to individual professional reporting or group practice reporting:

MECHANISM	AVAILABLE AS OPTION TO:
claims reporting	individuals
reporting through a qualified registry	individuals and groups of 2+ EPs
EHR (new for groups in 2014)	individuals and groups of 2+ EPs
GPRO web-based interface	groups of 25+ EPs
qualified clinical data registry (new for 2014)	individuals
certified survey vendor (new for 2014)	groups of 25+ EPs

5.3.10 Individual Eligible Professional PQRS Reporting

Individual EPs submitting PQRS data for the 2014 reporting year (2016 program year) may submit data using claims reporting, qualified registry, the QCDR reporting option, or through their EHR systems.

The Claims Reporting Option for Individual Eligible Professionals

- For claims reporting of PQRS, data is recorded and submitted through the Medicare Part B PFS professional-services claims, either through the paper-based CMS 1500 claim form or the equivalent electronic transaction claim, the 837-P.

- This method is readily available to all providers as part of a routine billing process and does not require any registration or CMS notification. CMS is alerted to provider intention to use the claims reporting option by the inclusion of QDC on the service lines of the PFS claim. The claims reporting option is the most widely used method of PQRS reporting with more than 70 percent of PQRS participants opting for this method of measures reporting.[234]

- Providers submit claims using their individual National Provider Identifier (NPI) and PQRS data is extracted by CMS and routed through the CMS national claims history (NCH) file to a designated analysis contractor for processing. EPs will be provided confidential feedback reports by CMS on incentive qualification.

- For 2014, 111 individual measures (of 284) are available for claims reporting (versus 151 measures out of 259 for 2013). However, beginning in 2014, measures groups reporting will no longer be available through the claims option and will only be possible through the QCDR reporting option.

- It is important that EPs using this option consult the most current CMS Specification Manual to ensure that claims reporting is available for the measures they select.

- All claims for services that occur during a calendar year must be processed and submitted by no later than the last Friday of the second month after the end of the reporting period. For all claims occurring through December 31, 2014, data submission must be made by February 27, 2015.

- CMS will provide confirmation of receipt for PQRS data submission to providers via use of the remittance advice (RA)/explanation of benefits (EOB) denial code N365. This denial code reads: "This procedure code is not payable. It is for reporting/information purposes only." When a

[234] http://www.facs.org/ahp/pqrs/2013/2011_Experience_Report.pdf

QDC is reported satisfactorily (by the individual EP), the N365 indicates that the claim will be used for calculating incentive eligibility.

- PQRS participants selecting claims reporting may elect to be evaluated under four different options:

  - Each option has different reporting requirements regarding numbers of measures and numbers or percentage of patients that must be reported on.

  - All options allow for reporting of individual measures and no option is available for measures groups reporting for 2014.

  - Each claims reporting option requires a twelve-month reporting period.

  - Each option is discussed below.

For more information on claims reporting, see Medicare Quality Reporting Incentive Programs Manual Chapter 1—The Physician Quality Reporting System 50.1—Claims-based Reporting Mechanism at:

http://www.cms.gov/Regulations-and-Guidance/Guidance/Manuals/downloads/qri122c01.pdf

The following lists the claims reporting options for CY2014 to qualify for the +.5 percent 2014 incentive and avoid the 2016 payment adjustment of 2.0 percent:[235]

Table 2: CY2014 PQRS Individual EP Claims Reporting Options for 2014 Incentive Qualification:

Note: Meeting these requirements will also avoid the 2016 payment adjustment.

---

[235] *Pages 803–804, Tables 47–48, CMS-1600-FC: Centers for Medicare & Medicaid Services Regulation #: CMS-1600-FC; Display Date: 2013-11-27; Publication Date: 2013-12-10; Calendar Year: 2014; Regulation Type: Final Rule with Comment ... http://www.cms.gov/Medicare/Medicare-Fee-for-Service-Payment/PhysicianFeeSched/PFS-Federal-Regulation-Notices-Items/CMS-1600-FC.html*

REPORTING PERIOD	MEASURE TYPE	REPORTING MECHANISM	SATISFACTORY REPORTING CRITERIA/SATISFACTORY PARTICIPATION CRITERIA
12-month CY2014	individual measures	claims	Reporting to earn the 2014 incentive payment and avoid the 2016 payment adjustment: • Report at least nine measures covering at least three NQS domains *and* report each measure for at least 50 percent of the Medicare Part B FFS patients seen during the reporting period to which the measure applies. Measures with a 0 percent performance rate would not be counted. OR • If fewer than nine measures covering at least three NQS domains apply to the EP, report 1–8 measures covering 1–3 NQS domains *and* report each measure for at least 50 percent of the Medicare Part B FFS patients seen during the reporting period to which the measure applies. Measures with a 0 percent performance rate would not be counted.* *For an EP who reports fewer than nine measures covering three NQS domains via the claims-based reporting mechanism, the EP will be subject to the MAV process, which would allow CMS to determine whether an EP should have reported QDC for additional measures and/or covering additional NQS domains.*

Table 3: CY2014 PQRS Individual EP Claims Reporting Options for Avoidance of 2016 Payment Adjustment

REPORTING PERIOD	MEASURE TYPE	REPORTING MECHANISM	SATISFACTORY REPORTING CRITERIA/SATISFACTORY PARTICIPATION CRITERIA
12-month CY2014	individual measures	claims	Reporting to avoid 2016 payment adjustment *and* earn 2014 incentive of +.5% • Report at least nine measures covering at least three NQS domains *and* report each measure for at least 50 percent of the Medicare Part B FFS patients seen during the reporting period to which the measure applies. Measures with a 0 percent performance rate would not be counted. OR • If fewer than nine measures covering at least three NQS domains apply to the eligible professional, report 1–8 measures covering 1–3 NQS domains *and* report each measure for at least 50 percent of the Medicare Part B FFS patients seen during the reporting period to which the measure applies. Measures with a 0 percent performance rate would not be counted.* *For an EP who reports fewer than nine measures covering three NQS domains via the claims-based*

				reporting mechanism, the EP will be subject to the MAV process, which would allow CMS to determine whether an EP should have reported QDC for additional measures and/or covering additional NQS domains.
				Reporting to avoid 2016 payment adjustment *only* **(does not qualify participant for 2014 incentive payment):** • Report at least three measures *and* report each measure for at least 50 percent of the EP's Medicare Part B FFS patients seen during the reporting period to which the measure applies. Measures with a 0 percent performance rate will not be counted. **OR** • If fewer than three measures apply to the EP, report 1–3 measures* *and* report each measure for at least 50 percent of the EP's Medicare Part B FFS patients seen during the reporting period to which the measure applies. Measures with a 0 percent performance rate will not be counted. Subject to MAV evaluation.

Qualified Registry Reporting For Individual Eligible Professionals

• A "registry" is a CMS-approved data vendor that is able to report PQRS data to CMS, on behalf of individual EPs and for group practices using the GPRO.

• As reported in the 2011 PQRS Experience Report (published in March 2013), 16 percent of PQRS-participating providers used qualified registries to submit individual measures data and 4 percent reported measures groups using registry reporting.[236]

• For 2014 reporting, a qualified registry must be able to collect all needed data elements and transmit to CMS the data at the TIN/NPI level for at least nine measures covering at least three of the NQS domains.

• Only the registry reporting method provides an option for a twelve-month or six-month reporting period, for measures groups only (1/1/13–12/31/13 or 07/01/13–12/31/13).

---

[236] http://www.facs.org/ahp/pqrs/2013/2011_Experience_Report.pdf

- Registry-based reporting of measures groups can include non-Medicare patients. However, the **majority** must be Medicare Part B patients.

- Each registry has the capability to report on some or all registry-reportable individual measures or measures groups and must be certified by CMS to report on those measures.

- Selection of a registry should be made based on the specific needs of an individual practice, based on the measures the practice selects to report.

- From the 2014 listing of 284 individual measures, 200 may be reported using the registry method.[237]

- The use of a qualified registry is the only method allowed, beginning in 2014, for the reporting of measures groups.

- CMS reports that EPs using registry-based PQRS reporting have been more successful in achieving satisfactory reporting of data as opposed to the claims-based reporting method. In the CY2014 Final PFS Rules, CMS reported that 88 percent of those using the registry method of reporting successfully met PQRS requirements.

- For CMS to approve a registry for PQRS reporting, each registry must undergo an annual certification process that includes a self-nomination process and a qualification process, regardless of whether the registry was qualified for the previous program year. Registry self-nomination must occur via web by 5:00 PM EST on January 31 for the year in which the registry wishes to submit PQRS data.

- As part of the qualification process, registries are required to provide at least **one** feedback report to participants for a given reporting period in a program year (twelve-month or six-month option). Registry qualification requirements may be viewed on pages 69179-69180 FR 77

  http://www.gpo.gov/fdsys/pkg/FR-2012-11-16/pdf/2012-26900.pdf

- Once qualified, CMS includes the registry in an annual listing of approved registries. For 2013 reporting, CMS has approved 71 registry

---

[237] Page 839, Table 52, CMS-1600-FC: Centers for Medicare & Medicaid Services, http://www.cms.gov/Medicare/Medicare-Fee-for-Service-Payment/PhysicianFeeSched/PFS-Federal-Regulation-Notices-Items/CMS-1600-FC.html

vendors for PQRS reporting. A listing of these approved registries and their capabilities can be viewed at:

http://www.cms.gov/Medicare/Quality-Initiatives-Patient-Assessment-Instruments/PQRS/Registry-Reporting.html

Note: CMS will publish a final list in the summer of each program year to allow for election/changes to be made by October 15.

- Some of the approved registry vendors are also able to submit eRx incentive program data on behalf of individual EPs and GPRO group practices.

Individual Eligible Professional Registry Reporting of PQRS[238]

To earn the 2014 PQRS +.5 percent incentive using registry reporting, individual EPs should:

- identify measures most applicable to medical demographics of practice

- consult the appropriate specifications manual (Individual measures/measures groups) for data reporting requirements

- select one of the registry reporting options (below) that is applicable to the selected individual measures/measures groups

- select registry vendor based on the vendor's ability to report on relevant measures

- submit data as required

---

[238] *Pages 803–804, Tables 47–48, CMS-1600-FC: Centers for Medicare & Medicaid Services Regulation #: CMS-1600-FC; Display Date: 2013-11-27; Publication Date: 2013-12-10; Calendar Year: 2014; Regulation Type: Final Rule with Comment ...*
http://www.cms.gov/Medicare/Medicare-Fee-for-Service-Payment/PhysicianFeeSched/PFS-Federal-Regulation-Notices-Items/CMS-1600-FC.html

Table 4: CY2014 Individual EP Registry Reporting Options for 2014 +.5% PQRS Incentive Payment[239]

REPORTING PERIOD	MEASURE TYPE	REPORTING MECHANISM	SATISFACTORY REPORTING CRITERIA/SATISFACTORY PARTICIPATION CRITERIA
12-month CY2014	individual measures	qualified registry	**Reporting to earn 2014 incentive of +.5%** • Report at least nine measures covering at least three NQS domains *and* report each measure for at least 50 percent of the Medicare Part B FFS patients seen during the reporting period to which the measure applies. Measures with a 0 percent performance rate would not be counted. **OR** • If fewer than nine measures covering at least three NQS domains apply to the eligible professional, report 1–8 measures covering 1–3 NQS domains *and* report each measure for at least 50 percent of the Medicare Part B FFS patients seen during the reporting period to which the measure applies. Measures with a 0 percent performance rate would not be counted.* ** For an EP who reports fewer than nine measures covering three NQS domains via the claims-based reporting mechanism, the EP will be subject to the MAV process, which would allow CMS to determine whether an EP should have reported QDC for additional measures and/or covering additional NQS domains.*
12-month CY2014	measures groups	qualified registry	• Report at least one measures group and report each measures group for at least 20 patients, a majority of which must be Medicare Part B FFS patients.
six-month (July 1–Dec. 31)	measures groups	qualified registry	• Report at least one measures group and report each measures group for at least 20 patients, a majority of which must be Medicare Part B FFS patients.

---

[239] *Pages 803–804, Tables 47–48, CMS-1600-FC: Centers for Medicare & Medicaid Services Regulation #: CMS-1600-FC; Display Date: 2013-11-27; Publication Date: 2013-12-10; Calendar Year: 2014; Regulation Type: Final Rule with Comment ...*
http://www.cms.gov/Medicare/Medicare-Fee-for-Service-Payment/PhysicianFeeSched/PFS-Federal-Regulation-Notices-Items/CMS-1600-FC.html

Using Registry Reporting of PQRS to Avoid the 2016 Payment Adjustment

Table 5: CY2014 Individual EP Registry Reporting Options for Avoidance of 2016 Payment Adjustment

REPORTING PERIOD	MEASURE TYPE	REPORTING MECHANISM	SATISFACTORY REPORTING CRITERIA/ SATISFACTORY PARTICIPATION CRITERIA
12-month CY2014	**individual measures**	**qualified registry**	• Report at least nine measures covering at least three NQS domains *and* report each measure for at least 50 percent of the Medicare Part B FFS patients seen during the reporting period to which the measure applies. Measures with a 0 percent performance rate would not be counted. **OR** • If fewer than nine measures covering at least three NQS domains apply to the eligible professional, report 1–8 measures covering 1–3 NQS domains *and* report each measure for at least 50 percent of the Medicare Part B FFS patients seen during the reporting period to which the measure applies. Measures with a 0 percent performance rate would not be counted.* ** For an EP who reports fewer than nine measures covering three NQS domains via the claims-based reporting mechanism, the EP will be subject to the MAV process, which would allow CMS to determine whether an EP should have reported QDC for additional measures and/or covering additional NQS domains.*
12-month CY2014	**individual measures**	**qualified registry**	• Report at least three measures covering at least one of the NQS domains *and* report each measure for at least 50 percent of the EP's Medicare Part B FFS patients seen during the reporting period to which the measure applies. Measures with a 0 percent performance rate would not be counted. **OR** • If fewer than three measures apply to the EP, report 1–2 measures covering at least one NQS domain for which there is Medicare patient data *and* report each measure for at least 50 percent of the EP's Medicare Part B FFS patients seen during the reporting period to which the measure applies. Measures with a 0 percent performance rate would not be counted. ** For an EP who reports fewer than three measures covering one NQS domain via the registry-based reporting mechanism, the EP will be subject to the MAV process, which would allow CMS to determine whether an EP should have reported on additional measures.*
12-month CY2014	**measures groups**	**qualified registry**	• Report at least one measures group *and* report each measures group for at least 20 patients, a majority of which must be Medicare Part B FFS patients.
six-month (July 1–Dec. 31)	**measures groups**	**qualified registry**	• Report at least one measures group *and* report each measures group for at least 20 patients, a majority of which must be Medicare Part B FFS patients.

Electronic Health Records (EHR) for Individual EP PQRS Reporting

- EHR—also called electronic medical records (EMRs)—allow providers to record patient information electronically, instead of using paper-based charting systems. Additionally, many such systems have reporting functionality as a core capability.

- As of April 30, 2013, HHS reported that its 2013 goals for EHR adoption by physicians had been exceeded. A total of 263,446 physicians, including 11,117 participating in Medicare Advantage Plans, have adopted an EHR product.[240]

- However, very few providers are using EHR as a PQRS reporting option. In the 2011 PQRS Experience Report published in March of 2013, only 560 providers, or .15 percent, used EHR to submit PQRS data.

- When using EHR as a reporting option, EPs are limited to the reporting of 64 EHR-specific individual measures for 2014 and cannot report any of the 25 measures groups when using EHR as their reporting option.

- EPs who wish to report PQRS measures via the EHR process are required to indicate their choice within the EHR incentive program attestation module. View additional information on the Medicare EHR incentive program.

- During the completion of the attestation process, providers will be required to enter a CMS EHR certification ID or number, obtained by entering information on the certified EHR technology product to be used for reporting information (found at the certified health IT product list (CHPL) on the ONC website: http://healthit.hhs.gov/chpl

- There are two sets of EHR measures required for PQRS reporting. The first set consists of individual measures contained under the traditional PQRS reporting process. A second set of PQRS measures is required for reporting under the EHR incentive program. Reporting through the

---

[240] Deloitte Center for Health Solutions,
http://www.deloitte.com/view/en_US/us/Insights/centers/center-for-health-solutions/

EHR mechanism may be accomplished by reporting EHR-specific PQRS quality measures through one of three EHR reporting options:[241]

- o direct submission through EHR system by the provider— EHR direct reporting

- o use of a qualified EHR data submission vendor— direct EHR vendor reporting

- o through the PQRS-Medicare EHR incentive program— direct or vendor.

Note: All 2013 data files submitted through either EHR reporting mechanism must meet a data submission deadline of February 28, 2014, to be analyzed and used for 2013 PQRS EHR measure calculations.

EHR Direct Reporting

- EPs electing to use EHR for PQRS reporting may submit data to CMS directly from their EHR system for 2013 (EHR direct reporting) *only* if the system in use meets CMS standards of qualification:

  - o CMS and the **Office of the National Coordinator for Health Information Technology (ONC)** have established standards and other criteria for structured data that EHRs must use in order to qualify for PQRS reporting.

  - o To learn which EHR systems and modules are certified for the PQRS reporting process, view the CHPL on the ONC website: http://healthit.hhs.gov/chpl

- Beginning in 2014, CMS is discontinuing the qualification process and will require instead that a direct EHR product be certified by ONC as a Certified EHR Technology (CEHRT), and therefore meets the definition of CEHRT in ONC's regulations.[242]

- EPs using EHR direct reporting must also register for an **Individuals Authorized Access for CMS Computer Services (IACS)** account to

---

[241] http://www.cms.gov/Medicare/Quality-Initiatives-Patient-Assessment-Instruments/PQRS/Electronic-Health-Record-Reporting.html

[242] Page 69184 http://www.gpo.gov/fdsys/pkg/FR-2012-11-16/pdf/2012-26900.pdf

upload data files. For more information, see the Physician and Other Health Care Professionals Quality Reporting Portal at: http://www.qualitynet.org/PQRS

EHR Vendor Reporting

- EPs may elect to use the services of a PQRS "direct EHR vendor" to submit data on their behalf. CMS publishes a listing of PQRS direct vendors and their systems (including specific versions or releases) that have been "qualified" to submit quality data on behalf of EPs. View the

  - These vendors receive data on PQRS measures from an EHR product. The EHR data submission vendor then submits the PQRS measures data to CMS in the CMS-specified format(s) on the EP's behalf.

- View the 2013 list of qualified vendors.

  (**Note:** The CY2014 lists will be available through the same website when published.)

Direct or vendor PQRS reporting as part of the Medicare EHR incentive program:

- EPs participating in the Medicare EHR incentive program are able to successfully submit PQRS data to earn both the PQRS incentive and an EHR incentive by meeting more stringent requirements for reporting and EHR utilization. In addition, through successful participation in the EHR incentive program during 2014, EPs are able to avoid 2016 payment adjustments.

Using Electronic Health Records (EHR) for Traditional Reporting of PQRS

Steps to earn the 2014 PQRS incentive using EHR reporting:

- Confirm EP status for EHR reporting (Therapists and Practitioners are excluded). For more information, see: http://www.cms.gov/Medicare/Quality-Initiatives-Patient-Assessment-Instruments/PQRS/index.html?redirect=/pqrs

- Identify specific individual measures for reporting that are most reflective of practice patient population and ensure that selected measures are available for EHR reporting. For 2014, there are sixty-four measures available for EHR reporting and *no* measures groups may be reported via EHR. For a list of EHR measures, see the Zip file titled "EHR Documents for Eligible Professionals" under Related Links at: http://www.cms.gov/Medicare/Quality-Initiatives-Patient-Assessment-Instruments/PQRS/Electronic-Health-Record-Reporting.html

- Select either the direct EHR reporting method or use the services of a qualified EHR data submission vendor to submit required data to CMS:

If quality measure data is submitted directly from an EHR system, it must be a PQRS-qualified EHR. For questions about the capabilities of an EHR, contact the vendor or consult a CMS list of qualified EHR vendors and their product version(s), available as a downloadable document in the Electronic Health Record Reporting section.

Note: The EHR reporting requirements to earn the 2014 incentive payment of +.5 percent and avoid the 2016 payment adjustment **are the same** (see Table 6 below).

CY2014 Individual EHR Reporting Options for PQRS[243]

Table 6: CY2014 Individual EP EHR Reporting Options for 2014 +.5% Incentive Payment and Avoidance of the 2016 Payment Adjustment

REPORTING PERIOD	MEASURE TYPE	REPORTING MECHANISM	SATISFACTORY REPORTING CRITERIA/ SATISFACTORY PARTICIPATION CRITERIA
12-month CY2014	individual measures	direct EHR product that is CEHRT and EHR data submission vendor that is CEHRT	• Report nine measures covering at least three of the NQS domains. If an EP's CEHRT does not contain patient data for at least nine measures covering at least three domains, then the EP must report the measures for which there is Medicare patient data. • An EP must report on at least one measure for which there is Medicare patient data.

[243] *Pages 803–804, Tables 47–48, CMS-1600-FC: Centers for Medicare & Medicaid Services Regulation #: CMS-1600-FC; Display Date: 2013-11-27; Publication Date: 2013-12-10; Calendar Year: 2014; Regulation Type: Final Rule with Comment ...* http://www.cms.gov/Medicare/Medicare-Fee-for-Service-Payment/PhysicianFeeSched/PFS-Federal-Regulation-Notices-Items/CMS-1600-FC.html

CY2014 Individual EP Qualified Clinical Data Registry Reporting: New for 2014[244]

- Section 601(b) of the American Taxpayer Relief Act of 2012 (ATRA) (Public Law 112–240, enacted January 2, 2013) amends Section 1848(m)(3) of the Social Security Act to provide for a new standard for individual EPs to satisfy the PQRS beginning in 2014, based on satisfactory participation in a QCDR.

- Based on this change, an EP is considered as "satisfactorily reporting" data on quality measures if, in lieu of reporting measures under other PQRS mechanisms, the EP is "satisfactorily participating" in a QCDR for the year.

- CMS defines a QCDR as a CMS-approved entity that has self-nominated and successfully completed a qualification process that collects medical and/or clinical data for the purpose of patient and disease tracking to foster improvement in the quality of care provided to patients.

- The QCDR is much more robust than a traditional qualified registry and goes much further to drive care quality than simply reporting quality data measures for PQRS. The QCDRs must:

  - submit quality measures data or results to CMS for the purposes of demonstrating that, for a reporting period, its EPs have satisfactorily participated in PQRS. A QCDR must have in place mechanisms for the transparency of data elements and specifications, risk models, and measures

  - submit to CMS, for the purposes of demonstrating satisfactory participation, quality measures data on multiple payers, not just Medicare patients

  - provide timely feedback, at least four times a year, on the measures at the individual participant level for which the QCDR reports on the EP's behalf for the purposes of the individual EP's satisfactory participation in the clinical quality data registry

---

[244] *Pages 760–801, CMS-1600-FC: Centers for Medicare & Medicaid Services http://www.cms.gov/Medicare/Medicare-Fee-for-Service-Payment/PhysicianFeeSched/PFS-Federal-Regulation-Notices-Items/CMS-1600-FC.html*

      o   possess benchmarking capacity that measures the quality of care an EP provides with other EPs performing the same or similar functions.

To participate in the 2014 PQRS reporting year, a QCDR:

- must be in existence as of January 1, 2013

- must have at least fifty clinical data registry participants by January 1, 2013 (please note that not all participants would be required to participate in PQRS)

- must submit an acceptable "validation strategy" to CMS by March 31, 2014

- must meet all CMS requirements outlined in the CY2014 Final PFS Rule

- must perform the validation outlined in the strategy and send evidence of successful results to CMS by June 30, 2015

- must publicly post by March 31, 2014 (on the entity's website or other publication available to the public) a detailed description (rationale, numerator, denominator, exclusions/exceptions, data elements) of the quality measures it collects to ensure transparency of information to the public

- **2014 QCDR reporting requirements:**

  o   For the twelve-month 2014 reporting period:

       ▪ report at least nine measures available for reporting under the QCDR covering at least three of the NQS domains;

       ▪ or, if fewer than nine measures apply to the eligible professional, report one to eight measures;

       ▪ and report each measure for at least 50 percent of the EP's applicable patients.

       ▪ Of the measures reported via a qualified clinical data registry, the EP must report on at least one outcome measure.

  o   The QCDR would be required to submit this data no later than the last Friday occurring two months after the end of the respective reporting period (that is, February 27, 2015, for reporting periods occurring in 2014).

o Measures may be selected from: CG CAHPS, NQF-endorsed measures, current PQRS measures, measures used by boards or specialty societies, and measures used in regional quality collaboratives.

o QCDRs may submit any number of PQRS measures during a reporting year. However, CMS is capping the number of **non-PQRS measures** received from each QCDR at **20** for 2014 reporting.

• The HHS secretary will qualify applicable clinical data registries and publish an approved list prior to January 1, 2014. For more information on clinical data registries, see:

http://effectivehealthcare.ahrq.gov/index.cfm/search-for-guides-reviews-and-reports/?productid=401&pageaction=displayproduct

CY2014 Individual EP QCDR Reporting[245]

Table 7: CY2014 Individual EP Qualified Clinical Data Registry Reporting for 2014 +.5% Incentive

REPORTING PERIOD	MEASURE TYPE	REPORTING MECHANISM	SATISFACTORY REPORTING CRITERIA/ SATISFACTORY PARTICIPATION CRITERIA
12-month CY2014	measures selected by the QCDR	QCDR	• Report at least nine measures covering at least three NQS domains. **AND** • Report each measure for at least 50 percent of the EP's applicable patients seen during the reporting period to which the measure applies. Measures with a 0 percent performance rate would not be counted. • Of the measures reported via a QCDR, the EP must report on at least one outcome measure.

---

[245] Pages 803–805, CMS-1600-FC: Centers for Medicare & Medicaid Services http://www.cms.gov/Medicare/Medicare-Fee-for-Service-Payment/PhysicianFeeSched/PFS-Federal-Regulation-Notices-Items/CMS-1600-FC.html

Table 8: CY2014 Individual EP Qualified Clinical Data Registry Reporting for Avoidance of the 2016 Payment Adjustment

REPORTING PERIOD	MEASURE TYPE	REPORTING MECHANISM	SATISFACTORY REPORTING CRITERIA/ SATISFACTORY PARTICIPATION CRITERIA
12-month CY2014	measures selected by the QCDR	QCDR	• Report at least nine measures covering at least three NQS domains. **AND** • Report each measure for at least 50 percent of the EP's applicable patients seen during the reporting period to which the measure applies. Measures with a 0 percent performance rate would not be counted. • Of the measures reported via a QCDR, the EP must report on at least one outcome measure.
12-month CY2014	measures selected by the QCDR	QCDR	• Report at least three measures covering at least one NQS domain. **AND** • Report each measure for at least 50 percent of the EP's applicable patients seen during the reporting period to which the measure applies. Measures with a 0 percent performance rate would not be counted.

5.3.11 PQRS Group Practice Reporting Option (GPRO)

GPRO Background

As introduced in 2010 under Section 1848 (m)(3)(C)(i) of the SSA, CMS is continuing the GPRO for the 2013 PQRS.

- **Group practice definition:** A group practice under 2014 physician quality reporting is defined as having two or more EPs (as defined by their individual NPI) defined by a single TIN who have reassigned their billing rights to the TIN. Groups are classified by CMS according to the number of EPs billing under one TIN as follows:

  o **small:** groups that have 2–24 NPIs.

    ▪ Small groups may report for 2014 via qualified registry or EHR (direct or vendor). Such groups are not eligible to use the web-based reporting option for 2014 PQRS reporting.

- **medium:** groups that have 25–99 NPIs.

    - Medium groups may report via qualified registry, the CMS-certified survey vendor, EHR (direct or vendor), or web-based interface for 2014 PQRS reporting.

- **large:** groups with 100+ NPIs.

    - Large groups may use the GPRO web-based interface, CMS-certified survey vendor, EHR, or qualified registry reporting options for 2014 PQRS reporting.

- Group practices that satisfactorily report required physician quality reporting measures for assigned Medicare beneficiaries in 2014 are eligible to earn an incentive payment equal to .5 percent of the group's total estimated Medicare Part B PFS of allowed charges for covered professional services during 2014. In 2016 a payment adjustment of -2.0 percent will be applied to all EPs and group practices that do not satisfactorily report such quality data.

- Once a group practice (as identified by its TIN) has self-nominated or registered to participate in the PQRS GPRO, individual providers are not eligible to separately earn an individual PQRS incentive payment. In addition, 2014 has been designated as the performance year for the 2016 application of a value-based modifier for large groups with 10+ EPs.

- If a group does not seek to report quality measures as a group, CMS will calculate a group quality score if at least 50 percent of the EPs within the group report measures individually:[246]

    - At least 50 percent of EPs must successfully avoid the 2016 PQRS payment adjustment.

    - EPs may report on measures available to individual EPs via the following reporting mechanisms:

        - claims

        - CMS-qualified registries

---

[246] *CMS National Provider call: The Physician Value-Based Payment Modifier under the 2014 Medicare Physician Fee Schedule December 3, 2013*

- EHR
- QCDR (new for CY2014)

Accountable Care Organization (ACO) GPRO:

By definition, ACOs are group practices recognized by one common TIN and must report PQRS measures under the Medicare Shared Savings Program:

- No registration or self-nomination is required for ACO members that are EPs to earn a PQRS incentive or avoid the payment adjustment penalty under the Medicare Shared Savings Program.

- ACO members must participate under the ACO participant TIN as a group practice under the PQRS GPRO under the Medicare Shared Savings Program for purposes of the PQRS incentive or payment adjustment penalty and are not required to report separately.

- Such ACO members who are EPs may not seek to avoid the payment adjustment by reporting either as an individual under the traditional PQRS or under the traditional PQRS GPRO.

- ACO providers/suppliers who are EPs who bill under a non-ACO participant TIN during the year could and should participate under the traditional PQRS as either individual EPs or a group practice for purposes of avoiding the PQRS payment adjustment for the claims billed under the non-ACO participant TIN.

- For purposes of satisfactory reporting in 2014 to avoid the **2016 PQRS** payment adjustment penalty, ACOs are required to satisfactorily report the twenty-two GPRO web-based interface measures.[247]

Note: EPs participating in the Medicare Shared Savings Program or the Pioneer ACO model, in which all providers bill through a common TIN, may not separately participate in the PQRS GPRO and will not be subject to the value-based payment modifier evaluation during 2014 (FY2016 VBM program year).

[247] *Page 1139, CMS-1600-FC: Centers for Medicare & Medicaid Services http://www.cms.gov/Medicare/Medicare-Fee-for-Service-Payment/PhysicianFeeSched/PFS-Federal-Regulation-Notices-Items/CMS-1600-FC.html*

Group practice PQRS reporting selection requirements:[248]

To be considered for PQRS GPRO, participants must submit a self-nomination statement via the web to be received by **September 30 of the year in which the reporting period occurs** (that is September 30, 2014, for reporting periods occurring in 2014). In addition, a selected method of reporting must be identified by this date. The method may be changed at any time prior to September 30, 2014. To be selected for GPRO, participants must agree to comply with the following requirements:

- have Medicare Part B billing on or after January 1, 2014, and prior to December 31, 2014

- agree to have results on the performance of their PQRS measures publicly reported on the Physician Compare website

- have minimum requisite technical abilities such as standard PC image with Microsoft Office and Microsoft Access software installed and minimum software configurations

- be able to comply with a secure method for data submission

- provide CMS with access to Medicare beneficiary data supporting the PQRS GPRO submissions or provide copies of such information upon CMS request

- indication of group practice's 2014 eRx incentive program participation with intended reporting mechanism and/or request for hardship exemption for 2015 eRx payment adjustment

- indicate intent to participate in eRx and PQRS as individuals or as a GPRO

- provide CMS-requested information contained on the CMS Communication Support Page (CSP)

  http://www.cms.gov/Medicare/Quality-Initiatives-Patient-Assessment-Instruments/PQRS/Downloads/2013-PQRS-GPRO-Requirements.pdf

---

[248] *Page 731, CMS-1600-FC: Centers for Medicare & Medicaid Services*
http://www.cms.gov/Medicare/Medicare-Fee-for-Service-Payment/PhysicianFeeSched/PFS-Federal-Regulation-Notices-Items/CMS-1600-FC.html

Group practice reporting methods:

The following methods mechanisms are available for GPRO reporting during 2014:

- qualified registry reporting

- GPRO web-based interface reporting

- CMS-certified survey vendor

- EHR reporting (CEHRT direct or CEHRT vendor)

Group practice reporting by registry:

- A GPRO qualified registry is a CMS-approved entity:
  - o that captures, stores, and submits clinically related data on behalf of providers;
  - o and is the only reporting method available for group practice reporting that provides calculated reporting and performance rates to CMS.
  - o Data must be submitted via defined .xml specifications.
  - o Providers extract patient (EHR or paper chart) data from submitted Medicare Part B claims, provider EHR system, billing records, etc. Providers then submit their data to the registry via a secure web portal.
  - o Once received, the registry then validates data, formats it into .xml files, and ensures timely submission to CMS.

- A list of registries approved for 2013 GPRO, along with a list of the measures for which the registry is qualified to submit and cost information, may be viewed at: http://cms.gov/Medicare/Quality-Initiatives-Patient-Assessment-Instruments/PQRS/Registry-Reporting.html

- For 2014 reporting, there are 200 PQRS measures that are reportable by groups by the registry reporting option. These are listed in Table 52 of the CY2014 Final PFS Rule.

- Group Practices reporting 2014 measures via the registry reporting option should consult the 2014 Physician Quality Reporting System (PQRS) Measure Specifications Manual for Claims and Registry Reporting of Individual Measures, which may be viewed at: http://www.cms.gov/Medicare/Quality-Initiatives-Patient-Assessment-Instruments/PQRS/Index.html.

CY2014 Group Practice PQRS Registry Reporting[249]

Table 9: CY2014 Group Practice Qualified Registry Reporting to Qualify for 2014 +.5% Incentive

REPORTING PERIOD	REPORTING MECHANISM	GROUP PRACTICE SIZE	SATISFACTORY REPORTING CRITERIA
12-month CY2014	qualified registry	2+ EPs	• Report at least nine measures covering at least three of the NQS domains *and* report each measure for at least 50 percent of the group practice's Medicare Part B FFS patients seen during the reporting period to which the measure applies. Measures with a 0 percent performance rate would not be counted. **OR** • If fewer than nine measures covering at least three NQS domains apply to the group practice, report 1–8 measures covering 1–3 NQS domains for which there is Medicare patient data *and* report each measure for at least 50 percent of the group practice's Medicare Part B FFS patients seen during the reporting period to which the measure applies. Measures with a 0 percent performance rate would not be counted. • For a group practice that reports fewer than nine measures covering at least three NQS domains via the registry-based reporting mechanism, the group practice will be subject to the MAV process, which would allow CMS to determine whether a group practice should have reported on additional measures and/or measures covering additional NQS domains.

---

[249] *Tables 49–50, CMS-1600-FC: Centers for Medicare & Medicaid Services, http://www.gpo.gov/fdsys/pkg/FR-2013-12-10/pdf/2013-28696.pdf*

Table 10: CY2014 Group Practice Qualified Registry Reporting to Avoid 2016 Payment Adjustment

REPORTING PERIOD	REPORTING MECHANISM	GROUP PRACTICE SIZE	SATISFACTORY REPORTING CRITERIA
12-month CY2014	qualified registry	2+ EPs	• Report at least nine measures covering at least three of the NQS domains *and* report each measure for at least 50 percent of the group practice's Medicare Part B FFS patients seen during the reporting period to which the measure applies. Measures with a 0 percent performance rate would not be counted. OR • If fewer than nine measures covering at least three NQS domains apply to the group practice, report 1–8 measures covering 1–3 NQS domains for which there is Medicare patient data *and* report each measure for at least 50 percent of the group practice's Medicare Part B FFS patients seen during the reporting period to which the measure applies. Measures with a 0 percent performance rate would not be counted. • For a group practice that reports fewer than nine measures via the registry-based reporting mechanism, the group practice would be subject to the MAV process, which would allow CMS to determine whether a group practice should have reported on additional measures and/or measures covering additional NQS domains.
12-month CY2014	qualified registry	2+ EPs	• Report at least three measures covering at least one of the NQS domains *and* report each measure for at least 50 percent of the group practice's Medicare Part B FFS patients seen during the reporting period to which the measure applies. Measures with a 0 percent performance rate would not be counted. OR • If fewer than three measures covering one NQS domain apply to the group practice, report 1–2 measures covering one NQS domain for which there is Medicare patient data *and* report each measure for at least 50 percent of the group practice's Medicare Part B FFS patients seen during the reporting period to which the measure applies. Measures with a 0 percent performance rate would not be counted. • For a group practice that reports fewer than three measures covering one NQS domain via the registry-based reporting mechanism, the group practice would be subject to the MAV process, which would allow CMS to determine whether a group practice should have reported on additional measures.

GPRO Web-based interface reporting:[250]

- The GPRO web-based interface is a product developed by CMS that is used by group practices that are selected to participate in the GPRO to submit data on PQRS quality measures.

- The web-based interface PQRS reporting mechanism is reserved as an option only available as a GPRO for group practices having 25+ EPs (as identified by their NPI) practicing under the same TIN.

- The GPRO web-based interface was modeled after a CMS demonstration project, the CMS Physician Group Practice (PGP) Project. This demonstration project was intended for large group practices, which tended to be multi-specialty practices with more than twenty-four eligible professionals. The variety of reporting measures contained in the GPRO web-based interface were determined to be more reflective of the clinical demographics of patients seen by practices with 25+ EPs.

- In 2011, 101 group practices, representing more than 39,000 eligible providers, self-nominated for GPRO reporting. In that same year, 98 percent of participating practices successfully reported PQRS.

- The method for assigning a Medicare beneficiary to a specific group practice for the purposes of GPRO mirrors the process used for patient assignment under the Medicare Shared Savings Plan to assign beneficiaries to an ACO:

  o beneficiary must have received at least one primary service furnished by a primary care physician at the participating group practice *and* received more primary care services (measured by Medicare allowed charges) furnished by primary care physicians in the participating group practice than furnished by primary care physicians at any other group or solo practice;

  o or, for those beneficiaries who do not receive any primary care services from a primary care physician during the reporting period, beneficiary assignment is made to the participating group

---

[250] http://www.cms.gov/Medicare/Quality-Initiatives-Patient-Assessment-Instruments/PQRS/GPRO_Web_Interface.html

practice if the beneficiary has at least one primary care service furnished by any group practice physician (regardless of specialty) and more primary care services were furnished by participating group practice EPs than at any other group or solo practice.

Web-based interface reporting for group practices with 25+ EPs involves the utilization of a CMS-determined sample number of beneficiaries (based on the size of the group practice) assigned to the participating group practice for whom specific data is collected and reported.*[251] FOR GROUPS WITH 25–99 EPs:	
reporting period:	January 1, 2013–December 31, 2013
sample size:	218 (with over sample of 283)
reporting requirements:	Report on all PQRS GPRO measures in the web-based interface and complete required data fields for the first 218 consecutively ranked and assigned Medicare beneficiaries, in the order listed in the sample, for each module or patient care measure. If the sample includes fewer than 218 assigned beneficiaries, 100 percent reporting of the sample is required.

- CMS will provide an "over-sample" listing of beneficiaries to ensure that the minimum requirements are met with qualified beneficiaries.

FOR GROUPS WITH 100+ EPs:	
reporting period:	January 1, 2013–December 31, 2013
sample size:	411 (with over sample of 534)
reporting requirements:	Report on all PQRS GPRO measures in the web-based interface and complete required data fields for the first 411 consecutively ranked and assigned Medicare beneficiaries, in the order listed in the sample, for each module or patient care measure. If the sample includes fewer than 411 assigned beneficiaries, 100 percent reporting of the sample is required.

*Groups with 2–24 EPs are not eligible to use the web-based interface reporting option and must use the registry method and report measures associated with that method.

---

[251] http://www.cms.gov/Medicare/Quality-Initiatives-Patient-Assessment-Instruments/PQRS/Downloads/2013_GPRO_SamplingSupplement.pdf

2014 PQRS measures reportable by GPRO Web-based interface:[252]

The 2014 GPRO includes web-based interface reporting on a total of seventeen specific quality measures (twenty-two measures when accounting for two composite measures). Such measures are grouped into five **disease modules** and ten **patient care modules** as follows:

GPRO DISEASE MODULES	NUMBER OF MEASURES
coronary artery disease	2 measures as 1 composite
diabetes disease	1
diabetes composite: optimal diabetes care	5 measures as 1 composite
heart failure	1
hypertension	1
ischemic vascular disease	2

GPRO PATIENT CARE MODULES	NUMBER OF MEASURES
Care Coordination/Patient Safety (CARE)	2
Preventive (PREV) Care Measures:	8 measures individually sampled

- Breast Cancer Screening
- Colorectal Cancer Screening
- Influenza Immunization
- Pneumococcal Vaccination for patients 65 and older
- Body Mass Index (BMI) Screening and Follow-up
- Tobacco Use: Screening and Cessation Intervention
- Screening for High Blood Pressure and Follow-up Documented
- Screening for Clinical Depression and Follow-up Plan

---

[252] Page 1107, CMS-1600-FC: Centers for Medicare & Medicaid Services
http://www.cms.gov/Medicare/Medicare-Fee-for-Service-Payment/PhysicianFeeSched/PFS-Federal-Regulation-Notices-Items/CMS-1600-FC.html

Inclusion of CG-CAHPS results:

- In 2014, group practices of 100+ will be evaluated on the results of the Clinician and Group Consumer Assessment of Healthcare Providers and Systems (CGCAHPS) survey:

- CGCAHPS is a standardized tool used to measure patient perceptions of care provided by a physician in an office setting.

- For 2014, CMS will fund the administration of the CG-CAHPS survey for groups with 100+ EPs only.

- For 2014, CMS will use CG-CAHPS survey results from January–March 2015.

- The following CGCAHPS measures will be surveyed:
    - Getting Timely Care, Appointments and Information
    - How Well Your Doctors Communicate
    - Patients' Rating of Doctor
    - Access to Specialists
    - Health Promotion and Education
    - Shared Decision-Making
    - Courteous and Helpful Office Staff
    - Care Coordination
    - Between Visit Communication
    - Educating Patients About Medication Adherence
    - Stewardship of Patient Resources

Note: *GPRO web-based interface reporting requirements to qualify for the 2014 +.5 percent incentive payment and avoidance of the FY2016 payment adjustment* **are the same** *(see Table 11 below).*

CY2014 Group Practice Web-based Interface PQRS Reporting Options[253]

Table 11: CY2014 PQRS GPRO Web-based Interface Reporting for 2014 +.5% Incentive *and* to Avoid the 2016 Payment Adjustment

REPORTING PERIOD	REPORTING MECHANISM	GROUP PRACTICE SIZE	SATISFACTORY REPORTING CRITERIA
12-month CY2014	GPRO web-based interface	25–99 EPs	• Report on all measures included in the web-based interface. **AND** • Populate data fields for the first 218 consecutively ranked and assigned beneficiaries in the order in which they appear in the group's sample for each module or preventive care measure. • If the pool of eligible assigned beneficiaries is fewer than 218, then report on 100 percent of assigned beneficiaries.
12-month CY2014	GPRO web-based interface	100+ EPs	• Report on all measures included in the web-based interface. **AND** • Populate data fields for the first 411 consecutively ranked and assigned beneficiaries in the order in which they appear in the group's sample for each module or preventive care measure. • If the pool of eligible assigned beneficiaries is fewer than 411, then report on 100 percent of assigned beneficiaries. • In addition, the group practice must also report all CG-CAHPS survey measures via certified survey vendor.

The CMS-certified survey vendor reporting option for group practices:[254]

- In the CY2014 PFS Final Rule, CMS finalized a new reporting option for submitting CG-CAHPS survey results for groups of 25+ EPs. The creation

---

[253] *Pages 821–823, CMS-1600-FC: Centers for Medicare & Medicaid Services http://www.cms.gov/Medicare/Medicare-Fee-for-Service-Payment/PhysicianFeeSched/PFS-Federal-Regulation-Notices-Items/CMS-1600-FC.html*

[254] *Page 733, CMS-1600-FC: Centers for Medicare & Medicaid Services http://www.cms.gov/Medicare/Medicare-Fee-for-Service-Payment/PhysicianFeeSched/PFS-Federal-Regulation-Notices-Items/CMS-1600-FC.html*

341

of the CMS-certified survey vendor option allows group practices to submit measures information along with CG-CAHPS data.

- CMS defines the survey vendor as: a vendor that is certified by CMS for a particular program year to transmit survey measures data to CMS.

- Group practices that elect this reporting mechanism for submission of CG-CAHPS must select an additional group practice reporting mechanism in order to meet the criteria for satisfactory reporting for the incentive payments.

  o Because only groups of 100+ EPs are required to submit CG-CAHPS for 2014, CMS only encourages groups of 25–99 to also participate, but will not pay for the services of the survey vendor.

  o Groups using the survey vendor reporting option will have a reduced number of measures required for reporting as compared to other methods of reporting that do not include the use of the survey vendor.

  o For 2014, CMS will use CG-CAHPS survey results from January–March 2015.

  o The following CGCAHPS measures will be surveyed:

    ▪ Getting Timely Care, Appointments and Information
    ▪ How Well Your Doctors Communicate
    ▪ Patients' Rating of Doctor
    ▪ Access to Specialists
    ▪ Health Promotion and Education
    ▪ Shared Decision Making
    ▪ Courteous and Helpful Office Staff
    ▪ Care Coordination
    ▪ Between Visit Communication
    ▪ Educating Patients About Medication Adherence
    ▪ Stewardship of Patient Resources

*Note: The 2014 survey vendor reporting requirements to qualify for the 2014 +.5 percent incentive payment and to avoid the 2016 payment adjustment **are the same** (see Table 12 below).*

CY2014 Group Practice Survey Vendor Reporting Options for PQRS[255]

Table 12: CY2014 Survey Vendor Reporting for 2014 +.5% Incentive *and* to Avoid the 2016 Payment Adjustment

REPORTING PERIOD	REPORTING MECHANISM	GROUP PRACTICE SIZE	SATISFACTORY REPORTING CRITERIA
12-month CY2014	CMS-certified survey vendor + qualified registry, direct EHR product, EHR data submission vendor or GPRO web-based interface	25+ EPs	• Report all CG-CAHPS survey measures via a CMS-certified survey vendor. **AND** • Report at least six measures covering at least two of the NQS domains using a qualified registry, direct EHR product, EHR data submission vendor, or GPRO web-based interface.

2014 group practice EHR reporting option for PQRS

- EHR direct or EHR vendor reporting for group practices is new for 2014

- Available for 2+ EPs

- Reporting period: twelve-month (January 1–December 31)

- EHR requirement: direct EHR product that is CMS-certified electronic health record technology (CEHRT) or EHR data submission vendor's product that is CEHRT.

- Group must report nine measures covering at least three NQS domains. If the group practice's CEHRT does not contain patient data for at least nine measures covering at least three domains, then the group practice must report the measures for which there is patient data

- 2014 EHR and registry reporting options for GPRO do not require every EP in the group to report PQRS measures. The established criteria will

---

[255] *Pages 821–823, CMS-1600-FC: Centers for Medicare & Medicaid Services*
http://www.gpo.gov/fdsys/pkg/FR-2013-12-10/pdf/2013-28696.pdf

require the group to report on a specific percentage of its applicable patients; regardless of how many of the group practice's EPs participate in reporting the PQRS measures.[256]

Note: The 2014 EHR group practice reporting requirements for 2014 incentive qualification and avoidance of the 2016 payment adjustment *are the same* (see Table 13 below).

2014 Group Practice EHR Reporting for PQRS[257]

Table 13: CY2015 Group Practice EHR Reporting to Qualify for the +.5% 2014 Incentive *and* Avoid the 2016 Payment Adjustment

REPORTING PERIOD	MEASURE TYPE	REPORTING MECHANISM	SATISFACTORY REPORTING CRITERIA
12-month CY2014	measures selected by the QCDR	QCDR	• Report at least nine measures covering at least three NQS domains. **AND** • Report each measure for at least 50 percent of the EP's applicable patients seen during the reporting period to which the measure applies. Measures with a 0 percent performance rate would not be counted. • Of the measures reported via a qualified clinical data registry, the EP must report on at least one outcome measure.

---

[256] http://www.cms.gov/Regulations-and-Guidance/Legislation/EHRIncentivePrograms/Downloads/beginners_guide.pdf

[257] Pages 821–823, CMS-1600-FC: Centers for Medicare & Medicaid Services http://www.gpo.gov/fdsys/pkg/FR-2013-12-10/pdf/2013-28696.pdf

Section 5.4: Acronym Guide

ACA..............................Affordable Care Act

ACO ....Accountable Care Organization

AHA..............................American Hospital Association

AHRQ........................Agency for Healthcare Research and Quality

APRN........................Advanced Practice Registered Nurse

ARRA........................American Recovery and Reinvestment Act of 2009, Public Law 111–5

ATRA ....American Taxpayer Relief Act of 2012, Public Law 112–240

BBA..........................Balanced Budget Act of 1997, Public Law 105–33

BL..............................Bureau of Labor Statistics

CAH ....Critical Access Hospital

CAUTI......................Catheter-Associated Urinary Tract Infection

CERT ....Comprehensive Error Rate Testing

CEHRT ....Certified Electronic Health Records Technology

CFR..........................Code of Federal Regulations

CG-CAHPS..............Care-Giver Consumer Assessment of
                           Healthcare Providers and Systems

CHPL ....Certified Health IT Product List

CLABSI ....Central Line-Associated Bloodstream Infection

CMS..........................Centers for Medicare & Medicaid Services

CMSA........................Consolidated Metropolitan Statistical Area

CPT..........................Current Procedural Terminology

CRNA........................Certified Registered Nurse Anesthetist

CY ....Calendar Year

DRA ....Deficit Reduction Act of 2005, Public Law 109–171

DRG..........................Diagnosis-Related Group

DSH ....Disproportionate Share Hospital

EHR ....Electronic Health Record

EMR..........................Electronic Medical Record

E&M ....Evaluation and Management

EP ....Eligible Professional

eRx..............................ePrescribing

FAQ.........................Frequently Asked Questions

FFS ....Fee-For-Service

FFY ....Federal Fiscal Year

FR ....Federal Register

FTE ....Full-Time Equivalent

FY............................Fiscal Year

GPRO ....Group Practice Reporting Option

HAC ....Hospital-Acquired Condition

HAI ....Healthcare-Associated Infection

HCAHPS..................Hospital Consumer Assessment of
             Healthcare Providers and Systems

HCPCS ....Healthcare Common Procedure Coding System

HHS ....Department of Health and Human Services

HIPAA ....Health Insurance Portability and Accountability Act of 1996

HIS ....Health Information System

HIT ....Health Information Technology

HQA ....Hospital Quality Alliance

HQI...........................Hospital Quality Initiative

IACS.........................Individuals Authorized Access for CMS Computer Services

ICD-9-CM.................International Classification of Diseases, Ninth Revision,
             Clinical Modification

ICD-10-CM...............International Classification of Diseases, Tenth Revision,
             Clinical Modification

ICD-10-PCS.............International Classification of Diseases, Tenth Revision,
             Procedure Coding System

LTCH.........................Long-Term Care Hospital

MA............................Medicare Advantage

MAV ....Measures Applicability Validation

MCO.........................Managed Care Organization

MDH.........................Medicare-Dependent Hospital

MedPAC ....Medicare Payment Advisory Commission

MedPAR ....Medicare Provider Analysis and Review File

MIPPA......................Medicare Improvements for Patients and Providers Act
             of 2008, Public Law 110–275

MMA.........................Medicare Prescription Drug, Improvement, and Modernization Act of
             2003, Public Law 108–173

MOC.........................Maintenance of Certification

MS-DRG ....Medicare Severity Diagnosis-Related Group

MS-LTC-DRG ....Medicare Severity Long-Term Care Diagnosis-Related Group

NCH ....National Claims History

NCQA........................National Committee for Quality Assurance

NQF ....National Quality Forum

NQS ....National Quality Strategy

NCH ....National Claims History

NPI ....National Provider Identifier

ONC ....Office of the National Coordinator for Health Information Technology

PFP ....Physicians Feedback Program

PFS ....Physician Fee Schedule

PPS...........................Prospective Payment System

PS&R ....Provider Statistical and Reimbursement [System]

PQRI ....Physicians Quality Reporting Initiative

PQRS........................Physician Quality Reporting System

QDC..........................Quality Data Code

QCDR ....Qualified Clinical Data Registry

QIG ....Quality Improvement Group, CMS

QIO ....Quality Improvement Organization

RA/EOB ....Remittance Advice/Explanation of Benefits

RHC ....Rural Health Clinic

RHQDAPU ....Reporting Hospital Quality Data for Annual Payment Update

SCH ....Sole Community Hospital

SNF...........................Skilled Nursing Facility

TIN ....Tax Identification Number

VBM ....Value-Based Modifier

VBP...........................Value-Based Purchasing

Section 5.5: Appendix

5.5.1 Attachment A: 2014 PQRS Reporting Requirements Summary

Reporting Requirements for 2014 +.5 Percent Incentive Payment

Table 14: Individual EP Reporting

REPORTING PERIOD	MEASURE TYPE	REPORTING MECHANISM	SATISFACTORY REPORTING CRITERIA/ SATISFACTORY PARTICIPATION CRITERIA
12-month CY2014	individual measures	claims	• Report at least nine measures covering at least three NQS domains. OR • If fewer than nine measures covering at least three NQS domains apply to the EP, report 1–8 measures covering 1–3 NQS domains *and* report each measure for at least 50 percent of the Medicare Part B FFS patients seen during the reporting period to which the measure applies. Measures with a 0 percent performance rate would not be counted.* ** An EP who reports fewer than nine measures covering three NQS domains via the claims-based reporting mechanism will be subject to the MAV process, which would allow a determination of whether an EP should have reported QDC for additional measures and/or covering additional NQS domains.*
12-month (Jan. 1– Dec. 31)	individual measures	qualified registry	• Report at least nine measures covering at least three of the NQS domains. OR • If fewer than nine measures covering at least three NQS domains apply to the EP, report 1–8 measures covering 1–3 NQS domains for which there is Medicare patient data *and* report each measure for at least 50 percent of the EP's Medicare Part B FFS patients seen during the reporting period to which the measure applies. Measures with a 0 percent performance rate would not be counted.* ** An EP who reports fewer than nine measures covering three NQS domains via the registry-based reporting mechanism will be subject to the MAV process, which would allow a determination of whether an EP should have reported on additional measures and/or measures covering additional NQS domains.*

12-month (Jan. 1– Dec. 31)	individual measures	direct EHR product that is CEHRT and EHR data submission vendor that is CEHRT	• Report nine measures covering at least three of the NQS domains. If an EP's CEHRT does not contain patient data for at least nine measures covering at least three domains, then the EP must report the measures for which there is Medicare patient data. An EP must report on at least one measure for which there is Medicare patient data.
12-month (Jan. 1– Dec. 31)	measures groups	qualified registry	• Report at least one measures group and report each measures group for at least 20 patients, a majority of which must be Medicare Part B FFS patients.
six-month (July 1– Dec. 31)	measures groups	qualified registry	• Report at least one measures group and report each measures group for at least 20 patients, a majority of which must be Medicare Part B FFS patients.
12-month (Jan. 1– Dec. 31)	measures selected by QCDR	QCDR	• Report at least nine measures covering at least three NQS domains and report each measure for at least 50 percent of the EP's applicable patients seen during the reporting period to which the measure applies. Measures with a 0 percent performance rate would not be counted. • Of the measures reported via a qualified clinical data registry, the EP must report on at least one outcome measure.

Table 15: Group Practice Reporting

REPORTING PERIOD	REPORTING MECHANISM	GROUP PRACTICE SIZE	SATISFACTORY REPORTING CRITERIA
12-month CY2014	GPRO web-based interface	25–99 EPs	• Report on all measures included in the web-based interface. **AND** • Populate data fields for the first 218 consecutively ranked and assigned beneficiaries in the order in which they appear in the group's sample for each module or preventive care measure. If the pool of eligible assigned beneficiaries is fewer than 218, then report on 100 percent of assigned beneficiaries.
12-month (Jan. 1– Dec. 31)	GPRO web-based interface	100+ EPs	• Report on all measures included in the web-based interface. **AND** • Populate data fields for the first 411 consecutively ranked and assigned beneficiaries in the order in which they appear in the group's sample for each module or preventive care measure. If the pool of eligible assigned beneficiaries is fewer than 411, then report on 100 percent of assigned beneficiaries. In addition, the group practice must also report all CG-CAHPS survey measures via certified survey vendor.

349

12-month (Jan. 1–Dec. 31)	qualified registry	2+ EPs	• Report at least nine measures covering at least three of the NQS domains. **OR** • If fewer than nine measures covering at least three NQS domains apply to the group practice, report 1–8 measures covering 1–3 NQS domains for which there is Medicare patient data and report each measure for at least 50 percent of the group practice's Medicare Part B FFS patients seen during the reporting period to which the measure applies. Measures with a 0 percent performance rate would not be counted.* *For a group practice that reports fewer than nine measures covering at least three NQS domains via the registry-based reporting mechanism, the group practice will be subject to the MAV process, which would allow a determination of whether a group practice should have reported on additional measures and/or measures covering additional NQS domains.*
12-month (Jan. 1–Dec. 31)	direct EHR product that is CEHRT/ EHR data submission vendor that is CEHRT	2+ EPs	• Report nine measures covering at least three of the NQS domains. If a group practice's CEHRT does not contain patient data for at least nine measures covering at least three domains, then the group practice must report the measures for which there is Medicare patient data. A group practice must report on at least one measure for which there is Medicare patient data.
12-month (Jan. 1–Dec. 31)	CMS-certified survey vendor + qualified registry, direct EHR product, EHR data submission vendor or GPRO web-based interface	25+ EPs	• Report all CG-CAHPS survey measures via a CMS-certified survey vendor and report at least six measures covering at least two of the NQS domains using a qualified registry, direct EHR product, EHR data submission vendor, or GPRO web-based interface.

Reporting Requirements for 2016 Payment Adjustment Avoidance

Table 16: Individual Eligible Professional Reporting

REPORTING PERIOD	MEASURE TYPE	REPORTING MECHANISM	SATISFACTORY REPORTING CRITERIA/ SATISFACTORY PARTICIPATION CRITERIA
12-month CY2014	individual measures	claims	• Report at least nine measures covering at least three NQS domains. OR • If fewer than nine measures covering at least three NQS domains apply to the EP, report 1–8 measures covering 1–3 NQS domains and report each measure for at least 50 percent of the Medicare Part B FFS patients seen during the reporting period to which the measure applies. Measures with a 0 percent performance rate would not be counted.* * For an EP who reports fewer than nine measures covering three NQS domains via the claims-based reporting mechanism, the EP will be subject to the MAV process, which would allow us to determine whether an EP should have reported QDC for additional measures and/or covering additional NQS domains.
12-month (Jan. 1– Dec. 31)	individual measures	claims	• Report at least three measures. OR • If fewer than three measures apply to the EP, report 1–2 measures. AND • Report each measure for at least 50 percent of the EP's Medicare Part B FFS patients seen during the reporting period to which the measure applies. Measures with a 0 percent performance rate will not be counted.
12-month (Jan. 1– Dec. 31)	individual measures	qualified registry	• Report at least nine measures covering at least three NQS domains. OR • If fewer than nine measures covering at least three NQS domains apply to the EP, report 1–8 measures covering 1–3 NQS domains for which there is Medicare patient data. AND • Report each measure for at least 50 percent of the EP's Medicare Part B FFS patients seen during the reporting period to which the measure applies. Measures with a 0 percent performance rate would not be counted.* * For an EP who reports fewer than nine measures covering at least three NQS domains via the registry-based reporting mechanism, the EP will be subject to the MAV process, which would allow a determination of whether an EP should have reported on additional measures and/or measures covering additional NQS domains.

351

12-month (Jan. 1– Dec. 31)	individual measures	qualified registry	<ul><li>Report at least three measures covering at least one of the NQS domains.</li></ul> **OR** <ul><li>If fewer than three measures apply to the EP, report 1–2 measures covering at least one NQS domain for which there is Medicare patient data.</li></ul> **AND** <ul><li>Report each measure for at least 50 percent of the EP's Medicare Part B FFS patients seen during the reporting period to which the measure applies. Measures with a 0 percent performance rate would not be counted.*</li></ul> *For an EP who reports fewer than three measures covering one NQS domain via the registry-based reporting mechanism, the EP will be subject to the MAV process, which would allow us to determine whether an EP should have reported on additional measures.*
12-month (Jan. 1– Dec. 31)	individual measures	direct EHR product that is CEHRT and EHR data submission vendor that is CEHRT	<ul><li>Report nine measures covering at least three of the NQS domains. If an EP's CEHRT does not contain patient data for at least nine measures covering at least three domains, then the EP must report the measures for which there is Medicare patient data. An EP must report on at least one measure for which there is Medicare patient data.</li></ul>
12-month (Jan. 1– Dec. 31)	measures groups	qualified registry	<ul><li>Report at least one measures group.</li></ul> **AND** <ul><li>Report each measures group for at least 20 patients, a majority of which must be Medicare Part B FFS patients.</li></ul>
six-month (July 1– Dec. 31)	measures groups	qualified registry	<ul><li>Report at least one measures group.</li></ul> **AND** <ul><li>Report each measures group for at least 20 patients, a majority of which must be Medicare Part B FFS patients.</li></ul>
12-month (Jan. 1– Dec. 31)	measures selected by QCDR	QCDR	<ul><li>Report at least nine measures covering at least three NQS domains.</li></ul> **AND** <ul><li>Report each measure for at least 50 percent of the EP's applicable patients seen during the reporting period to which the measure applies. Measures with a 0 percent performance rate would not be counted.*</li><li>*Of the measures reported via a QCDR, the EP must report on at least one outcome measure.</li></ul>
12-month (Jan. 1– Dec. 31)	measures selected by QCDR	QCDR	<ul><li>Report at least three measures covering at least one NQS domain.</li></ul> **AND** <ul><li>Report each measure for at least 50 percent of the EP's applicable patients seen during the reporting period to which the measure applies. Measures with a 0 percent performance rate would not be counted.</li></ul>

Table 17: Group Practice Reporting

REPORTING PERIOD	REPORTING MECHANISM	GROUP PRACTICE SIZE	SATISFACTORY REPORTING CRITERIA
12-month CY2014	GPRO web-based interface	25–99 EPs	• Report on all measures included in the web-based interface. **AND** • Populate data fields for the first 218 consecutively ranked and assigned beneficiaries in the order in which they appear in the group's sample for each module or preventive care measure. If the pool of eligible assigned beneficiaries is fewer than 218, then report on 100 percent of assigned beneficiaries.
12-month (Jan. 1– Dec. 31)	GPRO web-based interface	100+ EPs	• Report on all measures included in the web-based interface. **AND** • Populate data fields for the first 411 consecutively ranked and assigned beneficiaries in the order in which they appear in the group's sample for each module or preventive care measure. If the pool of eligible assigned beneficiaries is fewer than 411, then report on 100 percent of assigned beneficiaries. In addition, the group practice must report all CG-CAHPS survey measures via certified survey vendor.
12-month (Jan. 1– Dec. 31)	qualified registry	2+ EPs	• Report at least nine measures covering at least three of the NQS domains. **OR** • If fewer than nine measures covering at least three NQS domains apply to the group practice, report 1–8 measures covering 1–3 NQS domains for which there is Medicare patient data. **AND** • Report each measure for at least 50 percent of the group practice's Medicare Part B FFS patients seen during the reporting period to which the measure applies. Measures with a 0 percent performance rate would not be counted.* *For a group practice that reports fewer than nine measures via the registry-based reporting mechanism, the group practice would be subject to the MAV process, which would allow a determination of whether a group practice should have reported on additional measures and/or measures covering additional NQS domains.*
12-month (Jan. 1– Dec. 31)	qualified registry	2+ EPs	• Report at least three measures covering at least one of the NQS domains. **OR** • If fewer than three measures covering one NQS domain apply to the group practice, report 1–2 measures covering one NQS domain for which there is Medicare patient data. **AND**

			• Report each measure for at least 50 percent of the group practice's Medicare Part B FFS patients seen during the reporting period to which the measure applies. Measures with a 0 percent performance rate would not be counted.* *For a group practice that reports fewer than three measures covering one NQS domain via the registry-based reporting mechanism, the group practice would be subject to the MAV process, which would allow a determination of whether a group practice should have reported on additional measures.*
12-month (Jan. 1– Dec. 31)	direct EHR product that is CEHRT/ EHR data submission vendor that is CEHRT	2+ EPs	• Report nine measures covering at least three of the NQS domains. If a group practice's CEHRT does not contain patient data for at least nine measures covering at least three domains, then the group practice must report the measures for which there is Medicare patient data. A group practice must report on at least one measure for which there is Medicare patient data.
12-month (Jan. 1– Dec. 31)	CMS-certified survey vendor + qualified registry, direct EHR product, EHR data submission vendor or GPRO web-based interface	25+ EPs	• Report all CG-CAHPS survey measures via a CMS-certified survey vendor. **AND** • Report at least six measures covering at least two of the NQS domains using a qualified registry, direct EHR product, EHR data submission vendor, or GPRO web-based interface.

5.5.2 Attachment B: Overview of the Physician Compare Website

- CMS was required by Section 10331 of the ACA of 2010 to establish the Physician Compare website. As a result, the site was launched on December 30, 2010. In its first iteration, Physician Compare used the existing Healthcare Provider Directory that was already part of Medicare.gov. Since that time, CMS has been working continually to enhance the site and its functionality, improve the information available, and include more and increasingly useful information about physicians and other health care professionals who take part in Medicare. This effort, along with the eventual addition of quality measures on the site, will help it serve its two-fold purpose:

- o to provide information for consumers to encourage informed health care decisions

- o to create explicit incentives for physicians to maximize performance

- Currently, Physician Compare is a website that allows consumers to search for physicians and other health care professionals who provide Medicare services. Some of the information on the site includes:

  - o physicians' and other health care professionals' names, addresses, phone numbers, specialties, clinical training, and genders

  - o whether physicians and other health care professionals speak languages other than English

  - o the hospitals that physicians and other health care professionals are affiliated with

  - o whether physicians and other health care professionals accept the Medicare-approved amount (patient will not be billed for any more than the Medicare deductible and coinsurance)

  - o group practice information, including: the practice's address and phone number; a map and directions to the practice; the practice's specialties; and a list of physicians and other health care professionals within that practice

- CMS uses feedback from the public and stakeholders through Town Hall meetings, Listening Sessions, email received at PhysicianCompare@Westat.com, and the rule-making process to define the scope and direction of Physician Compare. Through rule making, CMS proposes new policies—including what type of information will be publicly reported on Physician Compare in what years—and the public is provided the opportunity to comment on these proposals and give CMS its opinions.

- CMS has begun to implement a plan to make quality data available on Physician Compare. The ACA required the plan be established by January 1, 2013. The first step in this plan was outlined in the 2012 PFS Final Rule initiating a phased approach to public reporting. The second step as outlined in the 2013 PFS Final Rule furthers the plan to add quality data and other information to Physician Compare. According to this plan, CMS will post the first set of measure data on the site in CY2014, reflecting data collected no sooner than program year 2012. These data will include PQRS GPRO measures for group practices and ACOs.

- The plan for Physician Compare also includes publically reporting patient experience data, such as the Clinician and Group Consumer Assessment of Healthcare Providers and Systems (CG-CAHPS) measures, for ACOs and group practices of 100 or more EPs participating in the 2013 PQRS GPRO as soon as technically feasible, but not before CY2014.

5.5.3 Attachment C: QualityNet Website PQRS Feedback Reporting

https://www.qualitynet.org/portal/server.pt/community/pqri_home/212

- CMS provides online access to PQRS Feedback Reports via the QualityNet website.

- Provided reports, which detail participation in the PQRS and eRx incentive programs, are released at the TIN/NPI level.

- Data is presented for the PQRS and eRx health care delivery/reporting period from the following sources:

  o Medicare Part B claims

  o registries

  o EHR data submission vendors

  o EHR

  o MOC

  o GPRO

- Data contained in the reports is submitted as follows:
    - Registries submit data on behalf of EPs.
    - EHR data submission vendors submit data on behalf of EPs.
    - The MOC entity submits data on behalf of certified medical boards.
    - The GPRO participants submit data on behalf of group practices.
    - Providers using qualified EHR systems use the portal to submit their own data collected within the EHR.
    - Vendors of non-qualified EHR systems submit test data to qualify their systems.

CMS provides PQRS and eRx report user guides and portal use instructions through the following QualityNet link: https://www.qualitynet.org/portal/server.pt/community/pqri_home/212

CHAPTER 6

The Medicare Electronic Health Record (EHR) Incentive Program

Section 6.1: Flash Read!

Electronic health records (EHRs) have long been hailed as a critical step in boosting the quality of health care in America as well as bringing down costs. A vast majority of hospitals (85 percent) have demonstrated they are using EHRs in a meaningful way, but physicians and other providers lag behind. The Affordable Care Act (ACA) aims to change that and harness the full power of EHRs by using financial incentives and penalties to encourage participation. The Centers for Medicare & Medicaid Services (CMS) predicts that these mechanisms will generate a substantial increase in program participation, from 286,771 physicians in 2013 to 412,150 by 2019. In addition, the projected percentage of those successfully reporting for Meaningful Use (MU) is expected to rise to 67 percent by 2019.

- The Electronic Health Record (EHR) Incentive Program provides financial incentives and penalties to encourage the adoption and use of

EHR products, certified for a wide range of functionalities, by individual office-based physicians and hospitals.

- Separate Medicare and Medicaid EHR incentive programs have been established for individual eligible providers (EPs) and hospitals. EP participation is assessed on a calendar year (CY) basis and hospital participation is aligned with the fiscal year (FY).

- EPs include the following office-based physicians practicing individually or in a group practice (including EPs participating in the Pioneer Accountable Care Organizations (ACOs) or the Medicare Shared Savings Program ACOs): Doctor of Medicine or Osteopathy; Doctor of Podiatric Medicine; Doctor of Optometry; Doctor of Oral Surgery or Dental Medicine; and Doctor of Chiropractic.

- Participants have a one-time opportunity to change the election to participate in either the Medicare or Medicaid program. This option expires at the end of 2014.

- EHR program incentives are awarded and penalties imposed based on annual reporting that demonstrates participants are using EHR in a meaningful way—adopting technological functionality beyond simple record-keeping. Such use is defined as "Meaningful Use" (MU).

- Incentive payments are annual lump-sum payments paid for successful MU reporting and are paid only through 2016. Providers can enroll for incentive payments through 2014 and the total maximum incentive available for 2014 enrollees is $23,250 (-2.0 percent sequestration adjustment applied).

- The first year of penalty application for physicians is CY2015 and is based on CY2013 reporting.

- Through October 2013, more than half of physicians eligible for the Medicare EHR Incentive Program were enrolled. However, only 36 percent demonstrated MU and qualified for annual incentive payments, and 64 percent will receive payment adjustment penalties in 2015.

- Penalties are applied in the form of a payment adjustment made to Medicare Part B claims for covered professional services and are based on reporting that occurs two years prior.

- Penalty percentage application is cumulative for participants based on unsuccessful MU reporting. The CY2015 penalty is -1.0 percent, increasing to -2.0 percent for 2016, and -3.0 percent for CY2017. Beginning in CY2018, the secretary of the Department of Health and Human Services (HHS) can increase the penalty amount up to a maximum of -5.0 percent if less than 75 percent of participants are able to achieve MU.

- Providers subject to the 2015 penalty resulting from nonparticipation in the 2013 program may avoid penalties by registering in 2014 and meeting first-year reporting requirements.

- Reporting for the EHR incentive program is required for **all patients, regardless of payer**. An exception to this provision exists when reporting for dual credit with PQRS. Because PQRS requires reporting on clinical quality measures for Medicare beneficiaries, EPs must report required EHR incentive program data for Medicare patients only and submit data through the appropriate PQRS reporting mechanism.

- Three stages of MU participation have been established for the EHR Incentive Program, with increasing requirements for participation from stage to stage:

  o Stage 1: data capture and sharing

  o Stage 2: advanced clinical processes

  o Stage 3: improved outcomes and advanced patient engagement

- All providers begin participating by meeting the Stage 1 requirements for a ninety-day period in their first year of MU and a full year in their second year of MU. After meeting the Stage 1 requirements, providers will then have to meet Stage 2 requirements for two full years.

- Legislative action by CMS has extended the length of time of staged-reporting twice since 2011. (EPs with successful reporting since 2011 will have spent three years in Stage 1 and three years in Stage 2 by 2017.)

- In December 2013, CMS announced a delay until 2017 for implementation of Stage 3 requirements for participants with two years of successful Stage 2 MU reporting. As a result, some participants will spend a third year in Stage 2. This decision does not modify the beginning of Stage 2 reporting for EPs with two years of successful Stage 1 reporting.

- Progression between MU stages depends on when a Medicare provider begins participation in the program:

Timeline for Medicare EHR Incentive Program Reporting to Avoid Penalty

EP Payment Adjustment Year (Calendar Year)	For EPs beyond their first year of MU reporting: EPs must demonstrate MU during EHR reporting period two years prior to year of payment adjustment.	For an EP demonstrating MU for the first time in the year prior to the payment adjustment year, EHR reporting period is a continuous 90-day reporting period. OR beginning no later than:	apply or otherwise qualify for an exception no OR later than
2015	CY2013 (with submission no later than February 28, 2014).	July 3, 2014 (with submission no later than October 1, 2014).	July 1, 2015
2016	CY2014 (with submission no later than February 28, 2015).	July 3, 2015 (with submission no later than October 1, 2015).	July 1, 2016
2017	CY2015 (with submission no later than February 28, 2016).	July 3, 2016 (with submission no later than October 1, 2016).	July 1, 2017
2018	CY2016 (with submission no later than February 28, 2017).	July 3, 2017 (with submission no later than October 1, 2017).	July 1, 2018
2019	CY2017 (with submission no later than February 28, 2018).	July 3, 2018 (with submission no later than October 1, 2018).	July 1, 2019

- EHR incentive program reporting periods are for the full calendar year, with two exceptions:

  o **first-year reporting of Stage 1 MU**: The reporting period is for any ninety continuous days, beginning no later than July 3. Reporting must be accomplished via attestation no later than October 1 of the same year.

  o **2014 only:** All EHR products must be 2014 CMS-certified EHR technology (CEHRT) to meet annual reporting requirements. As of January 1, 2014, only 533 products meet CY2014 CEHRT requirements and may be used for 2014 reporting (as opposed to 4,208 CEHRT products available during 2013).

- To allow all participants sufficient time to upgrade their EHR systems to the 2014 edition CEHRT standard, CMS is allowing a reporting period during CY2014 of one calendar year quarter, for all EHR incentive program participants, regardless of a participant's stage of MU reporting.

- Annual reporting requirements for Stages 1 and 2 include defined criteria in two areas:

  1. **clinical quality measures (CQMs):** For 2014, there are sixty-four CQMs that are also contained within the 2014 Physician Quality Reporting System (PQRS).

  2. **health information technology objectives**: These objectives reflect the full range of technical functionality contained in CEHRT. Required use of advanced EHR functions escalates in complexity as participants move through the program stages.

- With the delay in Stage 3 implementation until CY2017, CMS has not yet established specific MU criteria. Stage 3 reporting metrics will be communicated through future CMS rule making.

- A variety of reporting options are available for EHR incentive program participants to meet annual requirements:

  o **attestation**: for first-year Stage 1 MU reporting and submission of health information technology objective attainment

  o **electronic options**:

    - **Option 1**: EHR incentive program only

    - **Option 2**: dual credit reporting for EHR incentive program and PQRS (for individual EPs and group practices)

Summary of 2014 Reporting Options for EHR Incentive Program

CATEGORY	DATA LEVEL	PAYER LEVEL	SUBMISSION OPTION	MU REPORTING REQUIREMENTS
EPs in first year of demonstrating MU	aggregate	all payers	attestation	Submit data on nine of 64 CQMs (includes list of recommended adult and pediatric CQMs) covering at least three of the six NQS domains. Reporting period is one quarter of CY2014.
EPs beyond first year of demonstrating MU				
Option 1	aggregate	all payers	electronic	Submit data on nine of 64 CQMs (includes list of recommended adult and pediatric CQMs) covering at least three of the six NQS domains. Reporting period is one quarter of CY2014.
Option 2	patient	Medicare only	electronic	Satisfy requirements of PQRS reporting options using CEHRT. Reporting period is full year CY2014.
group reporting (EPs beyond first year of MU reporting)	patient	Medicare only	electronic	Satisfy requirements of Medicare Shared Savings Program (MSSP) or Pioneer ACOs using CEHRT.
EPs satisfactorily reporting via PQRS group reporting options	patient	Medicare only	electronic	Satisfy requirements of PQRS group reporting options using CEHRT.

Section 6.2: Provider Perspectives

The electronic health record (EHR) and the things that come with it—electronic prescribing, the ability to exchange patient health information online, patient access to their own electronic records, and other related conveniences—is foundational to the entire effort to improve quality of care and reform the payment system. Without it, our ambitions toward improving the cost and quality of medical care, and the health of populations, would have to be far more modest. Until now, the information needed to mobilize the health system to higher performance has been locked away in file cabinets in the basement of hospitals and the back corridors of ambulatory clinics. The only way to get it out to where it can be useful for societal purposes is to digitize it.

6.2.1 Rationale

Most doctors and hospitals collect and manage health information pretty much the same way Hippocrates did 2,400 years ago. "We have substituted paper for tablet and papyrus, but most everything else is the same," wrote David Blumenthal, MD, and Anne-Marie J. Audet, MD, in The Commonwealth Fund blog.[258]

That's an exaggeration, but maybe less of one than we'd like to think. Many, but perhaps not most, physicians have been working with some form of health information technology in their practices for several years, in most cases starting with billing systems.

Sophisticated information systems for use in hospitals and doctors' offices have been available from a number of vendors since the 1980s, but they had relatively low penetration through the mid-2000s. Many practitioners regarded them as expensive, underpowered, hard to use, and just not worth the

---

[258] David Blumenthal, MD, and Anne-Marie Audet, MD, "Health Information Technology: The Gateway to Progress," The Commonwealth Fund blog, June 4, 2013. http://www.commonwealthfund.org/Blog/2013/Jun/Health-Information-Technology.aspx

investment and effort. Practicing medicine was difficult enough without adding the overlay of this cantankerous technology.

As the quality improvement movement proceeded by fits and starts to embrace the innovations in information technology, the federal government came to the realization that marketplace inertia was inhibiting adoption of these systems on the front line.

Many hospitals had installed some kind of computerized clinical information system, often built as an offshoot of a billing system (which brought its own limitations). These were frequently not functioning up to potential, but the investment at least had been made.

Physicians, however, were resistant. By 2008, ten years after the Institute of Medicine report that documented significant lapses in quality of care, only 17 percent of physicians and 12 percent of hospitals had a basic EHR system.[259] Without a full penetration into almost every physician's office and site of practice, and full-fledged adoption of the technology in hospitals and throughout the care continuum, it would not be possible for health care in the United States to attain the level of quality and accountability that the government and payers desired.

The government therefore decided to take action, in the form of a subsidy, to help providers make the switch from paper to electronic files. It also set predetermined thresholds of MU to ensure that providers would engage with the systems and effectuate the transformation that policy makers envisioned.

6.2.2 Summary

The Health Information Technology for Economic and Clinical Health Act (HITECH) was passed in February 2009, in the depths of the financial crisis, as part of the economic stimulus package formally known as the American Recovery and Reinvestment Act of 2009 (ARRA). Through this legislation, Congress and the administration attempted to enact programs to spur short-term growth as well as promote advancements that would work toward the

---

[259] David Blumenthal, MD, "Wiring the Health System—Origins and Provisions of a New Federal Program," New England Journal of Medicine, 2011; 365; 24. December 15, 2011. http://www.nejm.org/doi/full/10.1056/NEJMsr1110507

long-term benefit of the country.[260] Thus, the EHR subsidy program predates the ACA by about a year, although its intent and implementation are complimentary and simultaneous to the more comprehensive reform law. Congress allocated some $27 billion over ten years to reward providers for "meaningful use" of the devices that it helped purchase. That included a payment of as much as $44,000 to each physician that certified MU of the EHR.

The HITECH law also established the Office of the National Coordinator for Health Information Technology (ONC), gave it another $2 billion in discretionary funding, and tasked it with setting standards to facilitate the exchange of health information and with training a qualified health care IT workforce. Further, HITECH set up a network of sixty-two Regional Extension Centers, on the model of agricultural cooperative extension offices, to assist local providers with acquiring suitable IT and meeting the new requirements.[261]

While doctors may choose whether to participate in the subsidy program, they don't get to decide whether they'll be penalized for not meeting the MU requirements. Doctors who didn't satisfy MU requirements in 2013 will find their Medicare reimbursements reduced in 2015.

Doctors who haven't yet focused on EHR and MU may be in for an unhappy surprise in two years as their Medicare revenues get chipped down a notch. The penalties start at 1 percent and then go up another 1 percent for each succeeding year that MU is not attained, to a maximum of 5 percent after 2018. Whether doctors like it or not, or even know it or not, they are already deep into a systemic change that may reduce their income.

6.2.3 Current State

Take-up of the EHR accelerated with the federal encouragement. In early 2011, almost 34 percent of primary care and specialist physicians had a basic functioning EHR; by March 2012, 44 percent did. A basic EHR was defined as

---

[260] Blumenthal, NEJM, December 15, 2011.

[261] Adam Wright, et al., "Early Results of the Meaningful Use Program for Electronic Health Records," New England Journal of Medicine, 2013: 368; 779–780; February 21, 2013. http://www.nejm.org/doi/full/10.1056/NEJMc1213481

one that allowed doctors to see lab results, order prescriptions, look at X-rays, and record clinical notes, among other things.

Very few physicians met all 11 MU criteria in effect at that time, but many reported meeting most of them. Roughly 41 percent of primary care physicians said they met eight to ten MU functions. Primary care doctors were slightly more likely to have a basic EHR (45 percent) than specialists (41 percent), according to The Commonwealth Fund.[262]

That's consistent with the experience and perspective of Ross A. Slotten, MD, a family practitioner in Chicago in a three-doctor group. Primary care is likely to be the last part of the system to feel the punitive side of the regulations, he said. "The system is very dependent on having primary care people, whether they're physicians, physician assistants, or nurse practitioners," he said. "The whole system is engined by primary care. We're the critical point. I think we stand to gain, to some degree," at the expense of the specialists, who "are going to be the ones to feel it the most."[263]

The Commonwealth Fund study found that EHR systems with more advanced features were more challenging to integrate into clinical practice. Those features included data exchange with external physicians, the ability to create quality metrics, and the ability to give patients a summary of their visit. These are, of course, the higher-level uses of the EHR on which the future of quality reporting depends. Doctors may require additional training and assistance to reap all the intended benefits of the EHR, the study authors conclude.

The penetration of EHRs has continued apace. By the end of April 2013, more than 291,000 eligible professionals (EPs) and more than 3,800 hospitals had received incentive payments from Medicare or Medicaid for demonstrating at least the first stage of MU. That was more than 50 percent of physicians' offices and 80 percent of eligible hospitals, exceeding the department's goal.[264]

"We have reached the tipping point in adoption of electronic health records," HHS Secretary Kathleen Sebelius said in a statement. By August 2013, there were 405,000 active registrations for the MU program out of 533,000 providers.

[262] Catherine M. DesRoches, Anne-Marie Audet, MD, et al., "Meeting Meaningful Use Criteria and Managing Patient Populations: A National Survey of Practicing Physicians," Annals of Internal Medicine, 158(11): 791–99. June 4, 2013. http://annals.org/article.aspx?articleid=1692572

[263] Ross A. Slotten, MD, office interview, August 30, 2013.

[264] http://www.cms.gov/Newsroom/MediaReleaseDatabase/Press-Releases/2013-Press-Releases-Items/2013-05-22.html

By June 30, $15.5 billion had been paid out to 310,000 providers, according to the ONC.[265]

"Fundamentally, the federal government putting a mandate out to the industry—it has worked," said Mark Hagland, editor in chief of *Healthcare Informatics* magazine. "Has it worked out exactly as some people had hoped? No. It's turning out to be more complex than we thought."[266]

The EHRs are helping doctors to coordinate care, reduce duplicative tests and procedures, and keep patients healthier. Yet this revolution is about more than improving care for the individual patient. Once these data are organized and pulled together into meaningful form, they can contribute to an understanding of how well doctors, hospitals, and health systems are doing their work, compared to their cohort groups. Thus, health care IT is the essential piece to quality improvement (QI); without it, the QI movement in health care would never gain momentum, nor would we be able to conceptualize and implement a system of accountable care. In a more comprehensive iteration, these data can be used to evaluate medications, devices, and procedures across large populations and compare their effectiveness.

It all begins with data capture, said Jane Metzger, principal researcher at the Global Institute for Emerging Healthcare Practices. "Data capture is the foundation not just for informed care—that you have a medical record that's complete—but it's having the data that you need for measurement, and bringing that measurement into real time, so you can track patients, and if there are gaps in care, take care of those in real time," she said in an interview with *Healthcare Informatics*.[267]

Yet the EHR incentive program has received decidedly mixed reviews from physicians in practice. "These systems are wonderful information storage systems but fail to provide the benefit for which they were adopted," said Arthur E. Palamara, MD, a vascular surgeon in Broward County, Florida. "The simple vastness of individual medical information—without a search engine to present the recorded data in a rapid and comprehensible form—renders the information obscure and inaccessible." He thinks MU is largely a sham; checking the box

---

[265] Beth Walsh, *"MU Participants, Payments Continue to Climb," Clinical Innovation + Technology,* August 7, 2013.

[266] Mark Hagland, telephone interview, August 16, 2013.

[267] Mark Hagland, *"It's No Longer Just About Meaningful Use," Healthcare Informatics,* August 28, 2011. http://www.healthcare-informatics.com/article/its-no-longer-just-about-meaningful-use

attesting to MU is "just a formality that I participate in every time I see a patient. The step is not legitimate in my point of view."[268]

Michael Merry, MD, an internist and pediatrician with a group practice in Freeport, Illinois, said his productivity fell from twenty-five to thirty patients per day with paper records to twenty to twenty-four patients per day with the EHR system, in part because he is a "hunt-and-peck" typist.[269] Once he started using a scribe to type up his notes, his productivity improved.

Slotten, the family practice doctor in Chicago, echoes this frustration. He described the effort required to get histories of well-established patients into the EHR: "When was your last diphtheria-tetanus shot? Oops, I guess I never gave you one! Oh, yes, you had your gallbladder removed six years ago. Let's put that down in the surgical history section. I know you're 80, but can you tell me again what your mother died of, because Medicare insists that's meaningful data? A 15-minute visit stretched to 20 or more as I struggled to fill in all the fields. I started to get behind. I began to feel like an opera singer with a cold: I could perform, but sub-optimally. It made me irritable. I came to dread the patient I'd known and liked for 25 years with the 10-active-problems list. How do you record everything?"[270]

It felt to him as though the computerized input had increased, not decreased, his workload. "Overall, the system saves everyone time, except the doctor," Slotten said. "My current relationship with the electronic record is like dating someone that is good for me, smart and connected, but not particularly attractive. Maybe in another year I'll be in love."

Slotten wrote up those comments in early 2012, a few months after his practice installed an EHR system. By late 2013, his viewpoint was more nuanced; he is now more comfortable with the technology and sees its advantages. "The virtues that I see right now, it's a very nice way of organizing information. Now that I've got people in the system, there's certain information that's very easy to access. I think I know better what my patients are doing. The fact that you can do it on a

[268] Arthur E. Palamara, MD, telephone interview, August 25, 2013.

[269] Joseph Conn, "More docs get EHR help," Modern Healthcare, August 24, 2013. http://www.modernhealthcare.com/article/20130824/MAGAZINE/308249958#ixzz2dHAICQ40?trk =tynt

[270] Ross A. Slotten, MD, personal communication and interview, August 30, 2013.

computer is generally a good thing." It helps that he can touch-type; one of his partners who doesn't type has a harder time.

It's also easier to make decisions and execute them on the spot, Slotten reports. "I can be anywhere in the world and refill patients' prescriptions. I can say, 'Oh, this person saw me a month ago, here's their potassium.' I can do it on my cell phone, my laptop, or my tablet." He knows the last time the patient was seen in his office. If a patient is in the hospital, he can go to the hospital's website and find out everything he wants to know. Before the hospital's patient records were computerized, he spent his time chasing down consultants and paper files. Overall, he said, "Even though I started out whining, I actually like a lot of aspects" of the EHRs.

A survey of 1,200 providers by IT vendor AthenaHealth published in August 2013 showed a fair amount of skepticism among physicians. As doctors gain familiarity with the systems, their perspective darkens. Some 47 percent of respondents said EHRs were not designed with doctors in mind, up from 44 percent in 2012. More than two-thirds (69 percent) said they felt the system slowed them down during the patient encounter, up from 65 percent the year before. And 44 percent don't think the EHR achieves a measurable positive financial impact, up from 42 percent in 2012. Independent physicians are generally dourer on the outlook for EHRs than employed physicians. Nearly two-thirds of physicians expect the quality of patient care to decline in the next five years.[271]

The survey results send a number of warning signals. "Doctors are besieged by change and requirements and it's incredibly difficult for them to keep up," said Todd Rothenhaus, MD, chief marketing officer of AthenaHealth, in a statement. "We need to pay attention to the fact that doctors are overwhelmed and challenged in areas they shouldn't be … Physicians lack the time and, in too many cases, the resources to thrive through change. They need better support and need to know there are tools and services to remove the 'busy' work, so they can focus on patient care."[272]

---

[271] AthenaHealth, 2013 Physician Sentiment Index. http://www.athenahealth.com/physician-sentiment-index/future-of-medicine.php?intcmp=PSI/MEANINGFUL-USE-INCENTIVES.PHP&intcmp=I000859

[272] http://investors.athenahealth.com/phoenix.zhtml?c=213592&p=irol-newsArticle&ID=1846875&highlight=

The EHR "has the potential to work," Palamara said. "In some aspects it is extremely efficient. In other aspects, there are many deficiencies that do not help me practice medicine."

Electronic health records, even in their most advanced iterations, aren't immune to occasional lapses in service, especially as they are linked together across geographies and health systems. In 2010, an automatic antivirus software update caused the computers at a number of hospitals in Rhode Island to compulsively restart and lose their networking capability. The hospitals had to divert less serious emergencies and postpone elective surgeries.[273] On August 26, 2013, the $1 billion Sutter Health EHR system crashed, depriving physicians and nurses at the bedside of information on medication orders, allergies, and other patient data in the Northern California region. Alta Bates Summit Medical Center, Eden Medical Center, Sutter Modesto, Mills-Peninsula Hospital, and affiliated clinics were some of the locations affected.[274]

"I don't like it when the system goes down," Slotten said. "This morning, a patient had an MRI. I couldn't get results from the hospital. Some error message came up. It's infuriating."

Device failures and both natural and man-made disasters "are inevitable," wrote Dean F. Sittig and Hardeep Singh, MD, in the *New England Journal of Medicine*. "The potential consequences of an EHR failure becomes of increasing concern as large-scale EHR systems are deployed across multiple facilities within a health care system, often across a wide geographic area."[275]

The same capabilities that make them fast and convenient also make them vulnerable, not just in an isolated department or building, but across a community. Special care must be taken, Sittig and Singh argue, to ensure that patient safety goals are incorporated into EHR system planning and design, including minimizing downtime, reducing overload of clinical-decision support systems, and programming systems to detect underreported errors of omission.

Problem areas also include standardization of measures and data entry. Data elements may be entered inconsistently at different locations or in different

---

[273] *Dean F. Sittig and Hardeep Singh, MD, "Electronic Health Records and National Patient-Safety Goals," New England Journal of Medicine, 2012; 367:1854–60. November 8, 2012. http://www.nejm.org/doi/full/10.1056/NEJMsb1205420*

[274] *Erin McCann, "Setback for Sutter after $1B EHR crashes," Healthcare IT News, August 28, 2013. http://www.healthcareitnews.com/news/setback-sutter-after-1b-ehr-system%20crashes*

[275] *Sittig and Singh, NEJM, November 8, 2012.*

formats. Training and discernment are required to understand what are the appropriate denominators and numerators in the many measures that are expressed as a percent of a patient population. Using "incomplete, inaccurate or inconsistent data can lead to miscalculated denominators (e.g., patients eligible for a measure) and numerators (e.g., those eligible who received recommended care) and reduce the overall validity of the measure results," said a report by the ONC.[276]

Whether the EHR investments are worth the money is an open question in many physicians' minds. Respondents to the AthenaHealth survey were split on the cost/benefit question: 51 percent thought the financial benefits did not outweigh the costs. Yet 55 percent thought the benefits to patient care outweighed the costs. Here, the split between independent physicians and employed physicians was pronounced: 62 percent of employed physicians believed in the patient-care benefits, while only 45 percent of independent practitioners did.[277]

"It's hard or nearly impossible to justify the investment needed for a state-of-the-art EHR with hard-dollar savings," said Rick Hinds, the CFO of UC Health System in Cincinnati. "You have to look beyond that to the intangible benefits, the improvements in delivery of care, and positioning your organization to be competitive in the future."[278] Installing an EHR is a "have-to-do, not a want-to-do" if a health system wants to be viable in the long term, he told *HealthLeaders Media*.

There are a variety of ways to look at ROI, besides simple financial return, said Craig Richmond, associate CFO and vice president of MetroHealth in Cleveland. "You can look at ROI from a financial perspective. You can look at ROI from mitigating compliance risk. ... Don't even call it an ROI, but look at the value proposition associated with it."

For EHRs to really pay off, providers have to redesign patient-care processes around them. Otherwise, continuing in the same routines, with the same expectations, will lead to frustration and a failure to capture the underlying value

---

[276] *Office of the National Coordinator for Health Information Technology, Beacon Policy Brief, "Building a Foundation of Electronic Data to Measure and Drive Improvement," August 2013. http://www.healthit.gov/policy-researchers-implementers/briefs*

[277] *AthenaHealth, http://www.athenahealth.com/physician-sentiment-index/future-of-medicine.php?intcmp=PSI/MEANINGFUL-USE-INCENTIVES.PHP&intcmp=I000859*

[278] *Rene Letourneau, "ROI of Technology Systems Is More Than Financial," HealthLeaders, August 26, 2013.*

of the technology. Providers need to be able to move away from regarding the EHR as an electronic transcription machine for documentation and billing, to seeing it as a tool to generate real-time tracking of their clinical performance, experts say.

A report by the ONC on the Beacon Community Program—an initiative to invest $250 million in seventeen localities with leading-edge IT capabilities—notes that "QI strategies often focus on redesigning care processes, reforming payment systems, and/or increasing patient engagement. All of these approaches require an underpinning of data." This enables internal and external benchmarking and reporting, "which can be used to inform the decision making of hospitals, providers, insurers, patients, accreditors, and policy makers."[279]

For instance, at Inova, an integrated delivery system in Northern Virginia, Toyota Lean principles were applied throughout the system to unlock efficiencies and remove bottlenecks. Emergency department throughput was increased enormously after the newly installed EHR was used to measure all stages of the ED process at the system's five hospitals. Emergency department length of stay for discharged patients went from 215 to 135 minutes, time to see a doctor decreased from 55 to 22 minutes, time on diversion status dropped from 1,300 hours to 50 hours, and patient satisfaction rose considerably.[280]

Unfortunately, some doctors are not completely on board with the practice transformation concept, said Martin Love, CEO of the Humboldt-Del Norte Independent Practice Association in Eureka, California. Many doctors who have taken the government's incentive money either couldn't or wouldn't have installed an EHR on their own, and they're still dragging their feet. Many of the practices in Love's community put in EHRs but didn't particularly devote themselves to learning how to use them. Still, they somehow manage to meet the MU criteria.

"Most of the EHRs stink; they're not very good," Love said. "They're built around charge capture and up-coding. And if there's any group of people inflexible around work flows, it's doctors. So it's really heavy lifting."[281]

---

[279] Beacon Policy Brief, "Building a Foundation of Electronic Data to Measure and Drive Improvement," August 2013. http://www.healthit.gov/policy-researchers-implementers/briefs

[280] John S. Toussaint, MD, and Leonard L. Berry, "The Promise of Lean in Health Care," Mayo Clinic Proceedings, January 2013; 88(1):74–82. www.MayoClinicProceedings.org

[281] Martin Love, telephone interview, August 30, 2013.

In the long run, he believes, the EHR will prove to be a worthwhile investment. But first, one must define what the long run is and figure out how to keep the individual practices solvent until then. "I know a previously successful practice for which the cost of the EHR is ruining the practice," Love noted ruefully.

There's little connection between the cost of the EHR and its quality, he pointed out. Furthermore, the interoperability is not what it needs to be and there are too many offerings on the market. "The curse of this is every single practice in Humboldt County that has an EHR chose a different one." Many practices that selected inappropriate or less-than-fully functional systems are going to have to migrate to a different vendor, with attendant expense and headaches, he said.

6.2.4 The Road Ahead

Even though more than half of all providers have met the criteria for Stage 1 of MU, the road ahead is fraught with difficulties. Stage 2 of MU was planned to go into effect for hospitals on October 1, 2013, and for physicians on January 1, 2014. Many provider organizations petitioned the CMS to slow down and give practitioners a chance to catch their breath and evaluate how well-prepared they are to move to the next phase. In July 2013, the American Hospital Association (AHA) and the American Medical Association (AMA) wrote to HHS Secretary Kathleen Sebelius to express their concern that vendors were not fully ready to deliver what the government was requesting.

Stage 2 is considerably more complex than Stage 1. It requires physicians to be able to exchange data and communicate electronically with patients.

"For every Phase 2 MU requirement that is one line long, it has vast implications for what has to be changed," said Hagland, editor of *Healthcare Informatics.* "It is more complex than people expected, and more challenging, but it's where the industry has to go. The requirement that you have to supply patients with an electronic summary of their treatment—is that shocking? You have to be able to share live patient data with one provider not inside your enterprise."[282]

The bottom line for MU Stage 1 and MU Stage 2 is that "you have to be able to operate an EHR that gives patients access, that facilitates health information

---

[282] *Hagland, telephone interview, August 16, 2013.*

exchange, and that automatically gathers quality measures through the EHR," Hagland said. These requirements are "very basic," he added. "It's hard to argue that it is bizarre or excessive."

Practitioners don't necessarily agree. "The AMA is increasingly alarmed at the pace the Meaningful Use Program is moving ahead without a mechanism to correct the program," said AMA Immediate Past Chair Steven J. Stack, MD. "It is clear from the experience in Stage 1 that unless Stage 2 requirements are modified to allow greater flexibility for physicians, particularly specialists, not only will many physicians not qualify for incentives, they'll also be hit with a penalty."[283]

By July 17, 2013, only 11 EHR vendors for physician offices had met 2014 certification requirements for Stage 2, the associations stated, while 1,300 vendor products had been certified to meet Stage 1, according to *American Medical News.*[284] The associations were concerned that doctor groups and hospitals might have to junk their previous EHR system to meet the more strenuous requirements or fail to attain certification for Stage 2 MU and be forced to take Medicare penalties.

At a congressional hearing in July, Farzad Mostashari, MD, the national health care IT coordinator, declined to relax the deadlines. "I believe a pause in the program would stall the progress that's been hard-fought. … A pause would take momentum away from progress."

On August 22, 2013, the Medical Group Management Association asked HHS Secretary Sebelius to ease the burden on physicians. It requested an extension of one year and added flexibility on Stage 2 reporting. "HHS should immediately institute an indefinite moratorium on penalties for physicians that successfully completed Stage 1 meaningful use requirements," the letter from MGMA CEO Susan Turney, MD, said.[285]

Matters were thrown into further disarray when Mostashari announced in August 2013 that he would resign his post. This news came down on the same day a working group of CMS and ONC delivered a report on interoperability that left

---

[283] Charles Fiegl, "Doctors, hospitals unite to improve meaningful use stage 2," *American Medical News,* August 5, 2013.

[284] Fiegl, *American Medical News.*

[285] http://www.mgma.com/WorkArea/DownloadAsset.aspx?id=1375260

industry participants decidedly underwhelmed—all of this just seven weeks before providers were supposed to start implementing Stage 2 of MU.

But at the last minute, in December 2013, CMS gave the industry what appears to be a modest reprieve. The ONC announced a one-year extension of Stage 2 of the MU program, which started October 1, 2013, for hospitals and January 1, 2014, for physicians and other EPs. CMS's proposed rule change would mean that start dates for MU Stage 3 attestation would be extended by one year and begin in October 2016 for hospitals and January 1, 2017, for providers. However, it's important to note that this proposed rule has no effect on the start date and implementation requirements for the MU Stage 2 that began in 2014. Providers who attested to MU Stage 1 during 2011 and 2012 must attest to MU Stage 2 during 2014. Those attesting to Stage 1 in 2013 are still expected to attest to Stage 2 in 2015. The change in the start date for MU Stage 3 was proposed to accomplish two goals: first, to allow CMS and ONC to focus efforts on the successful implementation of the enhanced patient engagement, interoperability, and health information exchange requirements in Stage 2; and second, to use data from Stage 2 participation to inform policy decisions for Stage 3.

Later, in December 2013, the administration appointed Karen DeSalvo, MD, the health commissioner of New Orleans, to be the new national coordinator for health information technology.[286] DeSalvo helped establish a network of patient-centered medical homes in New Orleans after Hurricane Katrina. "She has deep experience with community health and likely will focus on safety, quality, and efficiency policy goals empowered by health care IT," said John Halamka, MD, chief information officer at Beth Israel Deaconess Medical Center in Boston, according to *Modern Healthcare*. "Her leadership in rebuilding health care post-Katrina is well-known in the industry."

In a video recorded at the 2013 Health Information and Management Systems Society conference in New Orleans, DeSalvo said, "We made a choice to go straight to electronic health records when we could, when these new clinics were forming. We didn't have to worry about restructuring work flow or getting rid of legacy systems. We were building from the ground."

---

[286] Andis Robeznieks, *"DeSalvo, known for using IT in public health, cheered as choice for ONC," Modern Healthcare, December 19, 2013.*
http://www.modernhealthcare.com/article/20131219/NEWS/312199959?

Without the EHR, she said, "We would not have had the success with medical homes. We knew, very specifically, that—if we wanted good quality primary care, to be medical homes—we would need that great, rich data and the support to do quality improvement that electronic health records would give us."

Section 6.3: Technical Appendix: Medicare Electronic Health Record (EHR) Incentive Program

Note: Information in this section is for the Medicare EHR incentive program for Eligible Professionals (EPs) only. View detailed information on hospital or Medicaid EHR incentive programs at CMS website.

6.3.1 Legislative Background

- Health care provisions contained in the **American Recovery and Reinvestment Act of 2009 (ARRA)** created opportunities for the HHS, its partner agencies, and the states to affect the quality of the nation's health care through the use of advanced health information technology (HIT).

- The combined provisions of Titles IV and XIII of the Recovery Act (cited together as the **Health Information Technology for Economic and Clinical Health Act or the HITECH Act**) statutorily require the use of health IT in improving the quality of health care, reducing medical errors, reducing health disparities, increasing prevention, and improving the continuity of care among health care settings.

- To achieve this goal, the HITECH Act authorized the promotion of the "meaningful use" of EHR through a process of incentives and payment adjustment penalties over time. The resulting initiative—The **EHR incentive program**—is designed to encourage the widespread adoption and increasingly sophisticated use of EHR capabilities by all health care providers, leading to improved patient care.

  o The HITECH Act specified the payment of incentives from 2011 through 2016 for EPs participating in the Medicare EHR incentive program who achieve annual criteria.

o Beginning with 2015, the HITECH Act mandated the initiation of payment adjustment penalties to physicians eligible for participation in the Medicare EHR incentive program who failed to meet annual requirements.

6.3.2 Electronic Health Records (EHR) Overview

Sometimes referred to as electronic medical records (EMR), EHR products are technological systems used by health care providers to record patient care information electronically instead of using paper records. During the past decade, significant advances have been made in the functionality of EHRs to perform a wide variety of care-related tasks well beyond electronic charting.

Basic EHR

- In addition to an electronic format for recording clinical notes, a basic system includes the capability to:
  - o maintain problem patient lists
  - o view laboratory results
  - o maintain a patient's active medication list
  - o order prescriptions electronically

Qualified EHR

- These systems build upon the fundamental capabilities of the basic EHR product with a greater interactive capability. Qualified EHR systems are electronic records of health-related information on an individual that:
  - o includes patient demographic and clinical information, such as medical history and problem lists
  - o has the ability to:

- provide clinical decision support

- support physician order entry

- capture and query information relevant to health care quality

- exchange and integrate electronic health information with other sources

Certified EHR Technology (CEHRT)

- As a specific requirement for successful reporting under the EHR incentive program, CMS requires the use of CEHRT systems that are qualified EHR systems that have undergone an extensive CMS testing and certification process to ensure that they have:

  o the ability to successfully report each of the Clinical Quality Measures (CQMs) for a specific program year

  o technological capabilities that meet the annual requirements for core technology objectives

  o the ability to automatically calculate measure attainment for each CQM for a given program year

  o the ability to aggregate and successfully transmit required information in the appropriate format for a given program year

  o CMS publishes a listing of all certified EHR products available for successful reporting for a given year at: http://www.healthit.gov/policy-researchers-implementers/certified-health-it-product-list-chpl

  Note: For 2013 reporting, there are 4,208 EHR products certified for EHR incentive program reporting. As of January 1, 2014, there are only 533 products certified for 2014 reporting. Because a large number of existing systems must be upgraded, tested, and certified, CMS has modified the reporting time period for 2014 to allow time for such changes to be made.[287]

---

[287] *http://www.healthit.gov/policy-researchers-implementers/certified-health-it-product-list-chpl*

6.3.3 Adoption of EHR by Physicians

Overview

- Under the provisions of the HITECH Act, an aspirational goal was established for all Americans to have an electronic health record by 2014. Achieving this requires all providers to adopt some form of EHR and actively use it for patient care-related processes. Since the passage of the act in 2009, significant progress has been made toward this goal in terms of overall EHR product adoption and enhancements to the technological capabilities of such systems.

- The determination of EHR adoption by individual physicians and group practices has been largely reliant upon voluntary reporting through numerous surveys:

    o The latest estimates indicate that some 80 percent of physicians in 2013 use some form of EHR in practice management.

    o Despite such a large usage rate, however, many providers are finding that their EHR systems are either underused or incapable of addressing the expanded functional requirements associated with successfully meeting the MU standards of the EHR incentive reporting program.

    o A significant number of physicians are faced with upgrading their existing EHR systems or acquiring new ones to be able to meet the CEHRT requirements of the EHR incentive program.

EHR Adoption Data: National Center for Health Statistics (NCHS)

- Each year since 2008, the CDC has funded the National Ambulatory Medical Care Survey (NAMCS) and the results are reported annually by the National Center for Health Statistics (NCHS). The NAMCS includes information on EHR adoption and usage rates and assesses physician readiness to meet MU criteria for a given year.

- In December 2012, the NCHS reported the result of the 2012 NAMCS survey and concluded that 72 percent of office-based physicians used some form of EHR—up from 48 percent in 2009—and may reach 80 percent by the end of 2013. However, only 40 percent of physicians reported using EHR that met criteria for a "basic system."[288]

- Sixty-six percent of physicians reported that they planned to apply or have already applied for MU incentives in 2012. Of these, only 27 percent had computerized systems (self-assessed) with the technical capability to support reporting of required information.

Note: *The self-assessment of system capability to report for MU was based on yes/no questions and did not specifically list functionality requirements needed to meet MU. This format may have led to an **over-estimation** of the percentage of EHR systems capable of meeting MU standards for 2012 because of a lack of physician understanding regarding MU reporting requirements.*

EHR Adoption Data: Independent Research

- A research article published in the *Annals of Internal Medicine* in June 2013 (Catherine DesRoches et al.) also relied on 2012 physician survey data analyzed by Mathematica Policy Research to draw conclusions concerning EHR systems capable of meeting 2012 MU reporting requirements.[289]

- The authors did not question the overall EHR adoption rate reported by the NCHS.

- By using a more stringent methodology to assess EHR capabilities, the research team came to different conclusions from those reported by the NCHS:

    o Instead of using yes/no questions about MU-capable systems, respondents were asked to answer questions about specific EHR functionality related to basic EHR systems and systems capable of meeting 2012 MU reporting requirements.

- Using this methodology, the researchers concluded:

---

[288] *NCHS Data Brief, Number 111, December 2012, Centers for Disease Control and Prevention* http://www.cdc.gov/nchs/data/databriefs/db111.pdf

[289] *Ann Intern Med. 2013; 158:791–799*

o The number of physicians having EHR systems in place that met basic system requirements was 40 percent (as compared to the NCHS-reported rate of 48 percent)

o Fewer than one in 10 (9.8 percent) physicians could meet MU criteria established for 2012 with their current EHR system (as compared to the NCHS-reported rate of 27 percent)

Note: In a similar survey conducted by DesRoches in 2007 (Catherine DesRoches et al., New England Journal of Medicine, July 3, 2008), 13 percent of physicians reported having a basic EHR system and 4 percent reported having an extensive, fully functional system.

EHR Adoption Summary

Despite an adoption rate approaching 80 percent, many physicians have EHR systems that are not capable of meeting the technological objectives of the EHR incentive program. Successful participation to avoid payment penalties and earn incentives will require many providers to significantly upgrade the functionality of existing EHR products or acquire new ones.

6.3.4 Medicare EHR Incentive Program Participant Eligibility

Overview

As required by the HITECH Act, the CMS established the EHR incentive program in 2011 to include individual office-based physicians and hospitals. Using metrics appropriate to the health care setting, CMS established annual requirements for reporting of CQMs and usage of specific core objectives related to technological usage of advanced EHR components.

Eligible and Excluded Professionals[290]

Eligible professionals:

- **EPs**: Unlike the listing of EPs eligible to participate in the PQRS reporting program, eligible participants in the Medicare EHR incentive program include only individual Medicare **physicians** (therapists and other practitioners are excluded). EPs for the EHR incentive program include the following:

    o Doctor of Medicine or Doctor of Osteopathy; Doctor of Podiatric Medicine; Doctor of Optometry; Doctor of Oral Surgery or Doctor of Dental Medicine; and Doctor of Chiropractic.

- **EPs in a group practice:** Incentive payments for EPs are based on individual practitioners. EPs who are part of a group practice may qualify for the EHR incentive payment if each individual EP in the practice successfully demonstrates MU of certified EHR technology. This definition also applies to EPs participating in:

    o the MSSP ACOs

    o the Pioneer ACO program

    o the Comprehensive Primary Care Initiative

Note: EPs who provide at least 80 percent of their Medicare services to Medicare Advantage Plan patients are excluded from the Medicare EHR incentive program, but may participate in the Medicare Advantage EHR incentive program.

- **EPs with multiple practice locations:** Each EP is only eligible for one EHR incentive payment per year regardless of how many practice locations they have.

Note: EPs may choose to participate in either the Medicare or Medicaid EHR incentive Programs. CMS allows an EP to change his or her election once during the life of the EHR incentive programs after making the initial election—2014 is the final year in which a change in program election can occur.

---

[290] http://www.cms.gov/Medicare/Quality-Initiatives-Patient-Assessment-Instruments/PQRS/Downloads/2013_PQRS_MedicareEHRIncentPilot_12192012.pdf

Excluded:

- **hospital-based professionals**: Defined by CMS as those who furnish at least 90 percent of their professional services in a hospital setting (i.e., inpatient or emergency room departments) in the year preceding payment year. Such individuals are **excluded** from participation in the Medicare EHR incentive program for EPs.

- **EPs participating in Medicare Advantage (MA) plans:** EPs that are either employed by a MA plan or who provide at least 80 percent of their Medicare services to MA patients and furnish at least 20 hours per week of patient care services are **excluded** from the Medicare EHR incentive program. Such individuals may participate in the Medicare Advantage EHR incentive program. However, any earned incentive payments will be made to the MA organization and not to individual EPs.[291]

Medicare EHR Incentive Program Participation Summary 2011–2013

- The participation rate in the EHR incentive program by individual Medicare providers has increased from 123,648 in 2011 to a total enrollment of 286,771 through October 2013.

- In part, because of physicians attempting MU reporting with inadequate EHR systems, the overall percentage of participants achieving MU has consistently been below 50 percent:[292]

TABLE 1: SUMMARY OF MEDICARE EHR ELIGIBLE PROFESSIONAL REPORTING 2011–2013

Calendar Year	Cumulative Number of Medicare EHR Incentive Program Enrollees	Number Achieving MU and Receiving Incentive Payments	Percentage Achieving MU and Receiving Incentive Payments
2011	123,648	57,573	47%

---

[291] http://www.cms.gov/Regulations-and-Guidance/Legislation/EHRIncentivePrograms/MedicareAdvantage.html

[292] http://www.cms.gov/Regulations-and-Guidance/Legislation/EHRIncentivePrograms/DataAndReports.html

| 2012 | 237,206 | 97,096 | 41% |
| 2013* | 286,771 | 104,140** | 36% |

*2013 numbers reflect enrollment and reporting through October 2013.

**These participants will also avoid the 2015 payment adjustment penalty.

Estimated Participation in the Medicare EHR Incentive Program 2014–2019

- With the cessation of incentive payments in 2016 and the application of payment adjustment penalties beginning in 2015 (2013 reporting year) for all eligible providers, CMS projects both a growth in participation and an increase in the percentage of successful MU reporting:
  - In the 2013 CMS Physicians Fee Schedule Final Rule, CMS projected that with the implementation of the payment adjustment penalty, EHR incentive program participation rates and the percentage of EPs achieving MU would rise from 37 percent to 67 percent between CY2014–CY2019.

TABLE 2: ESTIMATED MEDICARE EHR ELIGIBLE PROFESSIONAL REPORTING 2014–2019[293]

REPORTING YEAR	INCENTIVE YEAR	PENALTY YEAR	CMS-ESTIMATED MEDICARE EHR INCENTIVE PROGRAM ENROLLEES	ESTIMATED EPS ACHIEVING MU: (RECEIVING INCENTIVE/ AVOIDING PENALTY)	ESTIMATED EP PERCENTAGE ACHIEVING MU: (RECEIVING INCENTIVE/ AVOIDING PENALTY)
2014	2014	2016	397,500	145,100	37%
2015	2015	2017	396,900	184,200	46%
2016	2016	2018	397,150	206,500	52%
2017	NA	2019	402,300	229,311	57%
2018	NA	2020	407,300	252,500	62%
2019	NA	2021	412,150	276,100	67%

[293] Page 54140, Table 22: Federal Register/Vol. 77, No. 171/Tuesday, September 4, 2012 www.gpo.gov/fdsys/pkg/FR-2012-09-04/pdf/2012-21563.pdf

6.3.5 Incentives and Payment Adjustment Penalties

Overview

- The "value proposition" of the EHR incentive program is to encourage the adoption of electronic health technology to achieve specific benchmarks, resulting in better patient care and overall efficiency. Achieving these benchmarks is defined by CMS as demonstrating MU of EHR technology to use EHR in a meaningful way, outside simple record-keeping tasks.

- The achievement of MU during a given year determines the positive and negative financial incentives provided under the Medicare fee-for-service (FFS) EHR incentive program. CMS assigns annual MU criteria to participants based on their specific time period of participation. These reporting time periods are segmented into three MU "stages," as discussed below.

Incentives

- Since 2011, CMS has paid more than $3.9 billion in incentives to EPs participating in the Medicare and Medicaid EHR incentive programs.

- Incentive payments for the Medicare EHR incentive program are made only to individual providers, not to practices or medical groups. Although a provider can designate a practice to receive the incentive funds on its behalf, it is up to the provider to make this decision—the practice or medical group cannot claim the money or make the decision for the provider, even if the EHR belongs to the practice.

- Beginning in 2011, CMS provides for up to five continuous years of incentive payments to EPs who adopt an EHR product and meet annual MU criteria. The final year of incentive payments is 2016 and the final year to enroll for incentives is 2014.

- EHR incentive payment amounts are established as:

  o 75 percent of allowed Medicare Part B charges occurring in the reporting year, **up to** a published annual maximum amount for a given year of program participation:

  ▪ for example, a physician who joined the EHR incentive
    program in 2012 with $17,000 of allowed Medicare Part B
    charges is eligible for up to $12,750 in incentive payments,
    while a physician with $40,000 in allowed charges for the
    same time period would be eligible for the maximum annual
    incentive payment of $18,000.

- For those enrolling during 2011 and 2012 and meeting MU criteria each
  year, the maximum paid incentive totals $44,000 through 2016.

  o For 2013 and 2014 enrollment, the maximum incentive is reduced
    to $39,000 and $24,000, respectively.

- CMS did not design the EHR incentive program as a reimbursement
  program for purchasing, replacing or maintaining an EHR.

  o CMS estimates that the average adopt/implement/upgrade (AIU)
    cost for EHR is $54,000 per physician full-time equivalent (FTE),
    while annual maintenance costs average $10,000 per physician
    FTE.[294]

- Annual incentive payments from 2011 through 2016, based on
  participation dates, are as follows:*

**TABLE 3: MEDICARE EHR PROGRAM INCENTIVE PAYMENTS BY
MEANINGFUL USE STAGE[295]**

Maximum Total EHR Program Incentive Payment by Starting Calendar Year (CY)	ANNUAL INCENTIVE PAYMENT BY MEANINGFUL USE STAGE						
	2011	2012	2013	2014	2015	2016**	2017
2011 $43,720	Stage 1 $18,000	Stage 1 $12,000	Stage 1 $7,840 reduction ($160)	Stage 2 $3,920 reduction ($80)	Stage 2 $1,960 reduction ($40)	Stage 2 $0.00	Stage 3 $0.00
2012 $43,480		Stage 1 $18,000	Stage 1 $11,760 reduction ($240)	Stage 2 $7,840 reduction ($160)	Stage 2 $3,920 reduction ($80)	Stage 2 $1,960 reduction ($40)	Stage 3 $0.00
2013 $38,220			Stage 1 $14,700	Stage 1 $11,760	Stage 2 $7,840	Stage 2 $3,920	Stage 3 $0.00

[294] *Page 54139: Federal Register/Vol. 77, No. 171/Tuesday, September 4, 2012
www.gpo.gov/fdsys/pkg/FR-2012-09-04/pdf/2012-21563.pdf*

[295] *Medicare and Medicaid EHR Incentive Program Basics http://www.cms.gov/Regulations-and-
Guidance/Legislation/EHRIncentivePrograms/EducationalMaterials.html*

		reduction ($80)	reduction ($240)	reduction ($160)	reduction ($80)	
2014 $23,250			Stage 1 $12,000	Stage 1 $7,840 reduction ($160)	Stage 2 $3,920 reduction ($80)	**Stage 2 $0.00**

Amounts shown reflect the -2 percent sequestration adjustment as indicated.

**In December 2013, CMS announced a one-year delay in the start of Stage 3. Stage 2 will be extended through 2016 and Stage 3 will begin in 2017 for those providers who have achieved at least two years of successful Stage 2 reporting.*[296]

Note: *EPs participate in the program on the calendar years, while eligible hospitals and critical access hospitals (CAHs) participate according to the federal fiscal year.*

- Incentive payment modification:
  - **HPSA modification**: Incentive payments are increased by 10 percent for each year of participation for EPs who furnish services predominantly in an area designated by the HHS secretary as Geographic Health Professional Shortage Areas (HPSAs). Such areas are classified as those with a shortage of health professionals, based on the population-to-provider ratio and other factors.

  - **failure to meet MU criteria**: Participants who fail to achieve satisfactory MU criteria for a given year of participation will not receive the incentive payment for that year.

  - **sequestration modification**: Medicare EHR incentive payments are subject to mandatory reductions in 2013 federal spending, known as sequestration, mandated by the Budget Control Act of 2011. Under sequestration, EHR incentive payments will be reduced by 2 percent for all reporting periods ending on or after April, 1, 2013.

Note: *The sequestration reduction does not apply to **Medicaid** EHR incentive payments, which are exempt from the mandatory reductions.*

---

[296] *CMS Announcement of 2015 Policies: Progress on Adoption of Electronic Health Records http://www.cms.gov/ehealth/ListServ_Stage3Implementation.html*

Payment Adjustment Penalties

- Beginning in 2015, Medicare EPs who have not achieved MU in a specified reporting year will be subject to payment adjustment penalties.

  o The reporting year occurs two years prior to the payment adjustment penalty year. EPs earning an incentive payment in 2013 for successfully achieving MU will not be subject to the 2015 payment penalty.

  o Penalties are a per-claim percentage reduction in Medicare Part B-covered professional services furnished by the EP during the penalty year.

  o Beginning in 2015, **all** physicians who have been determined to be eligible for participation in the Medicare EHR incentive program during the reporting year of 2013 will be evaluated for penalty assessment, whether they participate or not.

- These payment adjustments will be applied beginning on January 1, 2015, for Medicare EPs.

  Note: Medicaid EPs who can only participate in the Medicaid EHR incentive program and who do not bill Medicare are not subject to these payment adjustments.

- Payment adjustment penalties finalized through CY2018 are as follows:

TABLE 4: MEDICARE EHR INCENTIVE PROGRAM PAYMENT ADJUSTMENT PENALTIES

REPORTING YEAR*	PAYMENT ADJUSTMENT YEAR	PAYMENT ADJUSTMENT PENALTY
CY2013	CY2015	-1.0% to -2.0%**
CY2014	CY2016	-2.0%
CY2015	CY2017	-3.0%
CY2016	CY2018	-3.0% to -5.0%***

For EPs beyond their first year of MU reporting. See exclusion for first-year reporting below.

*** Under HITECH Act Rules, EHR users who fail to achieve MU for 2015 (2013 reporting year) and were subject to the eRx penalty in 2014 (2013 reporting year) will receive a -2 percent EHR penalty in 2015.*

***For CY2018 (data available through October 1, 2017) and thereafter, if the HHS secretary determines that less than 75 percent of EPs meet EHR MU criteria, penalties can be increased by 1 percent per year, not to exceed a maximum of 5 percent.[297]

Note: *The payment adjustment is 1 percent per year, beginning in 2013, and is cumulative for every year that an EP is not a meaningful user.*

6.3.6 Meaningful Use (MU)[298]

Overview

- CMS defines MU as using a CEHRT in a "meaningful" way to more fully use the range of advanced capabilities inherent in such a system to enhance patient care.

  o In its 2010 Final Rule, CMS specified that meaningful use of CEHRT technology should result in health care that is "patient-centered, evidence-based, prevention-oriented, efficient, and equitable."

- To accommodate the expected evolution in EHR technology, CMS has established a phased definition of MU over time, with a three-stage approach.

  o Such a phased approach encompasses criteria for MU based on currently available technology capabilities and provider practice experience over specified time periods.

  o With the ultimate goal of improving population health through the use of existing and emerging technology, each stage builds up to a more robust definition of MU based on anticipated technology and capabilities development.

---

[297] *Page 54094, Federal Register/Vol. 77, No. 171/Tuesday, September 4, 2012* *www.gpo.gov/fdsys/pkg/FR-2012-09-04/pdf/2012-21563.pdf*

[298] *Page 44321, Federal Register/Vol. 75, No. 144/Wednesday, July 28, 2010/Rules and Regulations*

- To qualify for annual EHR incentives and avoid penalties (beginning in 2015), participants must meet CMS-established MU criteria for the appropriate stage of program participation, to include the following:

  - the use of a certified EHR in a meaningful manner by stage as defined by CMS

  - the use of certified EHR technology for electronic exchange of health information to improve the overall quality of health care

  - the use of certified EHR technology to submit information on CQMs and health IT objectives:

    - **health IT objectives (EP core objectives):** For 2014 reporting, there are twenty-four such objectives that focus on the use of specific basic and advanced EHR functions.

    - **CQM:** Such measures focus on processes and patient experience of care and/or outcomes of patient care, observations or treatment. For 2014 reporting, there are sixty-four CQMs for the EHR incentive program and they are the same as those used in the PQRS for EHR reporting.

Stage 1: Overview

- Stage 1 MU criteria are heavily focused on establishing the functionalities in a CEHRT product that will allow for future continuous quality improvement and ease of information exchange.

- Stage 1 focuses on electronically capturing health information in a structured format by:

  - using such information to track key clinical conditions and communicating that information for care coordination purposes

  - implementing clinical decision tools to facilitate disease and medication management

  - using EHR to engage patients and families

  - reporting CQMs and public health information

- Some functions of CEHRT are optional for use in Stage 1. However, through proactive adoption of all available functions in Stage 1, providers will be better-prepared for increased requirements of later MU stages.

- Stage 1 participation and reporting requirements:

  o For the first year that an EP applies for and receives an incentive payment, the EHR incentive program reporting period is ninety days for any continuous period beginning no later than July 3 with report submission via attestation no later than October 1 of the reporting year.

  o For years beyond the initial reporting year, participants are required to report for the full calendar year and report results electronically.

  o Participants that are beginning reporting in 2012 and later must successfully report Stage 1 for two years prior to moving to Stage 2. The exception is for those with an initial reporting year of 2011. Such participants will begin Stage 2 reporting in 2014 (three years of successful Stage 1 reporting).

    Note: In the 2014 Final PFS Rule, the reporting period for all participants in 2014 has been changed to reporting for any one calendar year quarter of 2014.

Stage 2: Overview

- Stage 2 expands upon Stage 1 criteria with a focus on ensuring that the MU of EHRs supports the six priorities of the NQS:

  o person and caregiver-centered experience and outcomes

  o patient safety

  o communication and care coordination

  o community and population health

  o efficiency and cost reduction

  o effective clinical care

    Note: For a detailed description of the NQS, please see Section 6.2 in Chapter 3.

- Stage 2 MU criteria encourages the use of health information technology for continuous quality improvement at the point of care and the exchange of information in the most structured format possible, such as the electronic transmission of orders entered using computerized provider order entry (CPOE).

- Stage 2 requirements include:

  - more demanding requirements for e-prescribing

  - incorporation of structured laboratory results (such as blood tests, microbiology, urinalysis, pathology tests, radiology, cardiac imaging, nuclear medicine tests, pulmonary function tests, genetic tests, genomic tests, and other such data needed to diagnose and treat diseases

  - an expectation that providers will electronically transmit patient care summaries with each other and with patients to support transitions in care

  - increased expectations for health exchange information to support the HITECH goal that information follows the patient

    Note: In the 2014 Final PFS Rule, the reporting period for all participants in 2014 only has been changed to reporting for any one calendar year quarter of 2014.

- Stage 2 reporting and participation requirements:

  - Almost all optional functional objectives for Stage 1 will be mandatory for Stage 2.

  - The HITECH Act specified that providers would be evaluated under Stage 3 criteria after completing two years of successful Stage 2 reporting.

  - In the Stage 1 MU regulations, CMS had established a timeline that required providers to progress to Stage 2 criteria after two program years under the Stage 1 criteria. This original timeline would have required Medicare providers who first demonstrated MU in 2011 to meet the Stage 2 criteria in 2013. However, Stage 2 requirements have been delayed. The earliest that the Stage 2 criteria will be effective is in CY2014 for EPs.

o Reporting of Stage 2 CQMs and health IT objectives will "ordinarily" be made for the full calendar year.

> **Note:** *In December 2013, CMS announced a one-year delay in the start of Stage 3, from 2016 to 2017. Stage 2 will be extended through 2016, with the result that some providers will have a third year of Stage 2 reporting. This ruling does not change the 2015 starting period for Stage 2 reporting for providers with two years of successful Stage 1 reporting.*[299]

Stage 3: Overview

- In December 2013, CMS announced a one-year delay in the start of Stage 3, from 2016 to 2017. Stage 2 will be extended through 2016 and Stage 3 will begin in 2017 for those providers who have achieved at least two years of successful Stage 2 reporting.

- For Stage 3, CMS intends to establish higher standards for meeting MU criteria by including every Stage 2 health IT objective. The MU criteria will focus on:

  o promoting improvements in quality, safety, and efficiency, leading to improved health outcomes

  o providing decision support for national high-priority conditions

  o providing patient access to self-management tools

  o providing access to comprehensive patient data through robust, secure, patient-centered health information exchange

  o improving population health

- Specific MU criteria for Stage 3 will be published through future rule making.

---

[299] *CMS Announcement of 2015 Policies: Progress on Adoption of Electronic Health Records*
http://www.cms.gov/ehealth/ListServ_Stage3Implementation.html

6.3.7 2014 Stage 1 and Stage 2 Meaningful Use Reporting Requirements

Stage 1 Meaningful Use Criteria 2014[300]

To qualify for 2014 incentive payments and avoid the 2016 payment adjustment penalty, participants reporting for Stage 1 MU must meet the following criteria:

TABLE 5: 2014 STAGE 1: REPORTING REQUIREMENTS SUMMARY

HEALTH IT OBJECTIVES: EP CORE OBJECTIVES	CQMS
EPs must meet and report on 19 of 24 IT objectives, consisting of: • 14 required core objectives; • and five additional objectives selected out of 10 from a menu set.	EPs must report on nine out of 64 total CQMs. For 2014 there are no "core" CQMs. Instead there are: • nine recommended adult measures;* • and nine recommended pediatric measures.* * Reporting on these is not required, but encouraged.

2014 Stage 1: Health Information Technology (IT) Objectives

14 Core EP objectives for Stage 1 MU 2014 Medicare FFS EHR incentive program:[301]

TABLE 6: 2014 STAGE 1: HEALTH INFORMATION TECHNOLOGY CORE OBJECTIVES

1.	Use CPOE for medication orders directly entered by any licensed health care professional who can enter orders into the medical record per state, local, and professional guidelines.
2.	Implement drug-drug and drug-allergy interaction checks.

---

[300] http://www.cms.gov/Regulations-and-guidance/Legislation/EHRIncentivePrograms/Recommended_Core_Set.html

[301] http://www.cms.gov/Regulations-and-Guidance/Legislation/EHRIncentivePrograms/Meaningful_Use.html

3. Maintain an up-to-date problem list of current and active diagnoses.

4. Generate and transmit permissible prescriptions electronically (eRx).

5. Maintain active medication list.

6. Maintain active medication allergy list.

7. Record all of the following demographics: (A) preferred language; (B) gender; (C) race; (D) ethnicity; and (E) date of birth.

8. Record and chart changes in the following vital signs: (A) height; (B) weight; (C) blood pressure; (D) calculate and display body mass index (BMI); (E) and plot and display growth charts for children 2–20 years, including BMI.

9. Record smoking status for patients 13 years old or older.

10. Report ambulatory CQMs to CMS or, in the case of Medicaid EPs, the states.

11. Implement one clinical decision support rule relevant to specialty or high clinical priority along with the ability to track compliance with that rule.

12. Provide patients with an electronic copy of their health information (including diagnostics test results, problem list, medication lists, and medication allergies) upon request

13. Provide clinical summaries for patients for each office visit.

14. Protect electronic health information created or maintained by the CEHRT through the implementation of appropriate technical capabilities.

Health IT

Ten EP menu objectives for Stage 1 MU 2014 Medicare FFS EHR incentive program:[302]

TABLE 7: 2014 STAGE 1: INFORMATION TECHNOLOGY MENU OBJECTIVES

1. Implement drug formulary checks.

2. Incorporate clinical lab test results into EHR as structured data.

3. Generate lists of patients by specific conditions to use for quality improvement, reduction of disparities, research, or outreach.

4. Send patient reminders per patient preference for preventive/follow-up care.

---

[302] http://www.cms.gov/Regulations-and-Guidance/Legislation/EHRIncentivePrograms/Meaningful_Use.html

5. Provide patients with timely electronic access to their health information (including lab results, problem list, medication lists, and allergies) within four business days of the information being available to the EP.

6. Use CEHRT to identify patient-specific education resources and provide those resources to the patient if appropriate.

7. The EP who receives a patient from another setting of care or provider of care or believes an encounter is relevant should perform medication reconciliation.

8. EPs who transition their patients to another setting of care or provider of care or refers their patients to another provider of care should provide summary care record for each transition of care or referral.

9. Capability to submit electronic data to immunization registries or immunization information systems and actual submission according to applicable law and practice.

10. Capability to submit electronic syndromic surveillance data to public health agencies and actual submission according to applicable law and practice.

2014 Clinical Quality Measures (CQMs) for Stage 1 Reporting

- For the 2014 EHR incentive program there are sixty-four CQMs available for MU Stage 1 reporting and these measures are the **same** as those listed in the PQRS as CQMs available for EHR reporting. Selected CQMs must cover at least three of the six NQS domains:

  ○ **patient and family engagement:** ensuring that each person and family is engaged as partners in their care

  ○ **patient safety**: making care safer by reducing harm caused in the delivery of care

  ○ **care coordination**: promoting effective communication and coordination of care

  ○ **population and public health**: working with communities to promote wide use of best practices to enable healthy living

  ○ **efficient use of health care resources**: making quality care more affordable for individuals, families, employers, and governments by developing and spreading new health care delivery models

○ **clinical processes/effectiveness**: promoting the most effective prevention and treatment practices for the leading causes of mortality, starting with cardiovascular disease

CQMs for 2014 Medicare FFS EHR incentive program

- 2014 Stage 1 MU CQM reporting standard:

    ○ EPs must report on nine out of sixty-four total CQMs.

    ○ For 2014 Stage 1 Reporting for MU, there are no "core" CQMs. However, CMS encourages reporting on measures contained in nine recommended adult measures and nine recommended pediatric measures.

2014 Stage 1 MU recommended adult and pediatric measures

TABLE 8: RECOMMENDED ADULT MEASURES FOR 2014 STAGE 1 REPORTING[303]

NQF NUMBER/NQS DOMAIN	CMS EMEASURE ID/PQRS NUMBER	MEASURE TITLE
0018 Effective Clinical Care	CMS 165v2 PQRS 236	Controlling High Blood Pressure
0022 Patient Safety	CMS 156v2 PQRS 228	Use of High-Risk Medications in the Elderly
0028 Community and Population Health	CMS 138v2 PQRS 226	Preventive Care/Screening: Tobacco Use: Screening/Cessation/Intervention
0052 Efficiency and Cost Reduction	CMS 166v3 PQRS312	Use of Imaging Studies for Low Back Pain
0418 Community and Population Health	CMS 2v3 PQRS 134	Preventive Care and Screening: Clinical Depression and Follow-Up Plan

---

[303] *https://www.cms.gov/ehrincentiveprograms/*

0419 Patient Safety	CMS 68v3 PQRS 130	Documentation of Current Medications in the Medical Record
0421 Community and Population Health	CMS 69v2 PQRS 128	Preventive Care and Screening: Body Mass Index (BMI) Screening/Follow-Up
TBD* Communication and Care Coordination	CMS 50v2 PQRS TBD*	Closing the Referral Loop: Receipt of Specialist Report
TBD* Person and Caregiver-Centered Experience and Outcomes	CMS 90v3 PQRS TBD*	Functional Status Assessment for Complex Chronic Conditions

* This measure is new to the PQRS and has been adopted for reporting beginning in CY2014.

TABLE 9: RECOMMENDED PEDIATRIC MEASURES FOR 2014 STAGE 1 REPORTING[304]

NQF NUMBER/ NQS DOMAIN	CMS EMEASURE ID/PQRS NUMBER	MEASURE TITLE
0002 Efficiency and Cost Reduction	CMS 146v2 PQRS 66	Appropriate Testing for Children with Pharyngitis
0024 Community and Population Health	CMS 155v1 PQRS 239	Weight Assessment and Counseling for Nutrition and Physical Activity for Children and Adolescents
0033 Community and Population Health	CMS 153v2 PQRS 310	Chlamydia Screening for Women
0036 Effective Clinical Care	CMS 126v2 PQRS 311	Use of Appropriate Medications for Asthma
0038 Community and Population Health	CMS 117v2 PQRS 240	Childhood Immunization Status
0069 Efficiency and Cost Reduction	CMS 154v2 PQRS 65	Appropriate Treatment for Children with Upper Respiratory Infection (URI)

[304] http://www.cms.gov/Regulations-and-Guidance/Legislation/EHRIncentivePrograms/Recommended_Core_Set.html

0108 Effective Clinical Care	CMS 136v2 PQRS TBD*	ADHD: Follow-Up Care for Children Prescribed Attention Deficit/Hyperactivity Disorder (ADHD) Medication
0418 Community and Population Health	CMS 2v3 PQRS 134	Preventive Care and Screening: Screening for Clinical Depression and Follow-Up Plan
TBD Effective Clinical Care	CMS 75v2 PQRS TBD*	Children Who Have Dental Decay or Cavities

This measure is new to the PQRS and has been adopted for reporting beginning in CY2014.

All 2014 CQMs for Stage 1 MU reporting

TABLE 10: ALL 2014 CQMS FOR STAGE 1 MEANINGFUL USE REPORTING[305]

NQF NUMBER/ NQS DOMAIN	CMS EMEASURE ID/PQRS NUMBER	MEASURE TITLE
0002 Efficiency and Cost Reduction	CMS 146v2 PQRS 66	Appropriate Testing for Children with Pharyngitis
0004 Effective Clinical Care	CMS 137v2 PQRS 305	Initiation and Engagement of Alcohol and Other Drug Dependence Treatment
0018 Effective Clinical Care	CMS 165v2 PQRS 236	Controlling High Blood Pressure
0022 Patient Safety	CMS 156v2 PQRS 238	Use of High-Risk Medications in the Elderly
0024 Community and Population Health	CMS 155v1 PQRS 239	Weight Assessment and Counseling for Nutrition and Physical Activity for Children and Adolescents
0028 Community and Population Health	CMS 138v2 PQRS 226	Preventive Care and Screening: Tobacco Use: Screening and Cessation Intervention
TBD	CMS 125v2 PQRS 112	Breast Cancer Screening

[305] Page 839, Table 52, http://www.cms.gov/Medicare/Medicare-Fee-for-Service-Payment/PhysicianFeeSched/PFS-Federal-Regulation-Notices-Items/CMS-1600-FC.html

NQF NUMBER/ NQS DOMAIN	CMS EMEASURE ID/PQRS NUMBER	MEASURE TITLE
Effective Clinical Care		
0032 Effective Clinical Care	CMS 124v2 PQRS 309	Cervical Cancer Screening
0033 Community and Population Health	CMS 153v2 PQRS 310	Chlamydia Screening for Women
0034 Effective Clinical Care	CMS 130v2 PQRS 113	Colorectal Cancer Screening
0036 Effective Clinical Care	CMS 126v2 PQRS 311	Use of Appropriate Medications for Asthma
0038 Community and Population Health	CMS 117v2 PQRS 240	Childhood Immunization Status
0041 Community and Population Health	CMS 147v2 PQRS 110	Preventive Care and Screening: Influenza Immunization
0043 Effective Clinical Care	CMS 127v2 PQRS 111	Pneumonia Vaccination Status for Older Adults
0052 Efficiency and Cost Reduction	CMS 166v3 PQRS 312	Use of Imaging Studies for Low Back Pain
0055 Effective Clinical Care	CMS 131v2 PQRS 117	Diabetes: Eye Exam
0056 Effective Clinical Care	CMS 123v1 PQRS 163	Diabetes: Foot Exam
0059 Effective Clinical Care	CMS 122v2 PQRS 1	Diabetes: Hemoglobin A1c Poor Control

NQF NUMBER/ NQS DOMAIN	CMS EMEASURE ID/PQRS NUMBER	MEASURE TITLE
0060 Effective Clinical Care	CMS 148v2 PQRS NA	Hemoglobin A1c Test for Pediatric Patients
0062 Effective Clinical Care	CMS 134v2 PQRS 119	Diabetes: Urine Protein Screening
0064 Effective Clinical Care	CMS 163v2 PQRS 2	Diabetes: Low Density Lipoprotein (LDL) Management
0068 Efficiency and Cost Reduction	CMS 164v2 PQRS 208	Ischemic Vascular Disease (IVD): Use of Aspirin or Another Antithrombotic
0069 Efficiency and Cost Reduction	CMS 154v2 PQRS 65	Appropriate Treatment for Children with Upper Respiratory Infection (URI)
0070 Effective Clinical Care	CMS 145v2 PQRS 7	Coronary Artery Disease (CAD): Beta-Blocker Therapy-Prior Myocardial Infarction (MI) or Left Ventricular Systolic Dysfunction (LVEF <40%)
0075 Effective Clinical Care	CMS 182v3 PQRS 241	Ischemic Vascular Disease (IVD): Complete Lipid Panel and LDL Control
0081 Effective Clinical Care	CMS 135v2 PQRS 5	Heart Failure (HF): Angiotensin Converting Enzyme (ACE) Inhibitor or Angiotensin Receptor Blocker (ARB) Therapy for Left Ventricular Systolic Dysfunction (LVSD)
0083 Effective Clinical Care	CMS 144v2 PQRS 8	Heart Failure (HF): Beta-Blocker Therapy for Left Ventricular Systolic Dysfunction (LVSD)
0086 Effective Clinical Care	CMS 143v2 PQRS 12	Primary Open Angle Glaucoma (POAG): Optic Nerve Evaluation
0088 Effective Clinical Care	CMS 167v2 PQRS 18	Diabetic Retinopathy: Documentation of Presence or Absence of Macular Edema and Level of Severity of Retinopathy
0089	CMS 142v2 PQRS 19	Diabetic Retinopathy: Communication with the Physician Managing Ongoing Diabetes Care

NQF NUMBER/ NQS DOMAIN	CMS EMEASURE ID/PQRS NUMBER	MEASURE TITLE
Effective Clinical Care		
0101 Patient Safety	CMS 139v2 PQRS 318	Falls: Screening for Future Fall Risk
0104 Effective Clinical Care	CMS 161v2 PQRS 107	Major Depressive Disorder (MDD): Suicide Risk Assessment
0105 Effective Clinical Care	CMS 128v2 PQRS 9	Anti-Depressant Medication Management
0108 Effective Clinical Care	CMS 136v2 PQRS NA*	ADHD: Follow-Up Care for Children Prescribed Attention Deficit/Hyperactivity Disorder (ADHD) Medication
0110 Effective Clinical Care	CMS 169v2 PQRS TBD*	Bipolar Disorder and Major Depression: Appraisal for Alcohol or Chemical Substance Use
0384 Person and Caregiver- Centered Experience and Outcomes	CMS 157v2 PQRS 143	Oncology: Medical and Radiation-Pain Intensity Quantified
0385 Effective Clinical Care	CMS 141v3 PQRS 72	Colon Cancer: Chemotherapy for AJCC Stage III Colon Cancer
0387 Effective Clinical Care	CMS 140v1 PQRS 71	Breast Cancer: Hormonal Therapy for Stage IC-IIIC Estrogen Receptor/Progesterone Receptor (ER/PR) Positive Breast Cancer
0389 Efficiency and Cost Reduction	CMS 129v3 PQRS 102	Prostate Cancer: Avoidance of Overuse of Bone Scan for Staging Low-Risk Prostate Cancer Patients
0403 Effective Clinical Care	CMS 62v2 PQRS TBD*	HIV/AIDS: Medical Visit
0405 Effective Clinical Care	CMS 52v1 PQRS 160	HIV/AIDS: Pneumocystis Jiroveci Pneumonia (PCP) Prophylaxis

NQF NUMBER/ NQS DOMAIN	CMS EMEASURE ID/PQRS NUMBER	MEASURE TITLE
TBD Effective Clinical Care	CMS 77v1 PQRS TBD*	HIV/AIDS: RNA Control for Patients with HIV
0418 Community and Population Health	CMS 2v3 PQRS 134	Preventive Care and Screening: Screening for Clinical Depression and Follow-Up Plan
0419 Patient Safety	CMS 68v3 PQRS 130	Documentation of Current Medications in the Medical Record
0421 Community and Population Health	CMS 69v2 PQRS 128	Preventive Care and Screening: Body Mass Index (BMI) Screening and Follow-Up
0564 Patient Safety	CMS 132v1 PQRS 192	Cataracts: Complications Within 30 Days Following Cataract Surgery Requiring Additional Surgical Procedures
0565 Effective Clinical Care	CMS 133v2 PQRS 191	Cataracts: 20/40 or Better Visual Acuity within 90 Days Following Cataract Surgery
0608 Effective Clinical Care	CMS 158v2 PQRS TBD*	Pregnant Women Who Had HBsAg Testing
0710 Effective Clinical Care	CMS 159v2 PQRS TBD*	Depression Remission at Twelve Months
0712 Effective Clinical Care	CMS 160v2 PQRS TBD*	Depression Utilization of the PHQ-9 Tool
TBD Effective Clinical Care	CMS 75v2 PQRS TBD*	Children Who Have Dental Decay or Cavities
1365 Effective Clinical Care	CMS 177v2 PQRS TBD*	Child and Adolescent Major Depressive Disorder: Suicide Risk Assessment
1401 Community and Population Health	CMS 82v1 PQRS TBD*	Maternal Depression Screening

NQF NUMBER/ NQS DOMAIN	CMS EMEASURE ID/PQRS NUMBER	MEASURE TITLE
TBD Effective Clinical Care	CMS 74v3 PQRS TBD*	Primary Caries Prevention Intervention as Offered by Primary Care Providers, including Dentists
TBD Effective Clinical Care	CMS 61v3 PQRS 316	Preventive Care and Screening: Cholesterol-Fasting Low Density Lipoprotein (LDLC) Test Performed
TBD Effective Clinical Care	CMS 64v3 PQRS 316	Preventive Care and Screening: Risk-Stratified Cholesterol-Fasting Low Density Lipoprotein (LDLC)
TBD Effective Clinical Care	CMS 149v2 PQRS 281	Dementia: Cognitive Assessment
TBD Effective Clinical Care	CMS 65v3 PQRS TBD*	Hypertension: Improvement in Blood Pressure
TBD Communication and Care Coordination	CMS 50v2 PQRS TBD*	Closing the Referral Loop: Receipt of Specialist Report
TBD Person and Caregiver- Centered Experience and Outcomes	CMS 66v2 PQRS TBD*	Functional Status Assessment for Knee Replacement
TBD Person and Caregiver- Centered Experience and Outcomes	CMS 56v2 PQRS TBD*	Functional Status Assessment for Hip Replacement
TBD Person and Caregiver- Centered Experience and Outcomes	CMS 90v3 PQRS TBD*	Functional Status Assessment for Complex Chronic Conditions
TBD Patient Safety	CMS 179v2 PQRS TBD*	ADE Prevention and Monitoring: Warfarin Time in Therapeutic Range

NQF NUMBER/ NQS DOMAIN	CMS EMEASURE ID/PQRS NUMBER	MEASURE TITLE
TBD Community and Population health	CMS 22v2 PQRS 317	Preventive Care and Screening: Screening for High Blood Pressure and Follow-Up Documented

* This measure is new to the PQRS and has been adopted for reporting beginning in CY2014.

Note: All 64 CQMS are reportable under one of 63 assigned PQRS codes:

- Two CQMs have been combined under one PQRS reporting code:

CMS 61v3 **PQRS 316**	Preventive Care and Screening: Cholesterol-Fasting Low Density Lipoprotein (LDLC) Test Performed
CMS 64v3 **PQRS 316**	Preventive Care and Screening: Risk-Stratified Cholesterol- Fasting Low Density Lipoprotein (LDLC)

- In the CY2014 Final PFS Rule, CMS specified that EPs electronically reporting quality measures must use the most recent Specifications Manual. For 2014 (until a revised manual is released), this means that the specifications manual dated June 2013 is to be used for 2014 reporting all measures, except:

  o CMS140v2, Breast Cancer Hormonal Therapy for Stage IC-IIIC Estrogen Receptor/Progesterone Receptor (ER/PR) Positive Breast Cancer (NQF 0387). Reporting for this measure must be accomplished using the December 2012 Specifications Manual.

Stage 2 Meaningful Use Criteria: 2014

To qualify for 2014 incentive payments and avoid the 2016 payment adjustment penalty, participants reporting for Stage 2 MU must meet the following criteria:

TABLE 11: 2014 STAGE 2: REPORTING REQUIREMENTS SUMMARY[306]

HEALTH IT OBJECTIVES: EP CORE OBJECTIVES	CQMs
Must report on the following: • seventeen core objectives; • and three objectives out of six from menu set.	**EPs must report on nine out of sixty-four total CQMs.** • EPs must select CQMs from at least three of the six key health care policy domains (priorities) recommended by the NQS.

2014 Stage 2 MU health IT objectives for EPs

Seventeen core IT objectives for 2014 EPs Stage 2 MU reporting

- MU reporting standard:
  - EPs must meet requirements for all seventeen core objectives and submit data for all core objectives.

TABLE 12: 2014 STAGE 2: HEALTH INFORMATION TECHNOLOGY CORE OBJECTIVES

1. **Computer Physician Order Entry (CPOE):** Use CPOE for medication, laboratory, and radiology orders directly entered by any licensed health care professional who can enter orders into the medical record per state, local, and professional guidelines.

2. **eRx Use:** Generate and transmit permissible prescriptions electronically (eRx).

3. **Record Patient Demographics:** Record the following demographics: preferred language, sex, race, ethnicity, and date of birth.

4. **Record Vital Signs:** Record and chart changes in the following vital signs: height/length and weight (no age limit); blood pressure (ages 3 and over); calculate and display body mass index (BMI); and plot and display growth charts for patients 0–20 years, including BMI.

5. **Record Smoking Status:** Record smoking status for patients 13 years old or older.

6. **Clinical Decision Support**: Use clinical decision support to improve performance on high-priority health conditions.

7. **Provide Patients with the Ability to View Online, Download, and Transmit their Health Information**: Provide ability within four business days of the information being available to the EP.

[306] http://www.cms.gov/Regulations-and-Guidance/Legislation/EHRIncentivePrograms/Stage_2.html

8. **Clinical Summaries:** Provide clinical summaries for patients for each office visit.

9. **Protect Electronic Health Information (EHI)**: Protect EHI created or maintained by the CEHRT through the implementation of appropriate technical capabilities.

10. **Clinical Lab Results:** Incorporate clinical lab test results into CEHRT as structured data.

11. **Generate Lists of Patients**: Generate lists by specific conditions to use for quality improvement, reduction of disparities, research, or outreach.

12. **Reminders for Follow-up Care**: Use clinically relevant information to identify patients who should receive reminders for preventive/follow-up care and send these patients the reminders, per patient preference.

13. **Patient-Specific Education Resources**: Use clinically relevant information from CEHRT to identify patient-specific education resources and provide those resources to the patient.

14. **Medication Reconciliation**: The EP who receives a patient from another setting of care or provider of care or believes an encounter is relevant should perform medication reconciliation.

15. **Summary Care Records**: EPs who transition their patients to another setting of care or provider of care or who refers their patients to another provider of care should provide a summary care record for each transition of care or referral.

16. **Electronic Data to Immunization Registries**: Capability to submit electronic data to immunization registries or immunization information systems except where prohibited and in accordance with applicable law and practice.

17. **Secure Electronic Messaging**: Use secured electronic messaging to communicate with patients on relevant health information.

- Six menu IT objectives for 2014 EPs Stage 2 MU[307]
  - MU standard: In addition to the seventeen core IT objectives, EPs are to select three additional menu objectives. Requirements must be met and data reported for each.

TABLE 13: 2014 STAGE 2: HEALTH INFORMATION TECHNOLOGY MENU OBJECTIVES

1. **Electronic Syndromic Surveillance Data**: capability to submit electronic syndromic surveillance data to public health agencies except where prohibited and in accordance with applicable law and practice.

2. **Electronic Notes**: Record electronic notes in patient records.

---

[307] http://www.cms.gov/Regulations-and-Guidance/Legislation/EHRIncentivePrograms/Stage_2.html

3. **Imaging Results**: Imaging results consisting of the image itself and any explanation or other accompanying information are accessible through CEHRT.

4. **Family Health History**: Record patient family health history as structured data.

5. **Identify and Report Cancer Cases**: capability to identify and report cancer cases to a public health central cancer registry, except where prohibited, and in accordance with applicable law and practice.

6. **Identify and Report a Specific Case**: capability to identify and report specific cases to a specialized registry (other than a cancer registry) in accordance with applicable law and practice.

2014 Clinical Quality Measures (CQMs) for Stage 2 Reporting (CQMs)[308]

For the CQM portion of 2014 Stage 2 MU reporting, the set of sixty-four CQMs available for Stage 1 selection are also available for Stage 2 MU reporting. These CQMS **are the same** as those listed in the PQRS as CQMs available for EHR reporting.

- 2014 Stage 2 CQM reporting standards:

    o EPs must report on nine out of sixty-four total CQMs

    o EPs must select CQMs from at least three of the six key health care policy domains recommended by the NQS

The alignment of the 2014 Stage 2 CQMs with the six domains of the NQS are as follows:

TABLE 14: SUMMARY OF CQM ALIGNMENT WITH NQS DOMAINS

NQS DOMAIN	DESCRIPTION	# OF ALIGNED CQMS
Person and Caregiver-Centered Experience and Outcomes	ensuring that each person and family is engaged as partners in their care	4
Patient Safety	making care safer by reducing harm caused in the delivery of care	5

[308] Page 839, Table 52, http://www.cms.gov/Medicare/Medicare-Fee-for-Service-Payment/PhysicianFeeSched/PFS-Federal-Regulation-Notices-Items/CMS-1600-FC.html

Communication and Care Coordination	promoting effective communication and coordination of care	1
Community and Population Health:	working with communities to promote wide use of best practices to enable healthy living	9
Efficiency and Cost Reduction	making quality care more affordable for individuals, families, employers, and governments by developing and spreading new health care delivery models	5
Effective Clinical Care	promoting the most effective prevention and treatment practices for the leading causes of mortality, starting with cardiovascular disease	40

2014 Stage 2 CQMs

- In the CY2014 Final PFS Rule, CMS specified that EPs electronically reporting quality measures must use the most recent Specifications Manual. For 2014 (until a revised manual is released) this means that the specifications manual dated June 2013 is to be used for 2014 reporting of all measures, except:

  - CMS140v2, Breast Cancer Hormonal Therapy for Stage IC-IIIC Estrogen Receptor/Progesterone Receptor (ER/PR) Positive Breast Cancer (NQF 0387). Reporting for this measure must be accomplished using the December 2012 Specifications Manual.

- The following list of the sixty-four CQMs available to meet 2014 Stage 2 MU criteria is aligned by NQS domain for ease of selection. For a more comprehensive definition of each measure, see: https://www.cms.gov/ehrincentiveprograms/

TABLE 15: STAGE 2: CQMS FOR 2014 REPORTING ALIGNED WITH NQS DOMAINS

NQF NUMBER/ NQS DOMAIN	CMS EMEASURE ID/PQRS NUMBER	MEASURE TITLE
0004 Effective Clinical Care	CMS 137v2 PQRS 305	Initiation and Engagement of Alcohol and Other Drug Dependence Treatment
0018 Effective Clinical Care	CMS 165v2 PQRS 236	Controlling High Blood Pressure

NQF NUMBER/ NQS DOMAIN	CMS EMEASURE ID/PQRS NUMBER	MEASURE TITLE
TBD Effective Clinical Care	CMS 125v2 PQRS 112	Breast Cancer Screening
0032 Effective Clinical Care	CMS 124v2 PQRS 309	Cervical Cancer Screening
0034 Effective Clinical Care	CMS 130v2 PQRS 113	Colorectal Cancer Screening
0036 Effective Clinical Care	CMS 126v2 PQRS 311	Use of Appropriate Medications for Asthma
0043 Effective Clinical Care	CMS 127v2 PQRS 111	Pneumonia Vaccination Status for Older Adults
0055 Effective Clinical Care	CMS 131v2 PQRS 117	Diabetes: Eye Exam
0056 Effective Clinical Care	CMS 123v1 PQRS 163	Diabetes: Foot Exam
0059 Effective Clinical Care	CMS 122v2 PQRS 1	Diabetes: Hemoglobin A1c Poor Control
0060 Effective Clinical Care	CMS 148v2 PQRS NA	Hemoglobin A1c Test for Pediatric Patients
0062 Effective Clinical Care	CMS 134v2 PQRS 119	Diabetes: Urine Protein Screening
0064 Effective Clinical Care	CMS 163v2 PQRS 2	Diabetes: Low Density Lipoprotein (LDL) Management
0070 Effective Clinical Care	CMS 145v2 PQRS 7	Coronary Artery Disease (CAD): Beta-Blocker Therapy-Prior Myocardial Infarction (MI) or Left Ventricular Systolic Dysfunction (LVEF <40%)
0075 Effective Clinical Care	CMS 182v3 PQRS 241	Ischemic Vascular Disease (IVD): Complete Lipid Panel and LDL Control
0081 Effective Clinical Care	CMS 135v2 PQRS 5	Heart Failure (HF): Angiotensin Converting Enzyme (ACE) Inhibitor or Angiotensin Receptor Blocker (ARB) Therapy for Left Ventricular Systolic Dysfunction (LVSD)
0083 Effective Clinical Care	CMS 144v2 PQRS 8	Heart Failure (HF): Beta-Blocker Therapy for Left Ventricular Systolic Dysfunction (LVSD)

NQF NUMBER/ NQS DOMAIN	CMS EMEASURE ID/PQRS NUMBER	MEASURE TITLE
0086 Effective Clinical Care	CMS 143v2 PQRS 12	Primary Open Angle Glaucoma (POAG): Optic Nerve Evaluation
0088 Effective Clinical Care	CMS 167v2 PQRS 18	Diabetic Retinopathy: Documentation of Presence or Absence of Macular Edema and Level of Severity of Retinopathy
0089 Effective Clinical Care	CMS 142v2 PQRS 19	Diabetic Retinopathy: Communication with the Physician Managing Ongoing Diabetes Care
0104 Effective Clinical Care	CMS 161v2 PQRS 107	Major Depressive Disorder (MDD): Suicide Risk Assessment
0105 Effective Clinical Care	CMS 128v2 PQRS 9	Anti-Depressant Medication Management
0108 Effective Clinical Care	CMS 136v2 PQRS NA*	ADHD: Follow-Up Care for Children Prescribed Attention Deficit/Hyperactivity Disorder (ADHD) Medication
0110 Effective Clinical Care	CMS 169v2 PQRS TBD*	Bipolar Disorder and Major Depression: Appraisal for Alcohol or Chemical Substance Use
0385 Effective Clinical Care	CMS 141v3 PQRS 72	Colon Cancer: Chemotherapy for AJCC Stage III Colon Cancer
0387 Effective Clinical Care	CMS 140v1 PQRS 71	Breast Cancer: Hormonal Therapy for Stage IC-IIIC Estrogen Receptor/ Progesterone Receptor (ER/PR) Positive Breast Cancer
0403 Effective Clinical Care	CMS 62v2 PQRS TBD*	HIV/AIDS: Medical Visit
0405 Effective Clinical Care	CMS 52v1 PQRS 160	HIV/AIDS: Pneumocystis Jiroveci Pneumonia (PCP) Prophylaxis
TBD Effective Clinical Care	CMS 77v1 PQRS TBD*	HIV/AIDS: RNA Control for Patients with HIV
0565 Effective Clinical Care	CMS 133v2 PQRS 191	Cataracts: 20/40 or Better Visual Acuity within 90 Days Following Cataract Surgery
0608 Effective Clinical Care	CMS 158v2 PQRS TBD*	Pregnant Women Who had HBsAg Testing
0710	CMS 159v2	Depression Remission at Twelve Months

NQF NUMBER/ NQS DOMAIN	CMS EMEASURE ID/PQRS NUMBER	MEASURE TITLE
Effective Clinical Care	PQRS TBD*	
0712 Effective Clinical Care	CMS 160v2 PQRS TBD*	Depression Utilization of the PHQ-9 Tool
TBD Effective Clinical Care	CMS 75v2 PQRS TBD*	Children Who Have Dental Decay or Cavities
1365 Effective Clinical Care	CMS 177v2 PQRS TBD*	Child and Adolescent Major Depressive Disorder: Suicide Risk Assessment
TBD Effective Clinical Care	CMS 74v3 PQRS TBD*	Primary Caries Prevention Intervention as Offered by Primary Care Providers, including Dentists
TBD Effective Clinical Care	CMS 61v3 PQRS 316	Preventive Care and Screening: Cholesterol-Fasting Low Density Lipoprotein (LDLC) Test Performed
TBD Effective Clinical Care	CMS 64v3 PQRS 316	Preventive Care and Screening: Risk-Stratified Cholesterol-Fasting Low Density Lipoprotein (LDLC)
TBD Effective Clinical Care	CMS 149v2 PQRS 281	Dementia: Cognitive Assessment
TBD Effective Clinical Care	CMS 65v3 PQRS TBD*	Hypertension: Improvement in Blood Pressure
0022 Patient Safety	CMS 156v2 PQRS 238	Use of High-Risk Medications in the Elderly
0101 Patient Safety	CMS 139v2 PQRS 318	Falls: Screening for Future Fall Risk
0419 Patient Safety	CMS 68v3 PQRS 130	Documentation of Current Medications in the Medical Record
0564 Patient Safety	CMS 132v1 PQRS 192	Cataracts: Complications Within 30 Days Following Cataract Surgery Requiring Additional Surgical Procedures
TBD Patient Safety	CMS 179v2 PQRS TBD*	ADE Prevention and Monitoring: Warfarin Time in Therapeutic Range
0002	CMS 146v2 PQRS 66	Appropriate Testing for Children with Pharyngitis

NQF NUMBER/ NQS DOMAIN	CMS EMEASURE ID/PQRS NUMBER	MEASURE TITLE
Efficiency and Cost Reduction		
0052 Efficiency and Cost Reduction	CMS 166v3 PQRS 312	Use of Imaging Studies for Low Back Pain
0068 Efficiency and Cost Reduction	CMS 164v2 PQRS 208	Ischemic Vascular Disease (IVD): Use of Aspirin or Another Antithrombotic
0069 Efficiency and Cost Reduction	CMS 154v2 PQRS 65	Appropriate Treatment for Children with Upper Respiratory Infection (URI)
0389 Efficiency and Cost Reduction	CMS 129v3 PQRS 102	Prostate Cancer: Avoidance of Overuse of Bone Scan for Staging Low Risk Prostate Cancer Patients
0024 Community and Population Health	CMS 155v1 PQRS 239	Weight Assessment and Counseling for Nutrition and Physical Activity for Children and Adolescents
0028 Community and Population Health	CMS 138v2 PQRS 226	Preventive Care and Screening: Tobacco Use: Screening and Cessation Intervention
0033 Community and Population Health	CMS 153v2 PQRS 310	Chlamydia Screening for Women
0038 Community and Population Health	CMS 117v2 PQRS 240	Childhood Immunization Status
0041 Community and Population Health	CMS 147v2 PQRS 110	Preventive Care and Screening: Influenza Immunization
0418 Community and Population Health	CMS 2v3 PQRS 134	Preventive Care and Screening: Screening for Clinical Depression and Follow-Up Plan
0421 Community and Population Health	CMS 69v2 PQRS 128	Preventive Care and Screening: Body Mass Index (BMI) Screening and Follow-Up

NQF NUMBER/ NQS DOMAIN	CMS EMEASURE ID/PQRS NUMBER	MEASURE TITLE
1401 Community and Population Health	CMS 82v1 PQRS TBD*	Maternal Depression Screening
TBD Community and Population Health	CMS 22v2 PQRS 317	Preventive Care and Screening: Screening for High Blood Pressure and Follow-Up Documented
0384 Person and Caregiver-Centered Experience and Outcomes	CMS 157v2 PQRS 143	Oncology: Medical and Radiation-Pain Intensity Quantified
TBD Person and Caregiver-Centered Experience and Outcomes	CMS 66v2 PQRS TBD*	Functional Status Assessment for Knee Replacement
TBD Person and Caregiver-Centered Experience and Outcomes	CMS 56v2 PQRS TBD*	Functional Status Assessment for Hip Replacement
TBD Person and Caregiver-Centered Experience and Outcomes	CMS 90v3 PQRS TBD*	Functional Status Assessment for Complex Chronic Conditions
TBD Communication and Care Coordination	CMS 50v2 PQRS TBD*	Closing the Referral Loop: Receipt of Specialist Report

* This measure is new to the PQRS and has been adopted for reporting beginning in CY2014.

6.3.8 Meaningful Use Reporting Timelines

Overview

CMS has established reporting timelines and reporting methods that are different between new participants (those in their first year of MU reporting) and those who are beyond their first year of MU reporting.

Participants in their First Year of Successful Meaningful Use Reporting

- **reporting period**: any continuous ninety-day time frame in the reporting year, starting no later than July 3.

- **reporting submission method/time period**: For the first year of MU reporting, participants must report via the attestation method no later than October 1 of the reporting year.

- **2014 reporting rules:** EPs who did not meet MU requirements in 2013 to avoid the 2015 penalty amount are provided with a second opportunity for penalty avoidance in 2014.

  - CMS allows participants meeting the continuous ninety-day reporting period for first-time MU reporting, in the year prior to a penalty year, to avoid the penalty and qualify for incentive payment:[309]

    - for example: an EP did not participate or was unsuccessful in meeting MU criteria for 2013. To avoid the 2015 penalty, qualify for the 2015 incentive payment, and avoid the 2016 penalty, the EP must successfully attest to Stage 1 MU in 2014.

    - This rule is illustrated in Table 16, below.

Participants Beyond their First Year of Successful Meaningful Use Reporting

- **reporting period:** a full calendar year for individual EPs or the fiscal year for participating hospitals

- **reporting submission method/time period:** attestation is required for the reporting of the health IT objectives and electronic reporting of CQMs is required. All reporting must be completed by February 28 of the year

---

[309] *Page 54096, Federal Register/Vol. 77, No. 171/Tuesday, September 4, 2012/Rules and Regulations 2013.*

following the reporting year (example: reporting for CY2014 must be completed by February 28, 2015).

- **2014 reporting rules:** successful MU 2014 reporting will qualify participants for the 2014 incentive payment and to avoid the 2016 payment adjustment penalty.

The reporting rules and timelines for avoiding the payment adjustment penalty in years 2015–2019 are listed below:

TABLE 16: TIMELINE FOR EHR INCENTIVE PROGRAM REPORTING TO AVOID PENALTY[310]

EP Payment Adjustment Year (Calendar Year)	For EPs beyond their first year of MU reporting: EPs must demonstrate MU during EHR reporting period two years prior to year of payment adjustment	OR	For an EP demonstrating MU for the first time in the year prior to the payment adjustment year, EHR reporting period is a continuous 90-day reporting period beginning no later than July 3, 2014 (with submission no later than October 1, 2014).	OR	apply or otherwise qualify for an exception no later than July 1, 2015**
2015	CY2013 (with submission no later than February 28, 2014).		–		–
2016	CY2014 (with submission no later than February 28, 2015).*		July 3, 2015 (with submission no later than October 1, 2015).		July 1, 2016
2017	CY2015 (with submission no later than February 28, 2016).		July 3, 2016 (with submission no later than October 1, 2016).		July 1, 2017
2018	CY2016 (with submission no later than February 28, 2017).		July 3, 2017 (with submission no later than October 1, 2017).		July 1, 2018
2019	CY2017 (with submission no later than February 28, 2018).		July 3, 2018 (with submission no later than October 1, 2018).		July 1, 2019

*In the 2014 PFS Final Rule, CMS modified the reporting period to a three-month quarter EHR reporting period to allow for updating to the 2014 Edition CEHRT Standard.[311]

**See "hardship exceptions" below.

---

[310] Page 54101, Table 22, *Federal Register/Vol. 77, No. 171/Tuesday, September 4, 2012* www.gpo.gov/fdsys/pkg/FR-2012-09-04/pdf/2012-21563.pdf

[311] Page 1136, http://www.cms.gov/Medicare/Medicare-Fee-for-Service-Payment/PhysicianFeeSched/PFS-Federal-Regulation-Notices-Items/CMS-1600-FC.html

Meaningful Use Hardship Exceptions for Medicare EPs[312]

- In recognition of conditions that may pose significant obstacles to the successful accomplishment of the criteria for MU, CMS allows EPs to apply for hardship exemptions to avoid the payment adjustments described above.

- Hardship exceptions will be granted only under specific circumstances and only if CMS determines that providers have demonstrated that those circumstances pose a significant barrier to their achieving MU.

- Information on how to apply for a hardship exception will be posted on the CMS EHR incentive program website in the future (www.cms.gov/EHRIncentiveProgram).

- **EPs can apply for hardship exceptions in the following categories:**

  - **infrastructure**: EPs must demonstrate that they are in an area without sufficient Internet access or face insurmountable barriers to obtaining infrastructure (e.g., lack of broadband). To avoid payment penalties, the EP is required to establish that the hardship existed two years prior to the penalty adjustment year.

  - **new EPs**: Newly practicing EPs who would not have had time to become meaningful users can apply for a two-year limited exception to payment adjustments (EPs who begin practice in CY2014 would receive an exception to the penalties in 2014 and 2015.)

  - **unforeseen circumstances**: examples may include a natural disaster or other unforeseeable barrier.

  - **characteristics of patient interaction**:

    - lack of face-to-face or telemedicine interaction with patients

    - lack of any need to follow-up with patients

    - multiple locations for practice

---

[312] *Page 54097, Federal Register/Vol. 77, No. 171/Tuesday, September 4, 2012*
www.gpo.gov/fdsys/pkg/FR-2012-09-04/pdf/2012-21563.pdf

- o **practice at multiple locations**: lack of control over availability of CEHRT for more than 50 percent of patient encounters.

6.3.9 Mechanisms for Meaningful Use Reporting

Overview

- To encourage greater participation in the Medicare EHR incentive program and reduce the related administrative burden, CMS allows a variety of methods by which required information may be submitted. When possible, reporting methods are aligned with requirements of other specific programs or initiatives, to minimize additional reporting.

- For EHR reporting periods during and after CY2014, **all** eligible providers must have EHR technology certified to meet the **2014 Edition CEHRT** criteria. This technology must meet a required base amount of functionality and then any other functionality needed to achieve MU criteria. EHR technology certified to the 2014 Edition CEHRT criteria will be able to support either MU Stage 1 or 2.

  - o Once tested and certified to successfully calculate and report results for a specific year, such EHR products are added to the certified health IT product list (CHPL).[313]

    - For 2013 EHR MU reporting, EHR products that met 2011 **or** 2014 CEHRT requirements could be used for 2013 EHR incentive program reporting.

      - For 2013 reporting there are 4,208 CEHRT products.

    - As of January 1, 2014, there are 533 products meeting CEHRT for 2014 reporting.

      - Because of the large number of EHRs requiring upgrades to meet 2014 CEHRT requirements, CMS

---

[313] http://www.healthit.gov/policy-researchers-implementers/certified-health-it-product-list-chpl

has modified the reporting time frame for 2014 for all participants to allow additional preparation time.

- Regardless of MU stage, all Medicare EHR incentive program participants for the reporting year of 2014 will have a ninety-day reporting period aligned with calendar year quarters. Completed reports still must meet the February 28, 2015, reporting deadline.

- Reporting under the EHR incentive program includes all patients, regardless of payer.

2014 Reporting Options

- Achievement of MU means meeting reporting requirements for health IT objectives and CQMs. Reporting options may be specific to the data reported, as well as the time period for achieving MU.

- For 2014, the following options are available for MU reporting:
  - Attestation method through CMS online system
  - electronic submission:
    - Option 1: EHR incentive program only
    - Option 2: EHR incentive program and PQRS:
      - individual EHR reporting
      - qualified clinical data registry reporting (QCDR)—new for 2014
      - GPRO EHR reporting
  - comprehensive primary care (CPC) initiative group reporting—new for 2014.

Attestation Reporting[314]

- Attestation is a legal statement that a participant in the EHR incentive program has met the thresholds and all of the applicable MU requirements of the Medicare EHR incentive program.

- It is the method to be used in the event that CMS "does not have the capacity to receive Clinical Quality Measures (CQM) data electronically" and is required for all EHR incentive program participants in their first year (Stage 1) of MU reporting.

- Attestation is also used to report health IT objective attainment for a given program year.

- Attestation can be completed immediately after the first year required ninety continuous day reporting period, but not later than October 1 of the reporting year.

- The process of attestation is made through an online CMS system that allows providers (or others acting on behalf of participating providers) to enter information on MU requirements through the same system used for EHR incentive registration. For additional information, select **CMS EHR Registration and Attestation Now** at: https://ehrincentives.cms.gov.

- During the attestation process, participants are required to enter data and answer yes/no questions on the required core objectives, menu objectives, and CQMs.

- An **Attestation Users Guide** is available that provides step-by-step directions on how to enter information and attest online. The Attestation User Guide also contains instructions for how a provider can allow a third party to complete attestation on his or her behalf. This guide can be accessed at:
  https://www.cms.gov/EHRIncentivePrograms/Downloads/EP_Attestation_User_Guide.pdf

- Participants will be notified immediately upon submission of the online attestation whether or not they have successfully achieved the core and menu objectives of the program:

---

[314] Attestation, https://www.cms.gov/ehrincentiveprograms/

- o For unsuccessful ratings, participants may edit any information that was entered incorrectly and resubmit—or participants may resubmit for a different ninety-day reporting period with new information.

- o If participants are successful, CMS will perform a number of internal checks to verify eligibility for payment, to be received in approximately four to eight weeks following attestation.

Electronic Submission Options Summary

- EPs participating in the EHR incentive program may electronically report the CQM) component of their stage of MU to meet the requirements of:

  - o the EHR incentive program only;

  - o or the EHR incentive program *and* the PQRS.

Electronic Submission Option 1: EHR Incentive Program Only

- Participants report CQMs appropriate to their stage of MU and according to the time periods established for the EHR incentive program:

  - o The modified EHR incentive program reporting time period for 2014 of one calendar year quarter is less than the required entire 2014 calendar year for PQRS reporting.

  - o Participants must use EHR that meets CEHRT 2014 edition requirements.

  - o This method requires participants to log in to a CMS-designated portal and submit, through an upload process, data payload based on specified structures, such as clinical data architecture (CDA), and accompanying templates produced as output from their CEHRT.

Electronic Submission Option 2: EHR Incentive Program and PQRS

- The PQRS is a voluntary pay-for-reporting program that is structured to provide incentive payments and payment adjustment penalties to EPs meeting submission requirements for specific CQMs that apply to Medicare Part B beneficiaries **only.** A variety of reporting methods are available for individual providers and group practices to report information:

    o Reporting to meet EHR incentive program requirements through a PQRS reporting option may be used by EPs **beyond** their first year of MU reporting.

    o Information is electronically submitted by EHR, which is CEHRT to 2014 edition standards, through the PQRS portal on the QualityNet website.

    o All CQMs reportable under the EHR incentive program are contained in the PQRS listing of individual quality measures reportable by EHR.

    o By meeting annual PQRS requirements, EPs also meet applicable EHR incentive program requirements for the reporting of CQMs.

    Note: For 2014, EPs would be required to meet the full calendar year PQRS reporting requirement, instead of the modified EHR incentive program 2014 one-quarter reporting period.

    o Although the EHR incentive program requires reporting CQMs for all patients, regardless of payer, participants must report required measures for their Medicare Part B beneficiaries *only* in order to report through the PQRS program:[315]

    o The following PQRS reporting mechanisms allow for EHR incentive program data reporting:*

---

[315] *Page 54058, Federal Register/Vol. 77, No. 171/Tuesday, September 4, 2012*
www.gpo.gov/fdsys/pkg/FR-2012-09-04/pdf/2012-21563.pdf

- individual EHR reporting

- QCDR—new for 2014

- GPRO EHR reporting

- GPRO web-based interface

  o EPs who are part of a group practice under the MSSP or Pioneer ACO may report for dual PQRS/EHR incentive credit using one of the PQRS reporting methods.

*Detailed information on each PQRS reporting option is provided in Chapter 5: Technical Appendix: The Physician Quality Reporting System (PQRS).

TABLE 17: SUMMARY OF 2014 REPORTING OPTIONS FOR EHR INCENTIVE PROGRAM

CATEGORY	DATA LEVEL	PAYER LEVEL	SUBMISSION OPTION	MU REPORTING REQUIREMENTS
EPs in first year of demonstrating MU	aggregate	all payers	attestation	Submit data on nine of 64 CQMs (includes list of recommended adult and pediatric CQMs) covering at least three of the six NQS domains. Reporting period is first quarter of CY2014.
EPs beyond first year of demonstrating MU				
Option 1	aggregate	all payers	electronic	Submit data on nine of 64 CQMs (includes list of recommended adult and pediatric CQMs) covering at least three of the six NQS domains. Reporting period is first quarter of CY2014.
Option 2	patient	Medicare only	electronic	Satisfy requirements of PQRS reporting options using CEHRT. Reporting period is full year CY2014.
group reporting (EPs beyond first year of MU reporting)	patient	Medicare only	electronic	Satisfy requirements of MSSP or Pioneer ACOs using CEHRT.
EPs satisfactorily reporting via PQRS group reporting options	patient	Medicare only	electronic	Satisfy requirements of PQRS group reporting options using CEHRT.

Comprehensive Primary Care (CPC) Initiative Group Reporting Option[316]

- The CPC initiative is a multi-payer initiative established under Section 3021 of the ACA. The goal of the CPC is to foster greater collaboration between public and private health care payers to strengthen primary care.

- CMS pays participating CPC primary care practices a care management fee to support enhanced, coordinated services.

- Simultaneously, participating commercial, state, and other federal insurance plans are also offering support to primary care practices that provide high-quality primary care.

- There are approximately 500 CPC participants across seven health care markets in the United States. More details on the CPC initiative can be found at:
  http://innovation.cms.gov/initiatives/Comprehensive-Primary-care-Initiative/index.html

- 2014 CPC reporting requirements:

  o CPC practice sites are required to report to CMS a subset of CQMs that were selected in the EHR incentive program Stage 2 Final Rule for EPs to report under the EHR incentive program beginning in CY2014.

  o For 2014, CMS has added a group reporting option for EPs who are part of a CPC site. All CPC site EPs will meet MU CQM reporting requirements if the CPC site successfully submits at least nine electronically specified CQMs covering three domains.

    ▪ Each of the EPs in the CPC practice site satisfies the CQM reporting component of MU for the relevant reporting period if the CPC practice site successfully submits and meets the reporting requirements of the CPC initiative.

---

[316] *CPC Page 1130 http://www.cms.gov/Medicare/Medicare-Fee-for-Service-Payment/PhysicianFeeSched/PFS-Federal-Regulation-Notices-Items/CMS-1600-FC.html*

- Only those EPs who are beyond their first year of demonstrating MU may use the CPC group reporting option.

- If a CPC practice site fails the requirements established for the CPC initiative, the EPs who are part of the site would still have the opportunity to report CQMs under the established 2014 EHR incentive program rules.

Detailed information on CPC reporting for the EHR incentive program may be viewed at: Comprehensive Primary Care Initiative, Instruction Guide.

Note: CPC practice sites must submit the CQM data in the form and manner required by the CPC initiative. Therefore, whether the CPC practice site requires electronic submission or attestation of CQMs, the CPC practice site must submit the CQM data in the form and manner required by the CPC initiative.

Section 6.4: Acronym Guide

ARRA.......................American Recovery and Reinvestment Act of 2009

ACA..........................Affordable Care Act

ACO ....Accountable Care Organization

ARRA.......................American Recovery and Reinvestment Act of 2009, Public Law 111–5

CAH ....Critical Access Hospital

CEHRT ....Certified Electronic Health Records Technology

CHPL ....Certified Health IT Product List

CMS.........................Centers for Medicare & Medicaid Services

CPC ....Comprehensive Primary Care Initiative

CQM.........................Clinical Quality Measure

CY ....Calendar Year

DRA ....Deficit Reduction Act of 2005, Public Law 109–171

EHR ....Electronic Health Record

EMR.........................Electronic Medical Record

EP ....Eligible Professional

eRx..........................Electronic Prescribing

FFS ....Fee-for-Service

FR ....Federal Register

FY.............................Fiscal Year

GPRO ....Group Practice Reporting Option

HIS ....Health Information System

HIT ....Health Information Technology

HITECH ....Health Information Technology for Economic and Clinical Health Act

HPSA ....Health Professional Shortage Area

MA............................Medicare Advantage

MIPPA......................Medicare Improvements for Patients and Providers Act of 2008, Public Law 110–275

MSSP.......................Medicare Shared Savings Program

MU ....Meaningful Use

NAMCS....................National Ambulatory Medical Care Survey

NQF ....National Quality Forum

NQS .... National Quality Strategy

NCHS .... National Center for Health Statistics

NPI .... National Provider Identifier

ONC .... Office of the National Coordinator for Health Information Technology (ONC)

PPACA .... Patient Protection and Affordable Care Act

PFS .... Physician Fee Schedule

PPS .... Prospective Payment System

PQRS .... Physician Quality Reporting System

QDC .... Quality Data Code

QCDR .... Qualified Clinical Data Registry

TIN .... Tax Identification Number

CHAPTER 7

The Physician Value-Based Payment Modifier (VBM) Program

Section 7.1: Flash Read!

The Physician Value-Based Payment Modifier (VBM) Program was mandated in the Affordable Care Act (ACA) of 2010 as a mechanism to encourage physicians to provide higher-quality care at a lower cost. The program uses quality-tiering to benchmark physicians against their peers and determine financial rewards or penalties based on their cost and quality.

- By collecting and comparing group practice-specific data on measures of *quality and cost,* Medicare will determine a VBM to be applied to each participating group of physicians.

- The payment modifier may result in an **increase, decrease** or **no change** to all physician reimbursements for physician services provided under Medicare Part B during a given VBM program year.

- The VBM for a given program year is based on data reported from a performance year occurring two years prior. For the 2016 VBM program year, 2014 is the performance reporting year.

- Performance data used to determine the VBM is culled from different sources and performance scoring is based on:
  - Participation in PQRS, which is mandatory for participation in the VBM program.
  - Outcomes Measures: CMS-extracted from Medicare claims
    - all-cause readmission
    - composite of Acute Prevention Quality Indicators for bacterial pneumonia, UTI's and dehydration
    - composite of Chronic Prevention Quality Indicators for COPD, heart failure and diabetes
  - Patient Experience of Care Measures: (Clinician Groups—Consumer Assessment of Healthcare Providers and Systems (CG-CAHPS) mandatory for groups of 100+ and optional for groups of 25+ physicians beginning January 2014 for program year 2016.
  - Cost Measures: CMS extracted from Medicare Part A and B claims
    - Total per capita costs measure (annual payment standardized and risk-adjusted Part A and Part B costs)
    - Total per capita costs for beneficiaries with four chronic conditions: COPD, Heart Failure, Coronary Artery Disease and Diabetes
    - Medicare Spending per Beneficiary measure
  - Data from Medicare Part D (prescription drugs) are not included in the VBM Program.
- The VBM program is being rolled out in phases to physician practices of different sizes:
  - Groups of 100 or more eligible professionals (EPs) were subject to the VBM in 2015 based on 2013 performance/reporting.
  - For the 2014 reporting year, all physician groups with **ten or more** EPs are **required** to participate in the VBM and will receive a VBM to be applied in 2016.

- For reporting year 2015 (2017 VBM program year), the ACA mandates that *all* physicians must participate in the VBM. However, for physicians just entering practice, CMS will exclude them from VBM evaluation for two years (the year they enter practice and the following calendar year).

- While penalties and incentives apply only to services provided by physicians, **group practice size is determined by the total number of EPs** (including physicians, physician assistants, nurse practitioners, clinical nurse specialists, certified registered nurse anesthetists, certified nurse-midwives, clinical social workers, clinical psychologists, registered dietitians, and nutrition professionals) in a given practice.

- →IMPORTANT! **The ACA allows the secretary of the Department of Health and Human Services (HHS) to include *all* EPs in the assessment of VBM penalties or incentives beginning with 2015 reporting. This decision has not yet been finalized.**

- Group practice size for the VBM is determined through: Tax Identification Number (TIN) analysis; Provider Enrollment, Chain, and Ownership System (PECOS) database query; and claims.

- For the 2016 VBM program year, CMS **will not apply** the VBM to physician groups participating in Accountable Care Organizations (ACOs) as part of the Medicare Shared Savings Program (MSSP), the testing of the Pioneer ACO Model, the Comprehensive Primary Care Initiative or other similar CMS Innovation Center initiatives.

- Attribution (assignment) of Medicare beneficiaries to a group practice participating in the VBM program is made through a two-step process for all quality measures:

    - Medicare first assigns beneficiaries who receive the plurality of their primary care services (in terms of allowed charges) from any *primary care physician* within the group practice, meaning the physician or group that provided more total allowed charges than anyone else for that patient.

    - Next, Medicare assigns beneficiaries who receive the plurality of their primary care services from *specialist physicians and certain non-physician practitioners* (Nurse Practitioners, Clinical Nurse Specialists, and Physician Assistants) within the group practice.

- **New for 2014 VBM reporting: the Medicare Spending Per Beneficiary (MSPB) cost measure:**
  - For 2014 VBM reporting, the MSPB is being added to cost measures for the individual chronic conditions of chronic obstructive pulmonary disease (COPD), heart failure (HF), coronary artery disease (CAD), and diabetes (DM).
  - The MSPB measures **all costs** associated with patient care occurring **three days prior to, during**, and **thirty days after** an index hospital admission.
  - The MSPB measure is expressed as a **total dollar amount** per physician group.
  - Attribution of beneficiaries is made based on physicians providing the plurality of Medicare Part B care **during** the index admission.

- **New for 2014 VBM reporting: application of a "specialty adjustment" to all cost measures:**
  - The specialty adjustment allows for peer-group comparisons while factoring in the mix of **specialty physicians**.
  - The specialty adjustment "levels the field" to allow for a more equal comparison of the risk-adjusted cost measures, against which groups of physicians of smaller size—which often have fewer or single-specialty composition—are evaluated.
  - The resulting adjusted cost measure results are used in determining national specialty-adjusted benchmarks and group-specific performance rates.

- The VBM is a budget-neutral initiative. Any increase in physician reimbursement rates must be offset by the reductions resulting from penalty adjustments. Funding for upward reimbursement adjustments will be composed of amounts withheld from reimbursements as a result of the VBM program **and** payment reductions resulting from PQRS penalties.

- Penalty application for the 2016 VBM is as follows:

2016 Value-Based Payment Modifier Amounts

COST/QUALITY	LOW QUALITY	AVERAGE QUALITY	HIGH QUALITY
Low Cost	+0.0%	+1.0x*	+2.0x*
Average Cost	-1.0%	+0.0%	+1.0x*
High Cost	-2.0%	-1.0%	+0.0%

* This includes groups of physicians eligible for an additional +1.0x to 2016 reimbursement rates if reporting PQRS quality measures and the average beneficiary risk score is in the top 25 percent of all beneficiary risk scores.

- CMS released practice-specific **Quality Resource and Use Reports (QRURs)** reflecting 2012 VBM data, based on metrics for the 2013 VBM reporting year, to all groups of twenty-five or more eligible professionals in December 2013.

  - These reports provide a "first look" for such practices on measures performance and how the value-based payment modifier could affect their payment in the future.

HIGHLIGHTS FROM AN ANALYSIS OF THE 2012 DATA CONTAINED IN THE DECEMBER 2013 QRURS:

- The 2012 data QRURs were distributed to **6,779** physician groups nationwide with twenty-five or more eligible professionals, covering some **400,000** physicians.
- Quality and Cost composite scores were able to be calculated for **3,876** groups
- **2,903** groups had insufficient data on which to compute performance measures.
- Beneficiaries that were attributed to a group of physicians received an average of five primary care services in 2012 of which, on average, **64.3** percent were provided by the group to which the beneficiary was **attributed**
- Reliability standards for quality and cost measures were **above 0.70** for groups with 25+ EPs, indicating that the measures determining overall quality and cost were highly reliable.
- For groups of 100 or more eligible professionals, measures reliability were:
  - 0.48 for the all-cause thirty-day readmission measure – moderately reliable
  - 0.98 for the total per capita cost measure – highly reliable
  - 0.94 for condition-specific cost measures – highly reliable

435

BASED ON THE 2013 VBM REPORTING METRICS:

- **80.7 percent** of all groups scored **average** in quality and cost and would not have received a payment adjustment.

- **8 percent** of all groups would have received an **upward VBM reimbursement adjustment.**

- **11 percent** of all groups would have received a **downward VBM reimbursement** adjustment

Section 7.2: Provider Perspectives

The Physician Value-Based Payment Modifier (VBM) Program is one of the most complex and least understood of all the payment reforms that aim to incentivize quality of care. Most physicians, overwhelmed with other parts of the improvement and payment-reform agenda, haven't thought much about it.

7.2.1 Rationale

The VBM program encapsulates the long-sought elusive goals of improving the quality of patient care while at the same time reducing the cost of care. It makes real and immediate certain concepts that had been introduced with mixed success in earlier legislation and rule making.

Under the traditional fee-for-service system, patients had no way of knowing whether the patient care delivered by hospitals or physicians was considered to be of high quality or low quality. Costs, too, were opaque and not a source of concern for the fully insured patient. Providers got paid whether they did a good job or not. In fact, under certain circumstances—such as hospital readmissions and higher volumes of care for patients who experience medical errors and hospital-acquired infections—they got paid more money if the care was less than successful. The new emphasis on transparency, public reporting, and value-based reimbursement has altered the landscape.

There is generally less awareness among physicians of these new payment incentives than policy makers and health economists would like. Yet physicians remain the essential players in this effort. It is they who must engage to make the system work, to induce the changes that the larger American polity is demanding. They're the people who determine how well the health delivery system operates and how well it serves patients' needs. Ultimately, whatever payment and quality reforms are devised must be actionable and affordable by physicians of good will.

"In simple terms, you have to report on quality," said William L. Rich III, MD, president of Northern Virginia Ophthalmology Associates in Falls Church, Virginia. "If you do, you get a gold star, you avoid the penalties."[317]

But there is also a cost side of the equation—and that's the hard part. The VBM rewards physicians if total costs for the beneficiaries assigned to them are low relative to the benchmark and penalizes them if the costs for their population are higher than the benchmark. The benchmark is the average cost of treating a Medicare patient by all physicians in the United States. This "average" cost is adjusted for severity of illness and geographical differences in costs.

"It's a profound change that I haven't seen people talk about as much as they should," said Chapin White, a senior health researcher at the Center for Studying Health System Change in Washington, DC. "It's setting a marker and saying physicians have some responsibility" and will be rewarded and penalized based on total spending for their beneficiary population. It uses the established Medicare fee-for-service (FFS) system as a basis.[318]

It may help to think of the VBM as one dimension of the government's multipronged effort to encourage hospitals and doctors to put quality and cost at the center of their concerns. For hospitals, the data are delivered to CMS via the Inpatient Quality Reporting (IQR) system (Chapter 1). The programs used to ascertain clinical quality include hospital-acquired conditions (HACs) (Chapter 4), readmissions (Chapter 3), and value-based purchasing (VBP) (Chapter 2). The metric of cost that accompanies the VBP program is the Medicare Spending Per Beneficiary (MSPB) efficiency ratio.

A similar framework obtains this information for physicians' practices. The sources of data include physicians' participation in electronic prescribing and electronic health records (Chapter 6) and the use of the PQRS (Chapter 5). Through the integration of developed quality and cost composites, the Value-Based Payment Modifier (VBM) program recognizes the provision of quality care in a cost-efficient manner.

With the introduction of the VBM, the quality of care incentives for hospitals and physicians are now aligned in three ways: physicians will be measured and incentivized for quality metrics aimed at reducing unnecessary admissions; improving care while in the hospital; and for coordination of care post

---

[317] *William L. Rich III, MD, telephone interview, September 17, 2013.*

[318] *Chapin White, telephone interview, September 13, 2013.*

discharge. CMS believes that this will encourage physicians and hospitals to collaborate more closely on patient care during the hospitalization and post discharge to avoid unnecessary readmissions. This holds the potential to improve the quality of care, reduce total cost of care, and avoid cost shifting between providers.

7.2.2 Summary

The program goes into effect in 2015 for medical groups of 100 or more EPs, using CY2013 as the initial performance period. Groups of 10 to 99 begin their performance period in 2014 for the 2016 program year. Like other pieces of the payment reform puzzle, the VBM is based on physicians' practice patterns in a period before they have been given full information about their own habits and preferences, and before they have any basis of comparison to their peers. The program will be applied to all physicians and groups by January 1, 2017. This means the performance period for FY2017 starts on January 1, 2015.

The only exemptions are physicians who practice at rural health clinics, federally qualified health centers, and critical access hospitals. For the first two years, physician groups in the Medicare shared savings ACO program, the Pioneer ACO pilot program, or the comprehensive primary care initiative will also be exempt.

The program is designed to be budget-neutral. To achieve that aim, Congress ordained that physicians be scored against each other; some will be winners and others will be losers. The advantage to that principle is that the effects of an external shock to outcomes, such as a shortage of a vaccine or an epidemic, won't count against an individual physician or against the profession as a whole. On the other hand, physicians don't really have a clear idea in advance how much improvement will be necessary to get a bonus or avoid the penalty.[319]

Of particular concern to physicians will be the fact that, at least for now, the upside of participation is unknown. Although Medicare has established a method for calculating incentive payments to groups achieving the twin goals

---

[319] Alyna T. Chien, MD, and Meredith Rosenthal, "Medicare's Physician Value-Based Payment Modifier—Will the Tectonic Shift Create Waves?" New England Journal of Medicine 369:22, November 28, 2013: 2076–78.

of providing high-quality patient care at average or low cost, the actual amount of incentives has yet to be determined. Specifically, the incentive pool for physicians will be funded by the penalties levied in the VBM program and the PQRS. Until that amount is known, the incentive to be earned can't be quantified for physicians. It's also unclear how large an incentive reward will be required to measurably affect physician performance.

To effectuate this change, CMS will divide the group practice universe into two categories for the 2014 reporting year (2016 program year):

- **Category 1** consists of groups of ten or more physicians that (a) have self-nominated or registered for the PQRS as a group or (b) will report PQRS as individuals in a group practice and have successfully met annual reporting requirements. For 2014 reporting, all Category 1 practices will be evaluated under a quality-tiering process and will have a value modifier calculated to be applied in the 2016 program year. First time participants (groups of 10–99), will be subject to upward or neutral adjustments only, while groups of 100+ will be subject to upward, downward or neutral adjustments in 2016.

- **Category 2** is everybody else who doesn't fit into (a) or (b) in Category 1. They will receive a value modifier of -2.0 percent.

Medical groups are required to register and choose their quality-tiering methodology by September 30, 2014. CMS will analyze claims for services given during the 2014 performance year through at least February 28, 2015. The agency intends to produce and send out Quality and Resource Use Reports (QRURs), also known as physician feedback reports, for 2014 performance in the fall of 2015 to all physicians.

7.2.3 Current State

Even though small practices and independent physicians are not required to participate at first, CMS recommends that they start familiarizing themselves with PQRS now, "because when we propose in future rule-making to apply the value modifier to smaller groups and solo practitioners, we anticipate basing the quality composite on PQRS quality data reported by such physicians," CMS said in an explainer document.

"The punch line is, the sooner you get involved the more benefit you have," said Bruce Bagley, MD, CEO of TransforMED, a consulting offshoot of the American Academy of Family Physicians. Those who don't report in 2014 will be assigned the negative modifier. "There's this built-in lag time. They have to have an entire year's worth of data for 2014 to be able to adjudicate who's going to get a little more and little less. They've got 2015 to do the calculation and make the adjustments for 2016 going forward."[320]

The 2 percent penalty is modest—"a nudge," White called it. Not a big dollar amount, but enough to send a message to physicians that they need to start considering how efficiently they practice medicine. But, he predicted, once physicians become more aware of the financial consequences of the treatments they recommend and the costs of specialty care, this opening move has the potential to affect the volume of services to patients and overall costs to Medicare. Because the VBM relies on data collected through PQRS, a practice that fails to participate in PQRS cannot successfully report information required for VBM. As a result, such practices will be subject to the -2.0 percent PQRS penalty, as well as the -2.0 percent VBM penalty. In addition, those who fail to participate in related programs supporting VBM, such as EHR, place at risk an additional 2 percent penalty for a total of 6 percent of their Medicare reimbursement.

In some ways, the VBM is still something of a sketch, a first draft showing the direction in which the government wants to move. It has not been much talked about or written about in scholarly journals. At the time of this writing, a citation search in *Health Affairs*, the premier journal for discussion of health policy and finance, yields just one passing reference to "value-based modifier." The archive of the *New England Journal of Medicine*, likewise, shows just one mention—by the same author. It wasn't until November 2013 that an article titled "Medicare's Physician Value-Based Payment Modifier—Will the Tectonic Shift Create Waves?" authored by Alyna T. Chein, MD, and Meredith Rosenthal, PhD, was published in the *New England Journal of Medicine*.[321]

---

[320] *Bruce Bagley, MD, telephone interview, September 14, 2013.*

[321] *Alyna T. Chen, MD, and Meredith B. Rosenthal, PhD, "Medicare's Physician Value-Based-Payment Modifier—Will the Tectonic Shift Create Waves," New England Journal of Medicine, November 28, 2013, 31:9, p. 2076. http://www.nejm.org/doi/full/10.1056/NEJMp1311957*

The concept is not only infrequently discussed; it has not even been thoroughly researched. We have found no pilot programs or trial rollouts in specific localities or multisite trials that have been described in the literature.

This is cause for consternation among physicians' organizations that are charged by their members with eyeballing these matters and heading off misconceived notions before they are enacted into law or laid down in regulations.

At the time the legislation was being drafted, "most of medicine said, 'This isn't going to have an impact,'" Rich said. "It turns out to be a big issue." Figuring out how to compare one physician's costs against another and risk-adjusting for variances in their respective patient populations is "very, very difficult," and CMS is struggling to find a suitable methodology, he said.

Rich is the medical director for policy at the American Academy of Ophthalmology and was previously the academy's secretary for federal affairs. For six years he served on the Relative Value Scale Update Committee (RUC), the American Medical Association's committee that determines the values and inputs that go into the Medicare physician fee schedule. He's been studying payment methodologies for decades.

While he's a supporter of the overall goals of the ACA, Rich thinks the implementation has been unsatisfactory. The new payment models "have not really worked out." He thinks too much emphasis was placed on short-term savings at the time the legislation was written, because Congress drew a line in the sand saying the new payment modalities had to be budget-neutral. No provision was made for a pilot.

"You don't know what's going to happen at the end of three years," he said. "Why would you go to the trouble to set up an infrastructure," such as what is required to generate the value-based modifier, "if you didn't know it was going to be successful? The entire construct and assumptions were flawed" because of lack of expertise on the part of CMS, he said.

Specialty societies are doing the real heavy lifting on deriving reliable quality indicators, Rich said. Using a registry developed by the ophthalmology society, he added, "I can press a button and compare my results to my group, my peers, the national benchmark, to see where I can improve."

Registries are the way to go, Bagley said. In his estimation, a standalone registry for diabetes will satisfy the basic requirements for PQRS and the modifier.

A registry has five essential characteristics, Bagley said:

1. It compiles a list of all the people with the condition, say, diabetes.

2. It gives a snapshot of every patient while the provider is seeing her or him or talking on the phone: "all the evidence-based recommended care and where they have gaps and where things are not in range."

3. It has to aggregate how you're doing with all the people on the list, so you have an idea whether your approach is better than somebody else's. "I have to see all my people with diabetes, so I get the average of all my patients. The patient sitting in front of you is an anecdote, an N of 1. If you have a set of 100, you have a picture of how all your patients are doing."

4. It has to support outreach. It gives a list of all those with diabetes who haven't had an eye exam or haven't had their A1c blood sugar checked.

5. It automatically generates the requested quality measures. "If you're watching the LDL of all your diabetics, to know what percent of them are under control, it's right there."

"The complexity of the way this is designed has created all kinds of confusion," said Keith M. Starke, MD, chief quality officer at Mercy Hospital St. Louis. "It's one of those things we're all striving to understand more effectively and do the right thing, yet the complexity makes it hard for physicians to get their hands around it."[322]

It's especially tough on small practices and solo operators, said Martin Love, CEO of the Humboldt-DelNorte Independent Practice Association in Eureka, Calif. Primary care practices may be more interested, he believes, as many of the payment reforms have the potential to boost their Medicare revenues, but they often lack the ability to make the investments required. "Specialists will just make a financial decision, 'Is this enough money to worry about?' It'll vary

---

[322] *Keith M. Starke, MD, telephone interview, September 12, 2013.*

from specialty to specialty and size of practice," Love added. "Larger practices will do it, smaller practices will not."[323]

7.2.4 The Road Ahead

While these changes to payment appear minimal at the start, they rapidly gather momentum and take on much more weight in a provider's final payment from Medicare. When the penalty or bonus is 1 percent or 2 percent of a practice's billings, "it sounds pretty optional," Bagley said. "What if it's 20 percent or 30 percent? Is it still optional? I believe that's where it's headed." In fact, legislative language contained in the ACA does not specify a maximum amount of penalties for the VBM program as long as physicians are "reimbursed differentially" for the quality and costs of provided care. It is the only program without a defined limit to the penalty. As a result, Medicare began with a 1.0 percent penalty for 2013, increased it to 2.0 percent for 2014, and will continue to increase it. "As we gain more experience with our value-based payment modifier methodologies, we will consider ways to increase the amount of payment at risk," CMS has said.

Health economist Paul B. Ginsburg also sees the system moving in that direction. Writing in *Health Affairs*, he prophesied that strategies that underlie ACOs and bundled payments that are introduced as voluntary "will become a mandatory part of fee-for-service physician payment … The risk borne by physicians will initially be very limited, but that may change later on through larger bonuses from a budget-neutral pool."[324]

Observers expect CMS to continue to move toward EHR and registry reporting and to diminish the importance of claims-based reporting. The agency is also looking into merging the reports from the VBM and PQRS. Each EP would receive a single comprehensive report showing VBM results and PQRS together.[325]

---

[323] *Martin Love, telephone interview, August 30, 2013.*

[324] *Paul B. Ginsburg, "Fee-For-Service Will Remain A Feature Of Major Payment Reforms, Requiring More Changes in Medicare Physician Payment," Health Affairs, September 2012 31:9, p. 1977. http://content.healthaffairs.org/content/31/9/1977.full*

[325] *http://blog.veicorp.com/2013/12/20/overview-of-the-2014-medicare-physician-fee-schedule-final-rule/*

In December 2013, CMS took a decisive step toward fulfilling the wishes of organized medicine by allowing specialty societies to select measures that are more meaningful to their work with patients and report them through qualified clinical data registries. CMS also aligned the quality measures among its various reporting requirements to reduce duplication of reports. Doctors may send in a metric once and be credited for meeting the needs of all relevant programs. Earlier iterations of the rule required specialists to use generalized quality measures that they believed were more applicable to primary care practices.[326]

A standalone clinical registry for diabetes "will give you all you need for PQRS or the modifier," Bagley said. "Building this stuff is good for patients and it's as easy as pushing a button."

To make these programs successful in the long run, he said, regulators, policy makers, and leaders in medicine must ultimately look beyond the measures available now, limited as they are, and keep their eye on how they improve outcomes for patients and populations. Building up the infrastructure to support primary care practices—adding care coordinators, establishing electronic registries, paying a complex care management fee, and the like—is likely to do more for population health and medical practice over time than prolonging the fee-for-service payment system beyond its useful life span, Bagley said.

"I believe in professionalism," Bagley said. "We have a tremendous sunk cost, a tremendous investment in how we've gotten this whole thing to work right now (with fee-for-service); to the point that we believe it's good medicine to work that way. It's been driven by the payment environment."

---

[326] Andis Robeznieks, "Specialists notch victory in new CMS rule on quality reporting," Modern Healthcare, December 4, 2013.
http://www.modernhealthcare.com/article/20131204/NEWS/312049948/specialists-notch-victory-in-new-cms-rule-on-quality-reporting

Section 7.3: Technical Appendix: The Physician Value-Based Payment Modifier (VBM) Program

7.3.1 Background:

Section 3007 of the ACA:

- The **VBM program** was mandated under Section 3007 of the ACA of 2010 as a method to *differentially* pay physicians and physician groups providing covered services to Medicare beneficiaries based on the *value* of care provided.

- Directed to be implemented as a budget-neutral initiative, the VBM evaluates patient care provided against metrics of *quality* and *cost* to determine a VBM for participants.

- Beginning with an initial program year of CY2105 (CY2103 performance period), the VBM program was to be implemented in a gradual fashion with a VBM to be applied to all physicians by CY2017 (2015 Performance Period). VBM performance reporting years and program years are aligned to the calendar year for the VBM program.

- The evaluation of individual group performance is made in a comparative fashion against established benchmarks to determine whether the VBM will have a positive, negative or neutral effect on annual Medicare reimbursement rates:

    o Unlike other CMS quality initiatives, the ACA does not specify a minimum or maximum penalty amount for a given VBM program year. The HHS secretary has been granted broad discretion to set penalties as deemed appropriate. Under Section 3007 of the

ACA, such decisions by the secretary are not subject to "legislative or administrative review."[327]

- o Funds made available through the imposition of negative payment modifiers will be used for incentive payments, in a budget-neutral manner.

- o For the 2016 VBM (2014 reporting year), the maximum VBM penalty is -2.0 percent.[328]

- As currently constructed, the VBM provides incentive and penalty adjustments for those group practices providing levels of patient care that have been determined to be "meaningfully different" from others.

  - o Based on an analysis of the CY2012 QRUR, released in September 2013: **80 percent** of group practices with 25 or more EPs were rated to receive a *neutral* VBM adjustment; **8 percent** were rated to receive an *upward* adjustment; and **11 percent** were rated to receive a *downward* adjustment.[329]

- →IMPORTANT! Section 3007(7) of the ACA also grants the HHS secretary the discretion of applying the VBM to all "eligible providers" on or after January 1, 2017:

  - o If implemented, a performance reporting period during CY2015 would be used to determine a VBM to be applied in CY2017.

  - o As defined under Section 1842(b)(18)(c) of the Social Security Act (SSA), this would extend the VBM program to include physicians and:

    - a Physician Assistant, Nurse Practitioner or Clinical Nurse Specialist

    - a Certified Registered Nurse Anesthetist

    - a Certified Nurse-Midwife

---

[327] *Page 670, Section 3007: Patient Protection and Affordable Care Act—US Government ..., http://www.gpo.gov/fdsys/pkg/BILLS-111hr3590enr/pdf/BILLS-111hr3590enr.pdf*

[328] *Pages 1177–1178: CMS-1600-FC, http://www.gpo.gov/fdsys/pkg/FR-2013-12-10/pdf/2013-28696.pdf*

[329] *Page 1171: CMS-1600-FC, http://www.gpo.gov/fdsys/pkg/FR-2013-12-10/pdf/2013-28696.pdf*

- a Clinical Social Worker

- a Clinical Psychologist

- a Registered Dietitian or Nutrition Professional

Section 3003 of the ACA:

- To support the quality and cost measurement objectives of the VBM program, Section 3003 of the ACA modified the **Physician Feedback Program** to include the collection and reporting of quality metrics and resource use involved in patient care. Such data is provided to physicians and physician groups in the form of a **QRUR**.

  Note: The QRUR is covered in detail in Section 7.3.11.

- CMS-extracted claims data from Medicare Part A (hospital) and Part B (physician services) are included in confidential QRUR reports to physicians, along with comparative data.

  *Note: Reflecting the integration of two initiatives, the VBM program is also referred to in subsequent rulemaking as the **Physician Feedback/Value-Based Modifier (PF-VBM) Program.***

7.3.2 VBM Guiding Principles:

- As part of CMS-directed value-based purchasing initiatives, the VBM program seeks to recognize and reward the provision of high-quality care and quality improvements. In addition, through encouraging the use of evidence-based measures, the VBM program is designed to result in more efficient and effective care with less fragmentation, duplication, and administrative burden.

- In the CY2013 PFS Final Rule, CMS established the following VBM implementation principles:[330]

  - **a focus on measurement and alignment**: Measures selected for the VBM will consistently reflect performance differences

---

[330] *Page 69307: CMS-1590-FC, http://www.gpo.gov/fdsys/pkg/FR-2012-11-16/pdf/2012-26900.pdf*

among physicians and physician groups. Such measures should account for a diverse range of services and be aligned with the NQS and other CMS quality initiatives, including the PQRS, the MSSP, and the Medicare EHR Incentive Program.

- **a focus on physician choice:** Physicians should be able to choose the level (individual or group) at which their quality performance will be assessed, reflecting physicians' choice over their practice configurations. The choice of level should align with the requirements of other physician quality reporting programs.

- **a focus on shared accountability:** The VBM can facilitate shared accountability by assessing performance at the group practice level and by focusing on the total costs of care, not just the costs of care furnished by an individual physician.

- **a focus on actionable information:** Quality and cost information related to patient care provided through **QRURs** should contain robust and actionable information to assist participants in identifying clinical areas in which they are doing well, as well as areas in which performance could be improved.

- **a focus on a gradual implementation**. The VBM should focus initially on identifying high- and low-performing groups of physicians. Beginning with groups of 100+ EPs evaluated in 2013 (2015 program year), CMS is expanding VBM assessment to groups of 10+ EPs during 2014 (2016 program year). By the 2017 program year (2015 performance reporting year), the VBM program will be expanded to all physicians. In addition, the HHS secretary has the discretion to extend the VBM program to all providers on or after January 1, 2017.

7.3.3 Overview of the 2016 VBM Program (2014 Performance Reporting)

With the end result of determining a VBM to be applied in 2016, based on 2014 performance reporting, the following process steps are required:

Figure 1: VBM Pathway

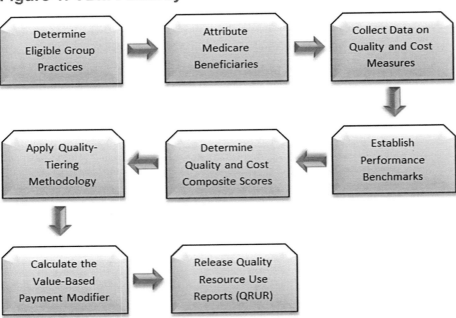

 ## 7.3.4 Step 1: Determine Eligible Group Practices for VBM Participation

For the 2016 VBM program year (2014 performance reporting year), CMS will develop a VBM for **all** group practices with 10+ EPs.[331]

Eligible Professionals (EPs)

- **VBM EPs**: EPs include specific physicians, practitioners, and therapists providing covered services to Medicare beneficiaries.

- As currently configured, the VBM program used total EP counts for determining group size. Incentives and penalties are **only** applied to

---

[331] *Page 1164: CMS-1600-FC, http://www.gpo.gov/fdsys/pkg/FR-2013-12-10/pdf/2013-28696.pdf*

covered professional services provided to Medicare beneficiaries by *physician* members of the group practice.

- For 2014 reporting, groups containing 10+ of the following EPs will be evaluated under the VBM program:[332]

    o **Medicare Physicians**: Doctor of Medicine; Doctor of Osteopathy; Doctor of Podiatric Medicine; Doctor of Optometry; Doctor of Oral Surgery; Doctor of Dental Medicine; and Doctor of Chiropractic.

    o **Practitioners**: Physician Assistant; Nurse Practitioner*; Clinical Nurse Specialist*; Certified Registered Nurse Anesthetist* (and Anesthesiologist Assistant); Certified Nurse Midwife*; Clinical Social Worker; Clinical Psychologist; Registered Dietician; Nutrition Professional; and Audiologists (*includes Advanced Practice Registered Nurse (APRN)).

    o **Therapists**: Physical Therapist; Occupational Therapist; and Qualified Speech-Language Therapist.

    *Note: CMS **will not apply** the VBM for 2015 and 2016 to groups of physicians that are participating ACOs as part of the MSSP, the testing of the Pioneer ACO Model, the Comprehensive Primary Care Initiative, or other similar CMS Innovation Center initiatives.*

CMS Determination of Eligible Group Practices for 2014 VBM Reporting:

- To meet its goal of all-physician VBM participation by the 2015 reporting year (2017 program year), CMS has lowered the required group practice size from 100+ EPs established for the 2013 reporting year to group practices with 10+ EPs for VBM participation during the 2014 reporting period (2016 program year):

    o CMS estimates that the 2014 VBM reporting requirement to include groups with 10+ EPs will cause approximately 17,000

---

[332] *http://www.cms.gov/Medicare/Medicare-Fee-for-Service-Payment/PhysicianFeedbackProgram/Background.html*

group practices and nearly 60 percent of physicians to be affected by the VBM in CY2016.[333]

- To ensure accurate selection of group practices eligible for VBM reporting during 2014, CMS employs a three-step process to confirm practice size before, during, and after the reporting period:[334]

  o Step 1: TIN review (before)

  o Step 2: PECOS database query (during)

  o Step 3: claims analysis (after)

Tax Identification Number (TIN) Review:

- CMS defines a group practice as an organization of EPs who practice through one TIN.

- To ensure continuity and reduce confusion, this definition was chosen in order to align with the PQRS reporting requirements for group practices.

- This approach also allows CMS to take advantage of the infrastructure and methodologies already developed for PQRS group-level reporting and evaluation.

- The VBM will be applied at the TIN level to *physicians* only, not to other EPs who also may bill under the TIN.

- If a physician moves to another TIN after the performance year of 2013, he or she will be subject to the 2015 VBM applied to the last TIN he or she practiced under.

---

[333] *Page 1160: CMS-1600-FC, http://www.gpo.gov/fdsys/pkg/FR-2013-12-10/pdf/2013-28696.pdf*

[334] *Pages 69308–60310: CMS-1590-FC, http://www.gpo.gov/fdsys/pkg/FR-2012-11-16/pdf/2012-26900.pdf*

PECOS Database Query:

- To confirm the number of EPs in a given practice, CMS has established a process of query through the **Provider Enrollment, Chain, and Ownership System (PECOS)** database:

  - PECOS is an Internet-based Medicare enrollment system through which providers and suppliers can: submit Medicare enrollment applications; view and print enrollment information; update enrollment information; complete the revalidation process; voluntarily withdraw from the Medicare program; and track the status of a submitted Medicare enrollment application.

- In the 2014 Physician Fee Schedule (PFS) Final Rule, CMS has established a PECOS query time frame to occur within ten days of the close of the group self-nomination/registration deadline of September 30, 2014, for participation in the PQRS:

  - The **PQRS** is a voluntary pay-for-reporting program that is structured to provide incentive payments and payment adjustments to EPs. A variety of reporting methods are available for individual providers and group practices to report information during 2014 on 284 individual quality measures and 25 measures groups. For more information on PQRS, see Chapter 5: Technical Appendix: The Physician Quality Reporting System (PQRS).

Claims Analysis:

- To ensure that identified groups had 10+ EPs during the *entire* performance period year, CMS will analyze the group's TIN claims submitted for the performance year, including at least a sixty-day claims "run-out" period following the end of a reporting year. For example, claims will be analyzed through at least February 28, 2015, for services provided during the performance year of CY2014.

- Based on the claims run-out period analysis, CMS will only **remove** groups from the eligibility list, if the group does not have at least 10+ EPs who billed under the group's TIN during the performance period.

- No additional groups will be added as a result of the claims run-out analysis process.

7.3.5 Step 2: Attribute Medicare Beneficiaries to Eligible Group Practices

Overview:

- In the calculation of performance under the VBM program, beneficiaries must be attributed (assigned) to a specific group of physicians.

- The same population of beneficiaries attributed to a medical group practice is used for calculating the denominators of all PQRS, and non-PQRS, quality and cost measures.

- To maintain consistency between CMS quality initiatives, the attribution methodology adopted for the VBM program is the same as used to attribute Medicare beneficiaries to ACOs by the MSSP and to the PQRS GPRO web-based interface.

- Based on an analysis of the 2012 Data Year QRUR, CMS attributed an average of 3,007 Medicare beneficiaries to each group practice with 25+ EPs.

Two-Step Attribution Process:

For all PQRS-reported quality measures and non-PQRS reported cost measures, beneficiaries will be assigned to physician groups in a two-step process, based on primary care services provided by the group, as captured in Medicare Part B claims.[335]

Note: A separate attribution process will be used in 2014 to determine the new MSPB cost measure. This process is described below:

- **The first step** assigns a beneficiary to a medical group practice (as identified by its TIN) if the beneficiary receives the plurality of his or her primary care services (in terms of allowed charges) from primary care physicians within the group practice:

---

[335] *Page 69320: CMS-1590-FC, http://www.gpo.gov/fdsys/pkg/FR-2012-11-16/pdf/2012-26900.pdf*

- o Primary care physicians are defined as those with one of four specialty designations: Internal Medicine; General Practice; Family Practice; and Geriatric Medicine.

- **The second step** only considers beneficiaries who have not had a primary care service furnished by *any* primary care physician either inside or outside the group practice:

  - o Under this second step, a beneficiary is assigned to a group practice if the beneficiary receives a plurality of his or her primary care services from specialist physicians and certain non-physician practitioners (Nurse Practitioners, Clinical Nurse Specialists, and Physician Assistants) within the group practice.

- Under this two-step attribution process, some large single-specialty groups (i.e., those limited to Emergency Medicine, Diagnostic Radiology, Pathology, and Anesthesiology) may not have any beneficiaries attributed to them.

  - o Under the VBM program, such groups would not have their payment adjusted. However, such groups must still participate in the PQRS program to avoid the -2.0 percent VBM penalty. CMS plans to address this issue in future rule making.

- Beneficiaries are not attributed to any medical group practice **if,** for any month in 2014, any of the following situations apply to them:

  - o they were enrolled in Part A only or Part B only

  - o they were enrolled in Medicare managed care

  - o they resided outside the United States, its territories, and its possessions

  - o they did not have any Medicare allowed charges in 2012

- Based on an analysis of 2012 data provided in QRURs released in September 2013, CMS found:[336]

---

[336] Page 1227: CMS-1600-FC, http://www.gpo.gov/fdsys/pkg/FR-2013-12-10/pdf/2013-28696.pdf

- o Beneficiaries attributed to a group of physicians using the two-step attribution process described above received an average of five primary care services in 2012.

- o On average, 64.3 percent of such services were provided by the group to which the beneficiary was attributed.

- o These results suggest that the adopted attribution approach attributes beneficiaries to those groups of physicians that deliver the plurality of a beneficiary's care and are well-positioned to oversee the beneficiaries' care.

7.3.6 Step 3: Collect Data on Quality and Cost Measures

Overview:

- Calculation of the VBM is made based on the determination of a **quality composite score** and a **cost composite score**.

- Composite scores for quality and cost are determined through individual measures performance assigned to equally weighted measures within each composite component.

- Data sources for calculation of the composite scores include individual or group practice PQRS-reported quality data and Medicare Part A and Part B claims cost data for non-PQRS quality measures and cost measures.

2014 VBM Measures Reliability Standards:[337]

- To ensure that the VBM is based on quality of care and cost composites that *reliably* measure performance, CMS uses a case-number reliability standard.

---

[337] *Page 1182: CMS-1600-FC, http://www.gpo.gov/fdsys/pkg/FR-2013-12-10/pdf/2013-28696.pdf*

- Statistical reliability is defined as the extent to which variation in the measure's performance rate is due to variation in the quality (or cost) furnished by the physicians (or group of physicians) rather than random variation due to the sample of cases observed.

- Potential reliability values range from zero to one, where one (highest possible reliability) signifies that all variation in the measure's rates is the result of variation in differences in performance across physicians (or groups of physicians).

- Generally, reliabilities in the 0.40–0.70 range are often considered moderate and values greater than 0.70 high. In the CY2013 Final PFS Rule, CMS adopted the twenty-case minimum as the reliability standard for the VBM program in order for a quality or cost measure to be included in the quality of care or cost composite.

  ○ In the 2012 data year QRURs released in September, CMS found that the reliability standards for quality and cost measures were above .70 for groups with 25+ EPs, indicating that the measures determining overall quality and cost were highly reliable.[338]

- If a group of physicians fails to meet the minimum number of twenty cases for a particular measure, the measure would not be counted and the remaining measures in the domain would be given equal weight.

- To the extent that CMS cannot develop either a reliable quality of care composite or cost composite because of a lack of reliable domain information, it would not calculate a VBM and payment would not be affected.

  ○ In the determination of cost measures, CMS will assign an "average" cost rating to those groups that, because of specialty concentration, do not have at least twenty beneficiaries attributed to them for calculation of cost measures.[339]

---

[338] Pages 1227–1228: http://www.gpo.gov/fdsys/pkg/FR-2013-12-10/pdf/2013-28696.pdf

[339] Page 1210: CMS-1600-FC, http://www.gpo.gov/fdsys/pkg/FR-2013-12-10/pdf/2013-28696.pdf

Quality Measures of the 2014 Reporting Year:

- Primary determination of the quality composite score is based on participation in the PQRS and providers will be evaluated for the 2016 VBM based on the PQRS quality measures they report during 2014. In addition, CMS has included three outcomes measures extracted from the 2013 administrative claims reporting option, for which data will be claims-extracted by CMS during 2014:

  - **The PQRS** is a voluntary pay-for-reporting program that is structured to provide incentive payments and payment adjustments to EPs. A variety of reporting methods is available for individual providers and group practices to report information during 2014 on 284 individual quality measures and 25 measures groups. For more information on PQRS, see Chapter 5: Technical Appendix: The Physician Quality Reporting System (PQRS).

- The determination of the group practice quality composite score for 2014 VBM reporting integrates data from the following sources:

  - **PQRS:**
    - includes 2014 quality measures reported through the PQRS process
    - also includes results from the Clinicians/Group Consumer Assessment of Healthcare Providers and Systems (CG-CAHPS) surveys. Reporting of such data is mandatory for groups of 100+ EPs for 2014

  - **Medicare Part A and Part B claims:**
    - Non-PQRS reported metrics used for three outcomes measures are CMS-extracted from claims.

Quality Measures Reported Through the Physician Quality Reporting System (PQRS):

- **Group practice PQRS registration requirements**:[340]

  - For the 2014 VBM performance reporting year 2014, group practices with 10+ EPs must register/self-nominate for the 2014 PQRS beginning May 1, 2014, and complete registration no later than September 30, 2014, using the Physician Value Quality Reporting System (PV-QRS) website.

  - Failure to meet this time line will result in the assessment of the - 2.0 percent VBM and the -2.0 percent PQRS payment adjustment to be applied in 2016.

    Note: For more information on the PV-QRS, see the CMS provider call information at:
    http://www.cms.gov/Outreach-and-Education/Outreach/NPC/National-Provider-Calls-and-Events-Items/2013-07-31-modifier.html?DLPage=2&DLSort=0&DLSortDir=descending

2014 PQRS Group Practice Reporting Options:

- For the 2014 VBM reporting period, group practices must satisfactorily meet PQRS reporting requirements associated with one of the following group practice reporting options:[341]

  - GPRO web-based interface

  - CMS-qualified registries

  - electronic health records (EHRs)

  - CMS-certified survey vendor (new for 2014 reporting and only available as an option for groups with 25+ EPs

    OR

---

[340] *http://www.cms.gov/Outreach-and-Education/Outreach/NPC/National-Provider-Calls-and-Events-Items/2013-07-31-modifier.html?DLPage=2&DLSort=0&DLSortDir=descending*

[341] *Table 48 and Table 50: CMS-1600-FC, http://www.gpo.gov/fdsys/pkg/FR-2013-12-10/pdf/2013-28696.pdf*

459

- EPs reporting PQRS individually through:
  - claims
  - EHR
  - CMS-qualified registries
  - CMS-qualified clinical data registry (QCDR), new for 2014

- Performance on any displayed GPRO quality indicators is based on a sample of beneficiaries who had at least two office or other outpatient visits with the medical group practice and for whom the medical group practice provided the plurality of all office and other outpatient services during 2014.

  Note: At least 50 percent of individual EPs in a group of physicians must meet PQRS reporting criteria to avoid the CY2016 PQRS payment adjustment in order to calculate a group quality score. Based on 2011 PQRS participation, CMS estimates that setting the satisfactory reporting requirement at a 50 percent threshold would result in 76 percent of groups of physicians with between 10–99 EPs would meet the 50 percent threshold and 45 percent of groups with 100+ EPs would meet the 50 percent threshold.[342]

PQRS and the Value-Based Payment Modifier:

- Because the performance determination of VBM program quality measures relies upon satisfactory PQRS reporting by eligible group practices of 10+ EPs in 2014 (for the 2016 VBM program year), CMS includes VBM penalties for eligible groups that fail to satisfactorily report PQRS.

- Groups are categorized into two categories for the 2014 reporting year, based on PQRS participation/satisfactory reporting:[343]

  - **Category 1:**
    - groups of 10+ EPs that self-nominate for 2014 PQRS reporting under the GPRO web-based interface, qualified

---

[342] *Page 1169: CMS-1600-FC, http://www.gpo.gov/fdsys/pkg/FR-2013-12-10/pdf/2013-28696.pdf*

[343] *Page 1169: CMS-1600-FC, http://www.gpo.gov/fdsys/pkg/FR-2013-12-10/pdf/2013-28696.pdf*

registries or EHR and satisfactorily report to avoid the 2016 PQRS payment adjustment

- groups of 10+ EPs that do not register to participate in the PQRS reporting under the GPRO web-based interface, qualified registries or EHR in CY2014, but elect individual EP reporting instead and avoid the 2016 PQRS payment adjustment:

  - Such groups must have at least 50 percent of the group's EPs meet the criteria for satisfactory reporting of data on PQRS quality measures as individuals for the CY2016 PQRS payment adjustment

    OR

  - In lieu of satisfactory reporting, satisfactorily participate in a PQRS-qualified clinical data registry to avoid the CY2016 PQRS payment adjustment.

- Category 1 groups are subject to mandatory quality-tiering to determine VBMs.

  - For 2014 VBM reporting (2016 program year), groups of 10–99 EPs will only have neutral or upward modifiers applied.

  - For 2014 reporting, groups of 100+ EPs will be subject to upwards, neutral or downward VBMs.

- Category 1 groups will also earn the +.5 percent PQRS incentive payment for satisfactory PQRS reporting during 2014.

- **Category 2:**

  - Category 2 groups are those physician groups with 10+ EPs that are subject to the CY2016 VBM and do not fall within Category 1, to include:

    - groups with 10+ EPs that that do not register for 2014 PQRS reporting via any of the group practice or individual EP reporting options

- groups with 10+ EPs that fail to avoid the 2014 PQRS payment adjustment penalty

  - Category 2 groups will have the -2.0 percent VBM **and** the -2.0 percent 2014 PQRS penalty applied to all Medicare Part B covered professional services provided by physicians. This modifier is applied at the TIN level.

2014 VBM PQRS Reportable Quality Measures:

- CMS uses risk-adjusted quality measures reported through the PQRS via the GPRO:[344]

  - differences in socioeconomic and demographic characteristics

  - ethnicity

  - health status of individuals

  - elimination of the effect of geographic adjustments in payments

- For 2014, there are 284 PQRS quality measures reportable by those group practices or EPs within a group practice that is reporting individually using one of the reporting options listed above. Each measure is reportable by one or more reporting options listed below. For additional information on specific quality measures, see:

  2014 PQRS Measure Group Specification, Release Notes, Getting Started with 2014 PQRS Measures Groups, 2014 Quality-Data Code Categories. and 2014 PQRS Measures Groups Single Source Code Master

---

[344] *Page 672, Section 3007: Patient Protection and Affordable Care Act—US Government ..., http://www.gpo.gov/fdsys/pkg/BILLS-111hr3590enr/pdf/BILLS-111hr3590enr.pdf*

TABLE 1: 2014 PQRS MEASURES REPORTABLE BY SUBMISSION OPTION[345]

REPORTING METHOD	NUMBER OF MEASURES REPORTABLE
claims	111
qualified registry	200
electronic health records (EHRs)	64
qualified clinical data registry (QCDR)	284*
GPRO web-based interface	22 (17 measures + two composite measures)
CMS certified survey vendor	variable according to associated reporting method**

*New for 2014 as an option for individual EP reporting, QCDR reporting can accommodate any of the PQRS quality measures, as well as up to 20 additional registry-specific measures.

**New for 2014, the certified survey vendor reporting option is for groups of 25+ EPs to use as a method to report CG-CAHPS survey results along with PQRS quality measures. Selection of this option also requires that the group specify a method to be used for measures reporting.

- For the purposes of the VBM program, CMS has aligned each of the 284 PQRS quality measures with one of the six domains of the NQS:[346]

TABLE 2: PQRS MEASURES ALIGNED WITH NQS DOMAINS

NQS DOMAIN	NUMBER OF ALIGNED QUALITY MEASURES
Effective Clinical Care	182
Patient Safety	30
Communication and Care Coordination	35*

---

[345] 2014 PQRS Measure Group Specification, Release Notes, Getting Started with 2014 PQRS Measures Groups, 2014 Quality-Data Code Categories. and 2014 PQRS Measures Groups Single Source Code Master, https://www.google.com/search?q=CMS-1600-FC+(PDF+version)&oq=CMS-1600-FC+(PDF+version)&aqs=chrome..69i57.439j0j9&sourceid=chrome&espv=210&es_sm=93&ie=UTF-8

[346] Table 52, Page 839: CMS-1600-FC, http://www.gpo.gov/fdsys/pkg/FR-2013-12-10/pdf/2013-28696.pdf

Person and Caregiver-Centered Experience and Outcomes	10
Efficiency and Cost Reduction	15
Community/Population Health	12
Total 2014 PQRS Quality Measures	**284**

In addition to the 35 2014 PQRS Communication and Care Coordination domain measures, CMS has assigned the three outcomes measures to this NQS domain for purposes of calculating the quality composite score.

Note: *For a detailed description of the NQS, see Chapter 2, Appendix: Attachment A.*

Clinician/Group Consumer Assessment of Healthcare Providers and Systems Survey (CG-CAHPS):

- Included as a measure under the Communication and Care Coordination domain, the CG-CAHPS is available for reporting by groups of 25+ EPs using the GPRO web-based interface or CMS-certified survey vendor reporting methods only.

- Inclusion of the CG-CAHPS is mandatory in 2014 for groups of 100+ EPs using the GPRO web-based interface or the CMS-certified survey vendor reporting options. Reporting of CG-CAHPS for groups of 25–99 EPs using these reporting methods is optional for 2014.[347]

Note: *The GPRO web-based interface and CMS-certified survey vendor PQRS reporting methods are available only to groups of 25+ EPs in 2014. Groups with 10–24 EPs will not have the option of reporting CG-CHPS in 2014.*

The following items are included in the 2014 CG-CAHPS:[348]

- Getting Timely Care, Appointments, and Information

- How Well Providers Communicate

- Patient's Rating of Provider

- Access to Specialists

---

[347] *Page 812: CMS-1600-FC, http://www.gpo.gov/fdsys/pkg/FR-2013-12-10/pdf/2013-28696.pdf*

[348] *Page 1113: CMS-1600-FC, http://www.gpo.gov/fdsys/pkg/FR-2013-12-10/pdf/2013-28696.pdf*

- Health Promotion and Education

- Shared Decision Making

- Health Status/Functional Status

- Courteous and Helpful Office Staff

- Care Coordination

- Between Visit Communication

- Helping You to Take Medication as Directed

- Stewardship of Patient Resources

2014 VBM Quality Outcomes Measures, Extracted from Medicare Claims[349]

- For the 2014 VBM Program, CMS has included three outcomes measures that were included in the 2013 administrative claims PQRS reporting option for group practices. Although administrative claims reporting option is not available to group practices for 2014 PQRS reporting, CMS will continue to extract data from claims for the outcomes measures for the 2014 VBM program:[350]

  - An outcome measure, as defined within the CMS Measures Management System Blueprint v10.0, indicates the result of the performance (or nonperformance) of functions or processes. It is a measure that focuses on achieving a particular state of health.

- **Outcome Measure 1: All-Cause Hospital Readmissions:**
  - The all-cause hospital readmissions measure is a medical group practice-specific all-cause thirty-day rate of acute care hospital readmissions:

---

[349] Page 1181: CMS-1600-FC, http://www.gpo.gov/fdsys/pkg/FR-2013-12-10/pdf/2013-28696.pdf
[350] Table 52, Page 69287: CMS-1590-FC, http://www.gpo.gov/fdsys/pkg/FR-2012-11-16/pdf/2012-26900.pdf

- All-cause thirty-day readmission is defined as an unplanned readmission for **any** cause within thirty days from the date of discharge of an index admission in 2014 for beneficiaries discharged from an acute care or critical access hospital.

  o The measure does not apply to:

  - attributed beneficiaries who were under age eighteen on January 1, 2012, discharged against medical advice, or transferred to another acute care hospital

  - beneficiaries who died within thirty days of discharge and those without continuous enrollment in Medicare Part A for at least one month following discharge

  - certain hospitalizations, such as those related to treatment of cancer or primary psychiatric disease, which are excluded from the set of index admissions considered

  o Index admissions are grouped into five specialty cohorts (surgery/gynecology, cardiorespiratory, cardiovascular, neurology, and medicine) based on the presumption that admissions treated by similar teams of clinicians are likely to have similar risks of readmission.

  o Readmissions are risk adjusted by estimation of a series of specialty-specific ratios of the number of readmissions predicted for a specific medical practice (adjusted for case mix) that are then compared to the number of readmissions expected among all medical group practices in the peer group with a similar case mix:

  - A case-weighted mean of these ratios is then determined and multiplied by the overall readmission rate for all beneficiaries across all groups.

  - For more information on readmissions risk-adjustment, see Chapter 3: The Hospital Readmissions Reduction Program (HRRP) or visit https://www.qualitynet.org/

    Select: *The Hospitals Inpatient/Readmissions Reduction/Readmission Measures Methodology Report.*

TABLE 3: OUTCOME MEASURE 1: ALL-CAUSE READMISSION

NQF #	MEASURE TITLE	DESCRIPTION
N/A	All-Cause Readmission	all-cause risk-adjusted readmissions for attributed Medicare beneficiaries occurring within 30 days of discharge from an index admission, expressed as a percentage of total attributed beneficiary admissions during a reporting period

- **Composite Measures of Ambulatory Care Sensitive Conditions (ACSCs):**[351]

  - ACSCs are conditions for which good outpatient care can prevent complications or more serious disease. The Agency for Healthcare Research and Quality (AHRQ) developed measures of potentially avoidable hospitalizations for ACSCs as part of a larger set of **Prevention Quality Indicators (PQIs)**.

  - PQI measures rely on hospital discharge data but are not intended to measure hospital quality—rather, high or increasing rates of hospitalization for these conditions in a defined population of patients may indicate inadequate access to high-quality ambulatory care.

  - The Care Coordination quality domain includes two PQI composite measures of hospital admissions for **acute** and **chronic** ACSCs:[352]

TABLE 4: OUTCOME MEASURE 2: COMPOSITE OF ACUTE PREVENTION QUALITY INDICATORS (PQIs)

NQF #	MEASURE TITLE	DESCRIPTION
0279	Bacterial Pneumonia	number of admissions for bacterial pneumonia per 100,000 population
0281	Urinary Tract Infections	number of discharges for UTI per 100,000 population age 18 years and older in a one-year period

---

[351] Page 1227: CMS-1600-FC, http://www.gpo.gov/fdsys/pkg/FR-2013-12-10/pdf/2013-28696.pdf

[352] Table 52, Page 69287: CMS-1590-FC, http://www.gpo.gov/fdsys/pkg/FR-2012-11-16/pdf/2012-26900.pdf

0280	Dehydration	number of admissions for dehydration per 100,000 population

TABLE 5: OUTCOME MEASURE 3: COMPOSITE OF CHRONIC PREVENTION QUALITY INDICATORS (PQIs)

NQF #	MEASURE TITLE	DESCRIPTION
0638	Uncontrolled Diabetes	number of discharges for uncontrolled diabetes per 100,000 population age 18 years and older in a one-year period
0272	Short-Term Diabetes Complications	number of discharges for short-term diabetes complications per 100,000 population age 18 years and older in a one-year period
0274	Long-Term Diabetes Complications	number of discharges for long-term diabetes complications per 100,000 population age 18 years and older in a one-year period
0285	Lower Extremity Amputations for Diabetes	number of discharges for lower-extremity amputation among patients with diabetes per 100,000 population age 18 years or older in a one-year period
0275	Chronic Obstructive Pulmonary Disease (COPD)	number of admissions for COPD per 100,000 population
0277	Congestive Heart Failure (CHF)	percent of the population with admissions for CHF

Cost Measures for 2014 VBM Reporting Year:

For the 2014 VBM performance period, CMS has adopted a total of six cost measures that are determined through claims analysis. Five of these measures are the total per capita cost measures used in the initial (2013 reporting) VBM performance year and the sixth measure, the MSPB, is new for 2014.

Per Capita Cost Measures:

All cost measures are "payment standardized" and "risk-adjusted:"[353]

- **cost measure risk adjustment**: Measures are risk-adjusted using Medicare's Hierarchical Condition Category (HCC) Model. This is the same Risk Adjustment Model used for physician feedback reporting. Risk adjustment under the HCC model includes:

  - assignment of prior year ICD-9-CM diagnosis codes to seventy high-cost clinical conditions (each with similar disease characteristics and costs) to capture medical condition risk

  - the HCC risk scores also incorporate patient age, gender, reason for Medicare eligibility (age or disability), and Medicaid eligibility status (to account, in part, for socioeconomic status)

  - the Risk Adjustment Model also includes the beneficiary's end-stage renal disease (ESRD) status

- **payment standardization of cost measures:** Cost measures are calculated on the basis of a *standardized* Medicare payment analysis. In determining the VBM, CMS will apply the same standardization methodology as in the 2011 Physician Feedback Reports and the MSPB measure that is used in CMS's feedback reports to hospitals.

  - This applied standardization methodology removes local or regional price differences that may cause cost variation that a physician cannot influence through practicing efficient care.

  - In effect, it "levels the field" among markets by excluding Medicare geographic adjustment factors, such as the geographic practice cost index (GPCI) and the hospital wage index. The standardized rates are updated annually.

---

[353] *http://www.cms.gov/Medicare/Medicare-Fee-for-Service-Payment/PhysicianFeedbackProgram/Downloads/122111_Slide_Presentation.pdf*

Cost Measure 1: Total Per Capita Costs Measure:[354]

- They include annual payment standardized and risk-adjusted Medicare Part A and Part B costs.

- Total per capita costs do not include Medicare payments under Part D for drug expenses.

- Medicare will use at least a sixty-day claims run-out (for example, claims paid through March 1 of the year following December 31, the close of the performance period) to calculate the total per capita cost measures.

Cost Measures 2–5: Total Per Capita Costs for Beneficiaries with Four Chronic Conditions:

- • For the 2014 VBM program, CMS has established individual cost measures for four specific chronic conditions:

    o chronic obstructive pulmonary disease (COPD)

    o heart failure (HF)

    o coronary artery disease (CAD)

    o diabetes (DM)

- The per capita costs for beneficiaries with each condition are computed in the same manner as the total per capita costs measure, except that expected costs for beneficiaries with a specific condition are computed based on a Risk Adjustment Model that includes *only* beneficiaries with that condition.

- These condition-specific per capita costs include all costs and are not limited to costs associated with treating the condition itself.

- The four chronic health conditions are not mutually exclusive. Beneficiaries with two or more conditions are counted (as are their per capita costs) within each of the condition subgroups. This means a patient with all four targeted conditions would be counted four times;

---

[354] *Template for groups that participated in 2012 Group Practice Reporting Option of the Physician Quality Reporting System, http://www.cms.gov/Medicare/Medicare-Fee-for-Service-Payment/PhysicianFeedbackProgram/Downloads/PY2012-GPRO-QRUR-Sample.pdf*

once per condition subgroup. However, cost measures are risk-adjusted to account for these sicker patients.

- For each chronic condition subgroup, the separate condition-specific Risk Adjustment Model estimated for that subgroup captures other chronic and acute comorbidities associated with beneficiaries in the particular subgroup.

Categories of Services for Per Capita Cost Measures:[355]

- Evaluation and Management (E&M) Services in All Non-Emergency Settings:
    - all E&M services provided by the participating group
    - all E&M services provided by other groups.

- Procedures in All Non-Emergency Settings:
    - all procedures performed by the participating group
    - all procedures performed by other groups

- Hospital Services (Excluding Emergency Outpatient)

- Emergency Services That Did Not Result in a Hospital Admission, including visits, procedures, laboratory, and other tests, and imaging services

- Services in Non-Emergency Ambulatory Settings

- Post-Acute Care Services, including: skilled nursing care; psychiatric, rehabilitation or other long-term facility care; and home health care

- all other Medicare-covered services not captured in other categories, such as anesthesia, ambulance services, chemotherapy, other Medicare Part B drugs, chiropractic, enteral and parenteral nutrition, vision services, hearing and speech services, and influenza immunization;

- other services billed by non-institutional providers

---

[355] *Template for groups that participated in 2012 Group Practice Reporting Option of the Physician Quality Reporting System, http://www.cms.gov/Medicare/Medicare-Fee-for-Service-Payment/PhysicianFeedbackProgram/Downloads/PY2012-GPRO-QRUR-Sample.pdf*

Beneficiary Attribution for Per Capita Cost Measures:[356]

- Beneficiaries are attributed to a group practice for evaluation of total per capita cost measures using the same two-step process used for VBM quality measures reporting (described above).

- This attribution process focuses on delivery of **primary care services** and as a result, groups not providing primary care services may have fewer than twenty attributed beneficiaries or none at all:

    o Commenters on the 2014 Final PFS Rule regarding attribution methodology for cost measures pointed out that many specialist physicians do not see *any* of the patients with the four chronic conditions and would have few, if any, attributed beneficiaries:

        ▪ As such, these groups would fail to achieve the reliability standard and CMS would be unable to calculate reliable cost measures for those groups of physicians.

        ▪ For 2014 VBM reporting, CMS would classify the cost composite score for groups with fewer than twenty attributed beneficiaries "average" under the quality-tiering methodology.

Cost Measure 6: Medicare Spending Per Beneficiary (MSPB) Cost Measure:[357]

- As a newly added cost measure for 2014 reporting, the MSPB includes all Medicare Part A and Part B costs incurred by a beneficiary during the three days **before** an inpatient index admission, **during** the admission, and thirty days **after** discharge.

    o **index admission**: An index admission is the admission with a principal diagnosis of a specified condition that meets the inclusion and exclusion criteria for the measure. For the VBM

---

[356] *Template for groups that participated in 2012 Group Practice Reporting Option of the Physician Quality Reporting System, http://www.cms.gov/Medicare/Medicare-Fee-for-Service-Payment/PhysicianFeedbackProgram/Downloads/PY2012-GPRO-QRUR-Sample.pdf*

[357] *Pages 1189, 1190, 1208: CMS-1600-FC, http://www.gpo.gov/fdsys/pkg/FR-2013-12-10/pdf/2013-28696.pdf*

program, index admissions include admissions for all medical conditions meeting this definition.

○ The MSPB only applies to admissions to hospitals reimbursed under the inpatient prospective payment system (IPPS) and does not include admissions to the following facilities:

- psychiatric hospitals

- rehabilitation hospitals

- long-term care hospitals

- children's hospitals

- cancer hospitals

- hospitals located in US territories

- critical access hospitals

Note: *For a detailed description of IPPS-reimbursed hospitals, see: Chapter 2: The Hospital Value-Based Purchasing (VBP) Program, Section 4.2.2 and Appendix: Attachment A: IPPS.*

- As a component of the hospital inpatient quality reporting (IQR) and VBP programs, CMS extended the MSPB measure to the VBM program for 2014 reporting to:

  ○ incentivize physicians to build stronger relationships with hospitals and better understand the providers and suppliers that furnish care for patients before, during, and after an acute care hospitalization

  ○ incentivize hospitals and physicians to furnish efficient, effective care during a hospitalization and to improve coordination of post-discharge care to avoid unnecessary services and preventable readmissions

  ○ increase shared accountability and alignment of incentives between hospitals and physicians to provide high-quality care at lower costs to Medicare

- For 2014 VBM reporting, CMS will use the MSPB total spending dollar amount as the measure's performance rate rather than converting it to a ratio as is done under the hospital IQR and VBP programs.[358]

- The payments included in the MSPB measure are adjusted according to the CMS price standardization methodology, located at: http://www.qualitynet.org. They are standardized to remove differences attributable to geographic payment adjustments and other payment factors.

Beneficiary Attribution for MSPB:[359]

As opposed to the two-step attribution approach used for the total cost per capita cost measures, CMS is using a single plurality attribution approach for the MSPB measure:

- Beneficiary attribution for the MSPB will be to a single group of physicians that provides the plurality of services (as measured by allowable charges) under the group's TIN for Medicare Part B services provided **during the index hospital admission only**.

- CMS defines "plurality of services" as the **highest total Medicare-allowed amount for Part B services billed by any group of physicians that provides Part B services** during the index admission period. This group may not necessarily be the group *billing the majority of charges*—rather, the group's *total **allowed** charges* must be greater than the total allowed changes of any other group of physicians for the index admission.

---

[358] *Page 1208: CMS-1600-FC, http://www.gpo.gov/fdsys/pkg/FR-2013-12-10/pdf/2013-28696.pdf*

[359] *Pages 1197–1198: CMS-1600-FC, http://www.gpo.gov/fdsys/pkg/FR-2013-12-10/pdf/2013-28696.pdf*

7.3.7 Step 4: Establish Quality and Cost Benchmarks

Overview

To determine group practice performance for PQRS-reported quality measures during a given VBM reporting year, CMS will establish national benchmarks for each quality measure, to include PQRS-reported measures and the CMS claims-extracted outcomes measures. Group performance as judged against these benchmarks is used to determine the quality and cost composite scores.

- National Quality Measure Benchmarks (to include outcomes measures) are established as the national mean of each measure's performance rate (as reported by all physician and physician groups) during the *year prior to the performance period.*

- National Cost Measures Benchmarks are calculated as the national mean of the performance rates (*during the current performance year*) among all groups of physicians to which beneficiaries are attributed and that are subject to the value-based payment modifier.

Comparison of PQRS-Reported Quality Measures against Benchmarks:

- Using reporting occurring in the year prior to the performance year, each physician and physician group will be assigned a weighted performance rate by dividing their reported (by any PQRS reporting option) performance rate by the total number of beneficiaries used to calculate the national performance rate. As a result, group performance is weighted appropriately in comparison to the national quality measure benchmark.

- To determine group practice performance against quality benchmarks, CMS will compare the weighted performance on each reported quality measure to the national performance rate benchmark at the TIN level.

  o The population of beneficiaries included in quality performance reporting is dependent on the method of PQRS reporting selected:

- Groups using the qualified registry or EHR PQRS reporting methods must report specific measures on at least 50 percent of Medicare beneficiaries attributed to the practice.

- For GPRO web-based interface reporting of PQRS, each participating medical group practice is required to report clinical data for at least the first 218 or 411 beneficiaries (depending on the group's size) on their list of assigned beneficiaries that the CMS has determined meet criteria for specific measures—or on 100 percent of the beneficiaries on their list for that measure, whichever is smaller.

- **Quality benchmarks are based on PQRS reporting that occurs in the year *prior* to the performance year**, so that physicians have information on national benchmarks before the end of the performance year. For example, benchmarks for the 2014 performance year will be based on 2013 PQRS reporting:

  o In the fall of 2014, CMS will disseminate QRURs containing: CY2013 quality and cost measures; measure performance and benchmarks used to score the composites; quality of care and cost composite scores; and the VBM amount.

- CMS will publish these measures benchmarks publicly to facilitate informed measures selection and reporting methods by physician groups for the applicable performance year. For the initial VBM performance year of 2013, CMS published the quality benchmarks (from 2012 PQRS reporting) in December 2013. For 2014 performance reporting, CMS intends to publish applicable benchmarks (from 2013) earlier in the performance year.

- For group practices reporting PQRS in 2012 via the GPRO, the benchmarks for the 2013 VBM performance year (2015 program year) are as follows:[360]

---

[360] *PY2013 Prior Year Benchmarks, Centers for Medicare & Medicaid Services, http://www.cms.gov/Medicare/Medicare-Fee-for-Service-Payment/PhysicianFeedbackProgram/Downloads/PY2013-Prior-Year-Benchmarks-.pdf*

TABLE 6: PQRS QUALITY INDICATORS FOR GROUPS VIA THE GROUP PRACTICE REPORTING OPTION (GPRO) *

PERFORMANCE MEASURE		2012 MEAN
CAD Composite (All-or-Nothing Scoring)		63.6%
	CAD-2 CAD: Lipid Control	54.1%
	CAD-7 CAD: ACE Inhibitor or ARB Therapy for Patient with CAD and Diabetes and/or LVSD	63.0%
Care-1	Medication Reconciliation: After Discharge from an Inpatient Facility	76.0%
Care-2	Falls: Screening for Future Fall Risk	32.6%
DM-2	DM: Hemoglobin A1c Poor Control in DM (> 9.0)	21.4%
	DM Composite (All-or-Nothing Scoring)	23.2%
	DM-13 DM: High Blood Pressure Control	66.8%
	DM-14 DM: LDL-C Control	54.0%
	DM-15 DM: Hemoglobin A1c Control (< 8.0)	65.3%
	DM-16 DM: Daily Aspirin Use for Patients with Diabetes and Ischemic Vascular Disease	70.8%
	DM-17 DM: Tobacco Non-Use	72.3%
HF-6 HF:	Beta-Blocker Therapy for LVSD	82.0%
HTN-2 HTN:	Controlling High Blood Pressure	65.0%
IVD-1 IVD:	Complete Lipid Profile and LDL-C Control	46.3%
IVD-2 IVD:	Use of Aspirin or Another Antithrombotic	62.4%
Prev-5 Prev:	Screening Mammography	48.3%
Prev-6 Prev:	Colorectal Cancer Screening	40.5%
Prev-7 Prev:	Influenza Immunization	38.9%
Prev-8 Prev:	Pneumonia Vaccination for Patients ≥ 65	45.4%
Prev-9 Prev:	BMI Screening and Follow-Up	49.1%
Prev-10 Prev:	Tobacco Use: Screening and Cessation Intervention	79.6%
Prev-11 Prev:	Screening for High Blood Pressure	90.6%
Prev-12 Prev:	Screening for Clinical Depression and Follow-Up Plan	22.3%

*Benchmarks are not available for measures for which fewer than 20 groups reported at least 20 cases.

Note: PQRS GPRO and ACO GPRO measures are the same in 2013. The full list of all 2012 measures benchmarks may be viewed at: http://www.cms.gov/Medicare/Medicare-Fee-for-Service-Payment/PhysicianFeedbackProgram/Downloads/PY2013-Prior-Year-Benchmarks-.pdf

- If a measure is new to the PQRS, CMS will be unable to calculate a benchmark and performance on that measure will not be included in the quality composite. In addition, if fewer than twenty groups report fewer than twenty cases for any quality measure, no benchmark will be calculated.

Comparison of Outcome Measures to Benchmarks:

- Using reporting occurring in the year prior to the performance year, each physician and physician group will be assigned a weighted outcomes measures performance rate by dividing their claims-extracted performance rate by the total number of beneficiaries used to calculate the national performance rate. As a result, group performance is weighted appropriately in comparison to the national outcomes measure benchmark.

- To determine group practice performance against outcomes benchmarks, CMS will compare the weighted performance for each outcomes measure to the national performance rate benchmark at the TIN level.

    o The population of beneficiaries used for performance comparison for claims-extracted outcomes measures includes all Medicare FFS beneficiaries attributed to the medical group practice.

Comparison of Cost Measures to Benchmarks: The Specialty Adjustment Process (New for 2014 Performance Reporting Year)[361]

Overview:

- To determine the 2016 VBM, CMS has adopted a **specialty adjustment** to be applied to group practice cost measure scores **before comparison to** national cost measures benchmarks.

---

[361] *Pages 1215–1218: CMS-1600-FC, http://www.gpo.gov/fdsys/pkg/FR-2013-12-10/pdf/2013-28696.pdf*

- The specialty adjustment allows for peer group comparisons while factoring in the mix of specialty physicians. The resulting adjusted cost measures allow for a more equal comparison of the risk-adjusted cost measures, against which groups of physicians of smaller size, which often have fewer specialist physicians or are composed entirely of a single-specialty:

  - This methodology creates one national benchmark for each cost measure.

  - The specialty adjustment accounts for the specialty composition of the group prior to the computation of the standardized score for each cost measure.

  - All groups of physicians (regardless of size) are assessed against the national cost measure benchmark in creating the group's standardized score. Although the calculations discussed may be very detailed, they are transparent and CMS intends to provide each group of physicians with information on how its costs were benchmarked in its QRUR.

- The specialty adjustment will be applied to all six cost measures (the five total per capita measures and the MSPB) for all groups and will be applied to risk-adjusted dollars.

- Specialty-adjusted benchmarks will be established using cost data from the VBM performance year, as opposed to using information from the year prior to the performance year (as done with quality benchmarks).

Three-Step Process to Determine the Specialty Adjustment:

The specialty adjustment is applied to all cost measures prior to scoring evaluation and involves a three-step methodology:

- **Step 1: Create a "specialty-specific expected cost:"**

  - Calculate the national average for each cost measure (referred to as the "national specialty-specific expected costs").

  - Beneficiaries are attributed to a group using the plurality of primary care services methodology for total per capita cost measures and the single attribution method for the MSPB.

- o **For each specialty**, CMS calculates the average cost of beneficiaries attributed to groups of physicians with that specialty, weighted by the number of EPs in each group.

- **Step 2: Calculate the "specialty-adjusted expected cost:"**

  - o The national specialty-specific expected costs are weighted by the group's specialty composition of Medicare Part B payments. That is, the specialty-adjusted expected cost for each group is the weighted average of the national specialty-specific expected cost of all the specialties in the group, for which the weights are each specialty's proportion of the group's Medicare Part B payments.

  - o The Medicare Part B payments for each specialty are determined based on the payments to each EP in the group. Each EP is identified with one specialty, based on its claims.

- **Step 3: Calculate the specialty-adjusted total per capita cost**

  - o Divide the total per capita cost by the specialty-adjusted expected cost to calculate a ratio.

  - o Multiply this ratio by the national average per capita cost to convert this ratio to a dollar amount (referred to as the "specialty-adjusted total per capita cost"). This dollar amount is then used as the measure standardized score (identified as the Z-score in statistical terms) to determine whether a group can be classified as high-cost, low-cost, or average for quality-tiering.

- The specialty adjustment for the MSPB cost measure is analogous to that described above for the total per capita cost measure, except that "number of beneficiaries" is replaced with "number of episodes" and "per capita cost" is replaced with "per episode cost." Thus, each cost measure will have its own set of specialty-specific expected costs.

- For a detailed example of how the specialty adjustment is calculated and applied to total per capita cost measures, see Appendix: 7.5.2 Attachment B: Example of Calculating Specialty-Adjusted Total Per Capita Cost.

National Cost Measures Benchmarks:

- After applying the specialty adjustment to all cost measures, CMS calculates the benchmark for each cost measure as the national mean of the specialty-adjusted performance rates among all groups of physicians to which beneficiaries are attributed and that are subject to the VBM.

- These individual measures national benchmarks are then used to determine the group practice cost composite scores.

7.3.8 Step 5: Determine Quality Composite and Cost Composite Scores[362]

Background:

- Section 1848(p)(2) of the SSA requires that quality of care be evaluated, to the extent practicable, based on a composite of measures of the quality of care furnished. In addition, Section 1848(p)(3) of the SSA requires that costs in the VBM be evaluated, to the extent practicable, based on a composite of appropriate measures of costs.

- Once appropriate quality and cost benchmarks have been established, CMS will determine individual measures scores and domain component scores to calculate the quality and cost composite scores used to determine the VBM.

Quality Composite Score Determination:

- The standardized score for each PQRS-reported and CMS claims-extracted quality measure is calculated by dividing the difference between the group's performance rate and the measure's benchmark (the national mean of the measure's performance rate from the previous year) by the measure's standard deviation.

---

[362] Page 43487: CMS-1600-P, http://www.gpo.gov/fdsys/pkg/FR-2013-07-19/pdf/2013-16547.pdf

- The standardized scores for each measure are classified into one of six domains based on the national priorities related to Clinical Care, Patient Experience, Population/Community Health, Patient Safety, Care Coordination, and Efficiency established in the NQS.

- Each measure is given equal weighting within the domain to determine a domain score.

- When a domain does not contain quality measures (for example, when a group chooses a reporting mechanism that does not contain measures in the domain), the remaining domains will be equally weighted to form the quality of care composite score. For example, if only three domains contain quality information, each domain will be weighted at 33.3 percent to form the quality composite score, while the remaining three domains will not be included. If a group only reports measures in a single domain, the domain will be weighted at 100 percent.

- The domains are then equally weighted and scores are added together to form the **quality composite score** used to determine the value-based payment modifier.

Cost Composite Score Determination:[363]

- In determining the 2014 VBM reporting period standardized scores for each of the six cost measures, CMS first performs the specialty adjustment (described above) and then calculates a standardized score by dividing the difference between the group's performance rate and the measure's specialty-adjusted national benchmark by the measure's standard deviation.

- Each of the six cost measures is assigned to one of two domains:

  o **Cost Domain 1**: Total per capita costs for all attributed beneficiaries (one measure)

  o and the MSPB measure (one measure).

---

[363] *Page 1208: CMS-1600-FC, http://www.gpo.gov/fdsys/pkg/FR-2013-12-10/pdf/2013-28696.pdf*

- ○ **Cost Domain 2:** Total per capita costs associated with the four chronic conditions of COPD, CAD, HF, and DM (four measures).

- Each cost measure is equally weighted within its domain. In those instances in which a specific cost measure cannot be calculated (for example, fewer than twenty cases) CMS will weight the remaining cost measures in the domain equally.

- Similar to the quality of care composite, each cost domain is weighted equally to form the cost composite—unless one of the domains contains no measures, in which case the remaining domain will be weighted at 100 percent.

- The weighted cost domain scores are totaled and added together to create the **cost composite score** used to determine the VBM amount.

Determining the VBM Amount:

- Using the calculated quality composite and cost composite scores, CMS determines the VBM amount using **quality-tiering**, as illustrated below:

FIGURE 2: INTEGRATION OF QUALITY AND COST COMPOSITES IN VBM DETERMINATION

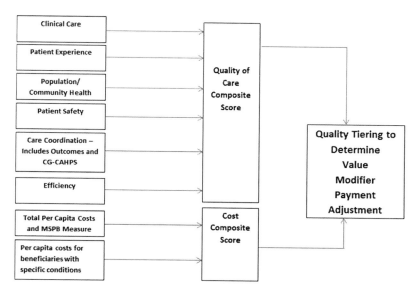

7.3.9 Step 6: Apply Quality-Tiering[364]

Overview:

- Quality-tiering is a transparent model used to determine a group practice-specific VBM based on a comparison of a group's quality of care composite score with its cost composite score. For the 2014 VBM performance year, **all** eligible groups (10+ EPs) will be subject to **mandatory quality tiering**:

  - Groups of between 10–99 EPs will be subject to upward or neutral adjustments only for determination of the 2016 VBM. Essentially, CMS is employing a "hold-harmless" policy for such groups participating in VBM for the first time.

  - Groups of 100+ EPs will be subject to upward, downward, or neutral VBM amounts.

Methodology:

- To make comparisons between the quality and cost composite scores, CMS first classifies each composite into "high, average or low" categories based on whether such scores are statistically above, not different from, or below the mean quality composite score of all participants in the VBM program for a given year:

  - To ensure that groups of physicians with composite scores classified as "low or high" have demonstrated performance that is meaningfully different from "average" performance, CMS requires that composite scores must be at least **one standard deviation above** the mean score to be classified as **"high"** and at least **one standard deviation below** the mean score to be classified as **"low."**

---

[364] *Page 69324: CMS-1590-FC, http://www.gpo.gov/fdsys/pkg/FR-2012-11-16/pdf/2012-26900.pdf*

- To ensure precision of the composite assessment, CMS requires a physician group score to be statistically different from the mean at a 95 percent confidence interval.

- Once the composite scores have been classified as high, not different from, or low, as compared to the national mean scores, CMS will determine the 2014 performance year VBM amount (to be applied in 2016) based on the following quality-tiering grid:[365]

TABLE 7: 2016 QUALITY-TIERING GRID

COST/ QUALITY	LOW QUALITY	AVERAGE QUALITY	HIGH QUALITY
Low Cost	+0.0%	+1.0x*	+2.0x*
Average Cost	-1.0%	+0.0%	+1.0x*
High Cost	-2.0%	-1.0%	+0.0%

*This includes groups of physicians eligible for an additional +1.0x to 2016 reimbursement rates if reporting PQRS quality measures and the average beneficiary risk score is in the top 25 percent of all beneficiary risk scores.

7.3.10 Step 7: Calculate the VBM Amount

2016 VBM Amounts:[366]

- Similar to the PQRS payment adjustment penalty, the VBM amount is applied to all physician-provided Medicare-covered professional services (at the TIN level) during a given program year:

  - CMS applies the VBM amount to the items and services billed by physicians under the TIN, not to other EPs who also may bill under the TIN.

---

[365] Page 1363: CMS-1600-FC, http://www.gpo.gov/fdsys/pkg/FR-2013-12-10/pdf/2013-28696.pdf

[366] Page 1362: CMS-1600-FC, http://www.gpo.gov/fdsys/pkg/FR-2013-12-10/pdf/2013-28696.pdf

Note: The VBM does not apply to any payments not made under the PFS, such as: rural health clinics; federally qualified health centers; and critical access hospitals (electing method II billing).

- ○ **downward payment modifier**: The maximum downward payment modifier is -2.0 percent for the 2016 VBM program year.

- ○ **upward payment modifier**: In order to meet VBM budget-neutrality requirements, amounts available for upward payment adjustments cannot be determined until the total amounts of penalty adjustments have been determined. Therefore, CMS includes an upward payment adjustment factor of "x," which is specified **after** the performance period has ended. For groups qualifying for the upward modifier, the value of "X" must be sufficient to fully offset penalty amounts.

- ○ **neutral payment modifier:** A 0.0 percent payment modifier is applied to groups that are rated as providing:

  - low quality at low cost

  - average quality at average cost

  - high quality at high cost

- Groups of physicians providing average or high-quality care at low cost for high-risk beneficiaries (average HCC risk scores in the upper 25 percent of all beneficiary risk scores) will receive an additional +1.0x upward payment adjustment. The quality-tiering grid for such groups is modified as follows:

Table 8: 2016 VBM Amounts for Groups Treating High-Risk Patients

COST/ QUALITY	LOW QUALITY	AVERAGE QUALITY	HIGH QUALITY
Low Cost	+0.0%	+2.0x*	+3.0x*

- →IMPORTANT! *The amount of "x" will be determined after calculation of penalty amounts, providing funding for the upward payment adjustments. All funds derived from the application of 2016 downward VBM adjustments **and** the 2016 PQRS downward 2.0 percent adjustment applied to groups that are eligible, but not participating, or unsuccessfully participating (category II groups), in PQRS reporting for 2014, will be available for all groups of physicians eligible for upward VBM adjustments.[367]

- Based on the CY2012 QRURs released in September 2013, of the 3,876 groups for whom the quality or cost composite could be calculated (2012 data):

   o more than 80 percent of the groups (**80.7 percent**) are in the **average** quality and average cost tiers under the quality-tiering methodology, and thus, would not receive a payment adjustment

   o approximately **8 percent** of groups are in tiers that would receive an **upward adjustment**

   o slightly **fewer than 11 percent** of groups are in tiers that would receive a **downward** adjustment

   o among the groups eligible for an upward adjustment, 11 percent would receive an additional +1X incentive payment due to treating high-risk beneficiaries

---

[367] *Page 1175: CMS-1600-FC, http://www.gpo.gov/fdsys/pkg/FR-2013-12-10/pdf/2013-28696.pdf*

7.3.11 Step 8: Quality Resource and Utilization Reports (QRURs)[368]

Overview:

QRURs evolved as part of the Physician Feedback Program and provide physician groups with measures data used to determine the VBM amount for a given VBM program year:

- Created under Section 131 of the Medicare Improvements for Patients and Providers Act of 2008 (MIPPA), the **Physician Resource Use Measurement and Reporting Program** was implemented with the goal of providing "confidential reports to physicians (and, as determined appropriate by the HHS secretary, to groups of physicians) that measure the **resources** involved in furnishing care to individuals" (SSA1848 (N). Resource use data was to be extracted from Medicare claims data in order to measure the costs of items and services on either an episode basis or per capita basis.

- In 2010 the ACA greatly expanded the scope of the **Physician Resource Use Measurement and Reporting Program** (now called the Physician Feedback Program) in Section 3003 to include quality reporting and data analysis for comparative use.

- CMS was directed under Section 3003 to establish appropriate data analytic methodologies to:

  o be able to attribute episodes of care, in whole, or in part, to individual physicians

  o identify methods for selection of physicians for comparison

  o aggregate episodes of care attributed to a physician into a composite measure

  o compare patterns of resource use (cost) among physicians and medical practices

---

[368] *Template for groups that participated in 2012 Group Practice Reporting Option of the Physician Quality Reporting System, http://www.cms.gov/Medicare/Medicare-Fee-for-Service-Payment/PhysicianFeedbackProgram/Downloads/PY2012-GPRO-QRUR-Sample.pdf*

- The Section 3003 modifications to the PFP were designed to produce information to encourage higher-quality and more efficient medical practice by aggregating data from multiple sources into confidential reports for individual physicians. Accordingly, the primary output of the PFP became known as the **QRUR**. In addition to providing physicians with meaningful and actionable practice-related information, the QRUR established a more transparent process for developing fair physician performance indicators that could later be used in value-based initiatives.

Goals of the QRUR:

- support physicians' efforts to provide high-quality care to their Medicare FFS patients in an efficient and effective manner

- display all report recipients' degree of involvement with all of their Medicare patients, based on claims submitted to Medicare

- to provide eligible physicians with quality-of-care and cost information that CMS expects to use in a given performance year to establish the VBM

Data Contained in the QRUR:

- Essentially, the QRUR "funnels" the clinical and quality data collected under the PQRS program *and* claims cost data from Medicare Parts A and B to consolidate data for individual physicians and group medical practices on *how* they can improve quality and efficiency. Such information is crucial in assisting providers to prepare for the application of the VBM, as CMS increasingly moves toward physician reimbursement that rewards overall *value* rather than service *volume*.

- The QRUR is a confidential report that provides information on:

  - the portion of a provider's Medicare FFS patients who have received indicated clinical services

  - how patients have used various types of services, such as inpatient hospital stays, outpatient visits to physicians, etc.

o how Medicare spending for their patients compares to average Medicare spending across a geographic region and clinical specialty

o the calculation of the VBM (beginning with CY2013 reports)

o Overall, QRURs provide information that allows physicians to view examples of the clinical care their patients receive and compare these examples to the average care and costs of other physicians' Medicare patients.

- The following snapshots of the 2012 QRUR report illustrate the format used within the QRUR for reporting measures performance and the aggregate feedback provided to physician groups of 25+ EPs:

FIGURE 3: FORMAT FOR QUALITY MEASURES FEEDBACK

Performance Measures	Your Medical Group Practice's Performance		Performance of All PQRS Participants Reporting the Measure		
				Average Range	
	Number of Eligible Cases	Performance Rate	Benchmark Rate	Benchmark –1 Standard Deviation	Benchmark +1 Standard Deviation
Chronic Obstructive Pulmonary Disease (COPD)					
COPD-1 COPD: Bronchodilator Therapy*	32	87.5%	Not Available	Not Available	Not Available
Coronary Artery Disease (CAD)					
CAD-1 CAD: Antiplatelet Therapy*	401	92.8%	82.8%	76.9%	88.8%
CAD-2 CAD: Lipid Control †	401	72.1%	88.8%	73.9%	100.0%
CAD-7 CAD: ACE Inhibitor or ARB Therapy for Patients with CAD and Diabetes and/or LVSD †	246	52.9%	69.0%	53.8%	84.1%
Diabetes Mellitus (DM)					
DM-2 DM: Hemoglobin A1c Poor Control in DM (>9.0)‡	519	38.2%	21.3%	8.9%	33.7%
DM-3 DM: High Blood Pressure Control in DM †	519	69.8%	69.0%	62.3%	75.7%
DM-5 DM: LDL-C Control in DM †	519	31.4%	56.2%	46.9%	65.6%

FIGURE 4: QUALITY COMPOSITE SCORING FEEDBACK

Quality Domain	Number of Quality Indicators	Standardized Score
Standardized Quality Composite Score	16	-0.13(Average)
Average Domain Score	16	-0.36
Clinical Process/Effectiveness	11	-0.80
Population/Public Health	1	-0.13
Patient Safety	1	-0.22
Care Coordination	3	-0.31

Note: The standardized quality composite score is a standardized average of equally-weighted domain scores indicating within how many standard deviations of the national mean a medical group practice's performance rate falls; positive scores reflect performance better than the mean, and negative scores reflect performance worse than the mean. Each domain-level performance score is an equally-weighted average of the standardized scores for all measures in the domain with at least 20 cases; the standardized score is the difference between the raw score and the peer group benchmark, divided by the peer group standard deviation. Domain scores are not computed for domains with no measure with at least 20 cases.

* Significantly different from the mean at the five percent level.

490

FIGURE 5: FORMAT FOR COST MEASURES FEEDBACK

Cost Categories	Your Medical Group Practice's Performance			Performance of All 1,032 Groups with at Least 100 Eligible Professionals		
	Number of Eligible Cases	Per Capita Costs Before Risk Adjustment	Per Capita Costs After Risk Adjustment	Benchmark Per Capita Costs (Risk-Adjusted)	Average Range	
					Benchmark −1 Standard Deviation	Benchmark +1 Standard Deviation
Per Capita Costs for All Attributed Beneficiaries (Domain Score = + 0.41)						
All Beneficiaries	1,351	$19,135	$10,898	$10,265	$8,722	$11,808
Per Capita Costs for Beneficiaries with Specific Conditions (Domain Score = - 0.03)						
Diabetes	373	$25,396	$14,732	$14,788	$12,379	$17,198
COPD	139	$36,685	$24,396	$24,153	$19,840	$28,466
Coronary Artery Disease	418	$26,036	$17,750	$17,265	$14,415	$20,115
Heart Failure	227	$34,857	$24,467	$26,013	$21,237	$30,788

Note: Per capita costs are based on payments for Medicare Part A and Part B claims submitted in 2012 by all providers (including medical professionals, hospitals, and post-acute care facilities) for Medicare beneficiaries attributed to a medical group practice. Outpatient prescription drug costs are not included.

FIGURE 6: COST COMPOSITE SCORING FEEDBACK:

Cost Domain	Standardized Score
Standardized Cost Composite Score	0.04(Average)
Average Domain Score	0.19
Per Capita Costs for *All* Attributed Beneficiaries	0.41
Per Capita Costs for Beneficiaries *with Specific Conditions*	-0.03

Note: The standardized cost composite score is a standardized average of equally-weighted domain scores indicating within how many standard deviations of the national mean a medical group practice's performance rate falls; positive scores reflect costs higher than the mean, and negative scores reflect costs lower than the mean. Each domain-level performance score is an equally-weighted average of the standardized scores for all measures in the domain with at least 20 cases; the standardized score is the difference between the raw score and the peer group benchmark, divided by the peer group standard deviation. Domain scores are not computed for domains with no measure with at least 20 cases.

* Significantly different from the mean at the five percent level.

FIGURE 7: AGGREGATE PERFORMANCE FEEDBACK AND VBM

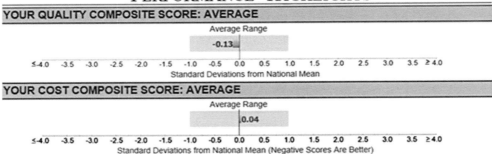

PERFORMANCE HIGHLIGHTS

YOUR QUALITY COMPOSITE SCORE: AVERAGE

Average Range

-0.13

≤-4.0 -3.5 -3.0 -2.5 -2.0 -1.5 -1.0 -0.5 0.0 0.5 1.0 1.5 2.0 2.5 3.0 3.5 ≥4.0

Standard Deviations from National Mean

YOUR COST COMPOSITE SCORE: AVERAGE

Average Range

0.04

≤-4.0 -3.5 -3.0 -2.5 -2.0 -1.5 -1.0 -0.5 0.0 0.5 1.0 1.5 2.0 2.5 3.0 3.5 ≥4.0

Standard Deviations from National Mean (Negative Scores Are Better)

YOUR BENEFICIARIES' AVERAGE RISK SCORE: 83RD PERCENTILE

- To account for differences in patient risk and reduce the influence of very high cost beneficiaries, the overall per capita costs of your beneficiaries were risk adjusted downward by 43.0 percent.

- Because your Medicare beneficiaries' average risk score is at or above the 75th percentile of all beneficiary risk scores, your group would be eligible for an additional upward adjustment under the quality tiering approach for serving high-risk beneficiaries.

YOUR QUALITY TIERING PERFORMANCE: AVERAGE QUALITY, AVERAGE COST

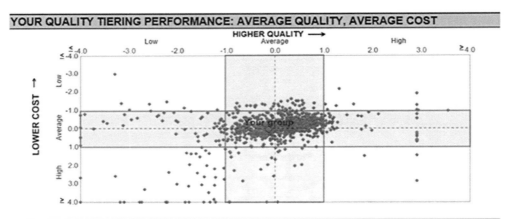

YOUR VALUE-BASED PAYMENT ADJUSTMENT BASED ON QUALITY TIERING

- Based on 2012 performance, electing the quality tiering approach would result in a payment adjustment of +0.0%.

Payment adjustments for each level of performance are shown below:

	Low Quality	Average Quality	High Quality
Low Cost	+0.0%	+2.0x%	+3.0x%
Average Cost	-0.5%	+0.0%	+2.0x%
High Cost	-1.0%	-0.5%	+0.0%

Note: x refers to a payment adjustment factor yet to be determined due to budget neutrality requirements.

Distribution of the QRUR to Physicians and Physician Groups:

The Physician Feedback Program began providing first reports to select physicians in 2009 and has expanded its scope in a phased manner since that time:

- Beginning in 2009, initial report distribution was limited to approximately 300 reports that included individual physician-level cost measures only.

- In 2010, modifications contained in the ACA required the HHS secretary to provide confidential information to physicians and groups of physicians about the quality of care furnished to Medicare beneficiaries compared to the cost of that care. The 2010 report distribution included reports to both individual physicians (about 1,700) and medical group practices (36). These QRURs included resource use information *and* selected quality measures extracted from PQRS metrics reporting.

- In fall 2011, QRURs were sent to each of the medical group practices participating in the 2010 PQRS using the GPRO (approximately 37,745 physicians in 54 group practices).

- In early 2012, approximately 24,000 QRURs were distributed to physicians who practiced in Iowa, Kansas, Missouri or Nebraska in 2010.

- Between December 2012 and April 2013, reports were made available to groups of 25+ EPs in nine states (California, Iowa, Illinois, Kansas, Michigan, Missouri, Minnesota, Nebraska, and Wisconsin) based on 2011 data:

  o Reports preview some value measurement information (PQRS and administrative claims measure comparisons to national benchmarks).

  o Reports contain the PQRS measures that physicians in these states submitted via any of the PQRS reporting methods, as well as information on 28 administrative claims measures included in the 2010 reports.

- In September, 2013 QRUR Reports based on 2012 data were provided to all groups of 25+ EPs and provided a "first look" at VBM program analytic methodologies:[369]

    o The 2012 data QRURs were distributed to 6,779 physician groups nationwide with 25 or more EPs, covering some 400,000 physicians.

    o These reports were available eight and one-half months from the close of the performance period (December 31, 2012) and five months from the close of the quality data submission period (March 31, 2013).

    o CY2012 QRURs contained detailed beneficiary-specific data on each group's attributed beneficiaries and their hospitalizations, and the group's associated EPs.

    o Three downloadable drill-down tables were included that provide information on each beneficiary attributed to the group and each EP billing under the group's TIN.

QRUR Reports for 2013 Data:

- The 2013 data reports will be **provided to all groups of physicians and solo practitioners** during the summer of 2014. Included in this QRUR release will be quality and cost measures as well as measure performance and benchmarks used to determine quality of care composite and cost composite scores and the VBM:

    o This report will also include performance on the MSPB measure and the peer group methodologies (new for 2014 reporting).

    o All physicians/TINs will be able to view how they would fare under the 2014 reporting policies used to determine the VBM:

        ▪ For groups with 10–24 EPs, the QRUR distributed in 2014 will be their *first* QRUR. Because the distribution of data is not until eight to ten months into the 2014 reporting year,

---

[369] http://www.cms.gov/Medicare/Medicare-Fee-for-Service-Payment/PhysicianFeedbackProgram/Downloads/PY2011-QRUR-Methods.pdf

these groups will be limited in their ability to make substantive changes, which will impact the VBM for 2016.

- Templates of current format for the QRUR (for individuals and group practices) may be viewed at: http://www.cms.gov/Medicare/Medicare-Fee-for-Service-Payment/PhysicianFeedbackProgram/ReportTemplate.html

How to Obtain the QRUR[370]

Overview:

Authorized representatives of groups can access the QRURs at https://portal.cms.gov using an individual's authorized access to the CMS computer services (IACS) account with one of the following group-specific Physician Value-Physician Quality Reporting System (PV-PQRS) registration system roles:

- Primary PV-PQRS Group Security Official
- Backup PV-PQRS Group Security Official
- PV-PQRS Group Representative

- If a group has already registered and selected its 2014 PQRS group reporting mechanism in the PV-PQRS registration system, then that same person who registered the group can access the group's QRUR using his or her IACS user ID and password.

- If a group does not yet have an authorized representative with an IACS account, then one person representing the group must sign up for an IACS account with the primary Group Security Official role.

- If a group has a representative with an existing IACS account, but not one of the three group-specific registration system roles listed above, then the group must ensure that the account is still active and add a group-specific registration system role to the representative's existing IACS account.

---

[370] Page 1224: CMS-1600-FC, http://www.gpo.gov/fdsys/pkg/FR-2013-12-10/pdf/2013-28696.pdf

- **CMS strongly encourages** representatives of groups to sign up for a new IACS account or modify an existing account at https://applications.cms.hhs.gov as soon as possible in order to be able to access the QRURs. Quick reference guides that provide step-by-step instructions for requesting each PV-PQRS registration system role for new or existing IACS account are available at:http://www.cms.gov/Medicare/Medicare-Fee-for-Service-Payment/PhysicianFeedbackProgram/Self-Nomination-Registration.html.

Section 7.4: Acronym Guide

ACA............................Affordable Care Act

ACO ....Accountable Care Organization

ACSC........................Ambulatory Care Sensitive Conditions

AHRQ.......................Agency for Healthcare Research and Quality

APRN........................Advanced Practice Registered Nurse

CAH ....Critical Access Hospital

CG-CAHPS...............Clinician/Group Consumer Assessment of Healthcare
        Providers and Systems

CMS.........................Centers for Medicare & Medicaid Services

CPC ....Comprehensive Primary Care

CPT..........................Current Procedural Terminology

CY ....Calendar Year

DRG.........................Diagnosis-Related Group

EHR ....Electronic Health Record

E&M ....Evaluation and Management

EP ....Eligible Professional

eRx...........................ePrescribing

FFS ....Fee-For-Service

FR ....Federal Register

GPCI ....Geographic Practice Cost Index

GPRO ....Group Practice Reporting Option

HHS ....Department of Health and Human Services

IACS.........................Individuals Authorized Access for CMS Computer Services

ICD-9-CM ....International Classification of Diseases, Ninth Revision,
        Clinical Modification

IPPS.........................Inpatient Prospective Payment System

IQR...........................Inpatient Quality Reporting

LTCH........................Long-Term Care Hospital

MA............................Medicare Advantage

MIPPA.....................Medicare Improvements for Patients and Providers
        Act of 2008, Public Law 110–275

MSPB........................Medicare Spending Per Beneficiary

MSSP........................Medicare Shared Savings Program

NQS ....National Quality Strategy

NPI ....National Provider Identifier

PECOS ....Provider Enrollment, Chain, and Ownership System

PFP ....Physician Feedback Program

PFS ....Physician Fee Schedule

PF-VBM ....Physician Feedback/Value-Based Payment Modifier

PPS...........................Prospective Payment System

PQRS........................Physician Quality Reporting System

PV-PQRS ....Physician Value-Physician Quality Reporting System

QCDR ....Qualified Clinical Data Registry

QRUR ....Quality Resource Use Report

TIN ....Tax Identification Number

VBM ....Value-Based Payment Modifier

VBP...........................Value-Based Purchasing

Section 7.5: Appendix

7.5.1: Attachment A: The Physician Value-Physician Quality Reporting System (PV-PQRS)[371]

- The PV-PQRS is a web-based registration system to support PQRS and VBM registration.

- For more information on registering through the PV-PQRS for the 2016 (2014 reporting) VBM program year, see: http://www.cms.gov/Outreach-and-education/Outreach/NPC/Downloads/2013-06-05-NPC.pdf

- An IACS account is required to access the PV-PQRS registration system:

  o Users are limited to one IACS account per person.

  o An existing IACS account cannot be transferred to another individual.

  o An account can be associated with multiple group practices (TINs) or individual EPs (TIN/National Provider Identifier (NPI)).

  o To confirm existing IACS account status, contact the QualityNet Help Desk

  o All IACS account holders are required to add a PV-PQRS registration system role to accounts. To add this, go to https://applications.cms.hhs.gov and select "Enter the CMS Applications Portal."

  o New sign-up for IACS may be accomplished at: https://applications.cms.hhs.gov/

---

[371] http://www.cms.gov/Outreach-and-education/Outreach/NPC/Downloads/2013-06-05-NPC.pdf

499

- The following group practices and EPs are **not required to register in PV-PQRS:**
  - group practices that participate in the MSSP (ACOs)
  - group practices that only provide care to Medicare beneficiaries who are enrolled in a Medicare Advantage Plan
  - group practices that only practice in a rural health clinic
  - group practices that only practice in a federally qualified health center
  - group practices that only practice in a critical access hospital (using method II billing)
  - individual EPs who want to participate in the PQRS in 2014 using a participating registry, claims, or electronic health records (EHRs)
- **Special PV-PQRS registration requirements for participants in a Pioneer ACO or comprehensive primary care initiative (CPCI):**
  - **must register in PV-PQRS:**
    - group practices of all sizes (2+ EPs) that include EPs who participate in a Pioneer ACO, where all of the EPs under the billing TIN have elected to participate in the PQRS as a group
    - group practices of all sizes (2+ EPs) that include comprehensive primary care (CPC) EPs, where all of the EPs under the billing TIN have elected to participate in the PQRS as a group
    - nonparticipating Pioneer ACO EPs who are part of a TIN that also includes Pioneer ACO EPs and want to participate in the PQRS as individuals using the CMS-calculated administrative claims reporting option
    - nonparticipating CPC EPs who are part of a TIN that also includes CPC EPs, and the participating CPC EPs have elected to receive credit for the PQRS reporting via a CPC waiver

- ○ **are not required to register in PV-PQRS:**
  - individual EPs who are part of a TIN that participates in a Pioneer ACO or the CPCI, but are nonparticipating Pioneer ACO or CPC EPs and want to participate in the PQRS as individuals using a participating registry, claims or EHR
  - individual EPs who are part of a TIN that participates in a Pioneer ACO or the CPCI *and* are participating Pioneer ACO or CPC EPs, and want to participate in the PQRS as individuals using a participating registry, claims or EHRs
  - CPC practice site EPs who have elected to obtain credit for their PQRS reporting by meeting all CPC clinical quality measure (CQM) reporting requirements successfully

7.5.2: Attachment B: Example of Calculating Specialty-Adjusted Total Per Capita Cost[372]

Below, three steps used in calculating the specialty adjustment to the standardized score are presented with an example:

Assumptions:

- Only two group practices identified by TINs exist: TIN 1 and TIN 2.
- Specialties are limited to two: Specialty A and Specialty B.
- Total per capita costs and specialty shares are as shown in Table 1.

---

[372] *Pages 1216–1218: CMS-1600-FC, http://www.gpo.gov/fdsys/pkg/FR-2013-12-10/pdf/2013-28696.pdf*

Table 1: Example of Calculating Specialty-Adjusted Total Per Capita Cost:

Assumptions

TIN	RISK-ADJUSTED PER CAPITA COST	NUMBER OF ATTRIBUTED BENEFICIARIES	NUMBER OF EPS IN TIN BY SPECIALTY TYPE A OR B	SPECIALTY SHARE OF EPS IN TIN	SPECIALTY SHARE OF PART B PAYMENTS IN TIN
TIN 1	$12,000	1,500	A: 10; B: 30	A: 25%; B: 75%	A: 35%: B: 65%
TIN2	$8,000	2,000	A: 21; B: 39	A: 35%; B: 65%	A: 60%; B: 40%

Step 1: Calculate the national specialty-specific expected cost:

To compute the national specialty-specific expected cost for a specialty across all TINs, the numerator is calculated first:

- **numerator:** the product of each TIN's total per capita cost times its weight (the number of attributed beneficiaries x that specialty's share of the TIN's EPs x the number of EPs of that specialty in that TIN), summed across all TINs. This sum is divided by the denominator.

- **denominator:** the sum across all TINs of the same weights that were used in the numerator.

- **For this example, the national specialty-specific expected cost for Specialty A is:**
  - ($12,000 x 1,500 x 25%*10 + $8,000 x 2,000 x 35%*21) / (1,500 x 25% x 10 + 2,000 x 35% x 21) = $8,813.
  - Similarly, the national specialty-specific expected cost for Specialty B is: ($12,000 x 1,500 x 75% x 30 + $8,000 x 2,000 x 65% x 39) / (1,500 x 75% x 30 + 2,000 x 65% x 39) = $9,599.

    National specialty-specific expected cost, by specialty (Step 1):
    Specialty A: $8,813   Specialty B: $9,599

Step 2: Calculate the specialty-adjusted expected cost for each group (TIN):

- Multiply the above national specialty-specific expected costs by each group's proportion of specialty-specific Medicare Part B payments.

- For each TIN, compute the product of the TIN's proportion of specialty-specific Medicare Part B payments, summed across all specialty types of the TIN.

- In this example, the specialty-adjusted expected cost for TIN 1 would be computed as:

- (35% x $8,813) + (65% x $9,599) = $9,324.

- Similarly, the specialty-adjusted expected cost for TIN 2 would be: (60% x $8,813) + (40% x $9,599) = $9,127.

Specialty-adjusted expected cost, by TIN (Step 2):
TIN 1: $9,324   TIN 2: $9,127

Step 3: Determine the adjusted per capita dollar amount:

- Divide the total per capita cost by the specialty-adjusted expected cost to obtain a ratio.

- Multiply the ratio by the national average per capita cost, to convert this ratio to a dollar amount.

- Assuming the national average per capita cost is $9,714, we can compute the specialty-adjusted

- total per capita cost for each TIN, as shown in Table 2.

Table 2: Example of Calculating Specialty-Adjusted Total Per Capita Cost: Calculations

Column	A	B	C	D
TIN	Total Cost Per Beneficiary	Specialty-Adjusted Expected Cost	National Average Per Capita Cost	Specialty-Adjusted Total per Capita Cost: ((Column A/ Column B) x Column C))
TIN 1	$12,000	$9324	$9714	$12,502
TIN 2	$8,000	$9127	$9714	$8,514

- The figure in column D is the specialty-adjusted total per capita cost that is used to compute a group's Z-score. The Z-score (aka, a standardized score) indicates how many standard deviations an element is from the mean. In the specialty adjustment, the Z-score determines average, high or low cost classification.

  o Multiply this ratio by the national average per capita cost to convert this ratio to a dollar amount (referred to as the "specialty-adjusted total per capita cost"). This dollar amount is then used as the measure standardized score (identified as the Z-score in statistical terms) to determine whether a group can be classified as high-cost, low-cost, or average for quality tiering.

- The specialty-adjusted total per capita cost for use in the standardized score is $12,502 for TIN 1 and $8,514 for TIN 2.

- CMS performs this specialty adjustment prior to computing the standardized score for all six cost measures included in the VBM: the total per capita cost measure, the four total per capita cost measures for beneficiaries with specific conditions, and the MSPB measure:

  o The specialty adjustment for the four condition-specific total per capita cost measures is identical to the total per capita cost measure that was described above.

  o The specialty adjustment for the MSPB cost measure is similar to that described above for the total per capita cost measure, except that "number of beneficiaries" is replaced with "number of episodes" and "per capita cost" is replaced with "per episode cost." Thus, each cost measure will have its own set of specialty-specific expected costs.

Note: *To illustrate the impact of the specialty-adjustment methodology, CMS examined the distribution, by specialty, of the overall specialty-adjusted total annual per capita cost measure based on 2011 claims for group of physicians with one or more EPs. The results of this analysis may be viewed in Table 66 of the CY2014 proposed Rule (78 FR 43498 through 43499): http://www.gpo.gov/fdsys/pkg/FR-2013-07-19/pdf/2013-16547.pdf*

PART 3

Care Coordination
Models Endorsed by
the Affordable Care Act

PART 3

Care Coordination
Models Endorsed by
the Affordable Care Act

CHAPTER 8

The Patient-Centered Medical Home (PCMH)

Section 8.1: Flash Read!

Recognizing the potential of patient-centered care and intensive care coordination as a means of enhancing patient care quality and reducing costs, the Affordable Care Act (ACA) mandated the creation of infrastructure to support widespread adoption of two voluntary models of coordinated care. The ACA has breathed new life into one of these models, the Patient-Centered Medical Home (PCMH), which dates back to the 1960s when it was first conceptualized in the field of pediatrics. The PCMH puts the relationship between a patient and his or her primary caregiver at the center of the health care universe, and a number of published reports have shown it is capable of improving health care quality while reducing costs. This model has also received endorsements from a variety of payers, including federal and state governments, commercial insurers, and large employers.

- The PCMH is more a *philosophy of care* than a physical place; it is focused on providing primary care services with direct coordination of additional services for the patient.

- The PCMH concept places emphasis on communication between patients and/or caregivers and the primary caregiver. It strives to give patients access to personalized, coordinated care based on communication, trust, respect, and shared decision-making.

- Some features of a PCMH model of care may include enhanced convenience for patients through: open scheduling, same-day appointments, and expanded hours; group visits for patients with the same health conditions; and various tools to boost patient engagement.

- A PCMH is identified by providers practicing under one Tax Identification Number (TIN).

- Under the ACA, state-level funding has been provided to back community-based interdisciplinary health teams, which support primary care providers in creating PCMHs. The health team may contract with, and reimburse, a number of providers or networks of providers for PCMH services.

- Financial incentives for PCMH participation are provided by commercial payers and through federal grants to include some, or all, of the following components:

  o A monthly care coordination payment for the physician and non-physician work that falls outside of a face-to-face visit and for the system infrastructure (e.g., heath information technologies) needed to achieve better outcomes.

  o A visit-based fee-for-service component that recognizes visit-based services that are currently paid under the present fee-for-service payment system and maintains an incentive for the physician to see the patient in an office-visit when appropriate.

  o A performance-based component that recognizes achievement of quality and efficiency goals.

  o A shared savings component to reward PCMH efficiency in providing patient care.

- In order to qualify for reimbursements from several payers, a PCMH must generally attain accreditation offered through one of several accrediting entities. The most widely provided accreditation is through the **National Committee for Quality Assurance (NCQA).**

- Many reimbursement models tie payments to the level of PCMH or individual provider accreditation. Currently more than 6,000 practices, involving more than 29,000 physicians, are NCQA qualified to one of three levels:

  - **Level 1: 35–59 points and all six must-pass elements**

  - **Level 2: 60–84 points and all six must-pass elements**

  - **Level 3: 85–100 points and all six must-pass elements**

- NCQA accreditation involves scoring against twenty-seven individual elements assigned to six standards:

  - Each element is scored through an assessment of related component factors.

  - Element scores are totaled for each standard.

  - Six elements (one for each standard) are "must-pass" elements requiring a successful level of performance to achieve accreditation.

  - Based upon achievement of the must-pass elements and the total of standard scoring points, the PCMH is assigned a level of accreditation.

- NCQA accreditation is valid for three years and the NCQA revises criteria for accreditation every three years (beginning with 2011):

  - In March 2014, new NCQA accreditation standards will be introduced:

    - June 30, 2014, is the final date that the 2011 accreditation survey tools may be ordered. They must be submitted by March 31, 2015.

    - March 31, 2014 is the first day that the revised accreditation survey tools may be ordered.

    - Between March 31, 2014, and March 31, 2015, participants seeking accreditation will be able to submit both 2011 and 2014 survey tool versions.

Section 8.2: Provider Perspectives

For years, primary care physicians have felt their field was undervalued, shunted aside while new medical graduates gravitated toward more remunerative subspecialties. Simultaneously, physician workforce experts have warned that the country is in danger of not producing enough primary care doctors to meet demand. The ACA takes on the challenge of reversing this long-term trend by strengthening primary care. It does this by expanding support for PCMHs, increasing payments to primary care, and giving extra assistance to historically underserved communities, which are less likely to have strong primary care physician relationships in place.

8.2.1 Rationale

"Physicians want to deliver coordinated, cost-effective care that improves patient outcomes, but the current payment system often penalizes the valuable services that make these improvements possible," said Peter W. Carmel, MD, in 2011, while serving as president of the American Medical Association (AMA).[373] That payment system has begun to change. Embedded in the ACA are a number of initiatives to alter reimbursements for the benefit of doctors who agree to take on the responsibility of coordinating care and reaching out past the office visit to help patients care for themselves. In most cases, this involves promoting primary care.

Included under the rubric "primary care" are general internists, family physicians, general practitioners, pediatricians, and geriatricians. These providers are often the initial point of contact for screening, assessing, and treating health issues, whether during annual physicals or other scheduled appointments.

---

[373] *http://www.ama-assn.org/ama/pub/news/news/ama-supports-cmmi-comprehensive-primary-care-initiative.page*

In 2010, there were 209,000 practicing primary care physicians in the United States, out of 624,434 physicians who spend the majority of their time in direct patient care, according to the Agency for Healthcare Research and Quality (AHRQ).[374] At the same time, physician burnout, retirements, and changing practice patterns are reducing access to primary care. Between 2008 and 2012, there was a 47 percent increase in the number of practices closed to new Medicare and Medicaid patients.[375] Many doctors are also tempted to toss out the insurance companies and public payers entirely and move to an all-cash practice or concierge service.

Fueling the trend is Medicare's fee-for-service (FFS) system, which has traditionally paid primary care doctors less than specialists and proceduralists. The disparity in compensation has, to a large extent, been ordained by the resource-based relative value scale (RBRVS) that determines physician compensation by Medicare. CMS relies on the advice of the AMA's Specialty Society RVS Update Committee (RUC) to evaluate and decide how much different services should be paid.[376]

The RUC has come under fire for allegedly favoring the interests of specialists and proceduralists. In a letter to the AMA's RUC in 2008, the acting commissioner of CMS wrote that Congress, MedPAC, and other stakeholders were concerned about the accuracy of pricing under the Medicare physician fee schedule, pointing out that "the presence of many overvalued procedures… disadvantages primary care services and creates distortion in our payment system."[377]

---

[374] http://www.ahrq.gov/research/findings/factsheets/primary/pcwork1/index.html

[375] http://www.mymdfast.com/news/Physician's%20Foundation%202012%20Medicare%20Medicaid%20survey%20results.pdf

[376] http://www.ama-assn.org/ama/pub/physician-resources/solutions-managing-your-practice/coding-billing-insurance/medicare/the-resource-based-relative-value-scale/the-rvs-update-committee.page

[377] Kerry Weems, acting administrator, CMS, June 19, 2008, letter to William L. Rich III, MD, found at http://www.ama-assn.org/ama/pub/physician-resources/solutions-managing-your-practice/coding-billing-insurance/medicare/the-resource-based-relative-value-scale/cms-applauds-ruc-efforts-improve-rbrvs.page

8.2.2 Summary

The CMS Center for Medicare & Medicaid Innovation (CMI) has implemented the Medicare Multi-Payer Advanced Primary Care Practice Demonstration (MAPCP), the Federally Qualified Health Center Advanced Primary Care Demonstration (FQHC APCP), and the Comprehensive Primary Care (CPC) Initiative.[378] CMS is also developing demonstration projects to evaluate advanced primary care practice, or PCMH, models of care delivery and payment.

CMS doesn't have an explicit strategy for PCMH-related work but is responding to the wishes of external stakeholders—primarily Congress and the administration. The MAPCP includes an extra monthly care management fee paid to physicians who provide advanced primary care to Medicare beneficiaries. The fee is expected to cover care coordination, improved access, patient education, and other services to support patients, especially those with chronic illnesses. It is hoped that the higher reimbursements will help retain doctors and recruit new ones to primary care. During the three-year period of the demonstration, more than 1,200 practices and almost 1 million beneficiaries are expected to participate.

The program includes intensive collaboration with eight states that are involved in multi-payer initiatives with Medicaid and private health plans. Linkages are being formed with state health promotion and disease prevention initiatives. The CMS project includes training and education modules for physicians and FQHCs, technical assistance, implementation advice, and evaluation of the success of the pilots.

8.2.3 Current State

There are several possible working definitions of a functioning PCMH. But the easiest, according to Donald Liss, MD, senior medical director at Independence Blue Cross in Philadelphia, is a primary care practice "that's able to show me its NCQA certification for achieving the standards." Liss is a recognized expert on the PCMH. Part of his job is determining which of the medical practices he contracts with are fully qualified PCMHs and therefore

---

[378] http://innovation.cms.gov/initiatives/

deserving of the extra payment that his health plan offers for coordinating care.[379]

The NCQA, which earlier created the Health Employer Data and Information Set (HEDIS) quality assurance system, has established a widely used PCMH accreditation program. In September 2013, it certified its 6,000th medical practice as a PCMH. Starting from 214 clinicians at 28 practices in 2008, when the program began, it now has 29,505 recognized clinicians in 49 states. The PCMH model has delivered "fewer costly emergency department and hospital admissions," said Margaret E. O'Kane, NCQA's founding president. "Patients get the access, personal attention, and care coordination from their primary doctor that they need and deserve."[380]

Asked to define a PCMH in plain English, Liss said it is "a practice that's organized itself and that's figured out how to keep track of patients not just when they're in the office for a 15-minute visit but across the care they're receiving. They're accessible; they've made arrangements with other parts of the delivery system, with specialty offices, hospitals, [and] other types of entities that deliver care. In an intentional way, the practice coordinates the care that its patients receive."

Liss was present in 2007 when a group of large employers made common cause with four medical societies—the American Academy of Pediatrics, the American Association of Family Physicians, the American College of Physicians, and the American Osteopathic Association—to produce a collaborative to advance primary care. The goal was to empower primary care offices to do a better job, and achieve better care delivery for populations and for patients with chronic illness.

Pilot programs around the country came out of this initiative, including one in southeast Pennsylvania involving Independence Blue Cross and Aetna, the two largest payers. At the time, Liss was a regional medical director at Aetna. The state of Pennsylvania acted as convener, averting antitrust issues among the commercial health plans and committing Medicaid participation. By 2008, thirty-three local medical practices had agreed to join. The payers gave the practices extra payments to create the infrastructure they needed to: get an NCQA certificate; hire and engage care managers and install the coordination

---

[379] *Donald Liss, MD, telephone interview, October 14, 2013*

[380] *http://www.ncqa.org/Newsroom/2013NewsArchives/NewsReleaseSeptember242013.aspx*

resources they needed to do population health; and reorganize how they delivered care.

"Lo and behold it worked, in terms of demonstrable impacts in quality of care measures," Liss said. The PCMH trial showed better treatment of diabetes and "even better outcomes:" better cholesterol management; tobacco cessation; and pediatric preventive care services. "It was HEDIS-type measures, the usual suspects. We showed that if you fund it, if you organized it, created the milieu in which practices can do this, they'll do it—at least some will. Early adopters. Some who were very frustrated being on the hamster wheel of primary care."

Richard J. Baron, MD, was one of those early adopters. First, he installed an electronic health record (EHR) in his practice, well before the CMS incentives were enacted for EHRs. Then, around 2007 and 2008, he started to hear talk of this mysterious PCMH. "They're like unicorns," he remembered. "I go to meetings all the time and people talk about them. I have never seen one." A medical director for Aetna whom he was friendly with—Donald Liss—indicated he would like to build a pilot in Philadelphia. Baron said, "We'd be happy to do it, but we need to understand the payment part, too." Liss asked him to work up a proposal for what additional resources would be required.[381]

Baron sat down with a spreadsheet and pretended he was applying for a grant. He had to make some assumptions. There is no work that the PCMH makes go away within the medical practice; it still has to do all that it was doing before, only now with additional services. What were the extra time and skills required to meet the insurance company's ideas of what it wanted?

Under the standard economic model of a primary care practice, roughly 60 percent of gross revenue goes to overhead: receptionists, medical assistants, rent, malpractice insurance, medications, supplies, and so forth. The remaining 40 percent covers the physicians' salaries, plus benefits, retirement, health insurance, and payroll taxes. For a doctor to give up half a day of revenue-generating patient care time to do the PCMH work means a huge hit to the gross revenue line. To make the PCMH model work, Baron's practice would have to ask the insurance company for a 30 percent bump-up in gross.

---

[381] *Richard J. Baron, MD, telephone interview, October 1, 2013*

"I came back to the next meeting with my heart in my mouth and said, 'This is a really big number.' They said, 'Go ahead, let's try to get there.'"

Today Baron is the president and CEO of the American Board of Internal Medicine and in a position to reflect on the complexities of introducing the medical home concept on a national scale. "That is part of why this has been difficult to change," he said. "Everybody is wedded to fee-for-service—and fee-for-service is cruel to all the activities that add value in the patient-centered medical home. All the things you do that don't generate revenue—phone outreach, hiring a health educator to do improved patient self-management— a lot of what's involved in PCMH is to get away from visit-based services. You're asking people to take on activities that by definition don't generate revenue. If you don't generate revenue, you shouldn't be surprised when people don't take that on."

It's going to take a lot of extra push to overcome the resistance in the field and the cost problem. Independent foundations, such as The Commonwealth Fund and the Robert Wood Johnson Foundation (RWJF), have concluded that this model bears further investment—and they have applied their considerable financial and intellectual resources toward making it work. RWJF's Aligning Forces for Quality program has developed a "primary care renewal initiative" to disseminate best practices at sixteen pilot sites around the country.[382]

Bruce E. Kessler, MD, runs an internal medicine practice in Eureka, California, that participates in the Aligning Forces project.[383] "We try to think in terms of population management and best practices," he said. With that in mind, he and his staff have reconfigured office protocols to be more responsive to patients. They have started tracking how many patients get to see their doctor on the same day they call and asking patients to take a more active role in their own care.[384]

"We're trying to do more with email and phone, to avoid office visits," he said. "The standard guideline for diabetes patients is to see them every three months. But if people are doing well with A1c (blood sugar levels) and are stabilized, it can be spaced out to four months or even six months. But you

---

[382] http://forces4quality.org/

[383] http://eimdoc.com/index.html

[384] Bruce E. Kessler, MD, office interview, June 25, 2013.

don't get a fee for it. You can't bill Medicare or Medicaid unless you actually see the patient. It's anachronistic."

8.2.4 The Road Ahead

The PCMH concept is yielding good results in early evaluations. A study of patients insured through Empire Blue Cross and Blue Shield published in the *American Journal of Managed Care* found that: PCMH adults and children had 12 percent and 23 percent lower odds of hospitalization; and required 11 percent and 17 percent fewer emergency department services, respectively, than non-PCMH patients. Costs were 8.6 percent lower for pediatric patients and 14.5 percent lower for adult patients.[385]

The medical home concept has even spread as far as selected specialty practices, with oncology leading the way. CMI awarded $19 million to implement medical home models in seven oncology practices around the country. A pilot study in Texas involving 184 cancer patients insured through Aetna found that patients in the pilot program had 39.8 fewer ER visits, 16.5 percent fewer inpatient admissions, and 35.9 percent fewer inpatient days in the first twelve months, compared to a control group in Texas. Physicians under this model showed lower costs than the year before.[386] An oncology practice in the Philadelphia region estimated that the medical home model saved payers $1 million per physician per year.

CMS is in the middle of a three-year rollout of support for PCMH. It's not clear whether the program and financial support for primary care physicians will continue once the demonstration project ends, although the extra payment for care coordination is already established in the Medicare reimbursement structure.

But if you ask Liss point blank whether the PCMH saved money for Aetna or Independence Blue Cross, he will hedge. "Five and a half years later, we can say, if we look at individuals with chronic conditions, the sick people being

[385] Andrea DeVries, et al, "Impact of Medical Homes on Quality, Healthcare Utilization, and Costs," *American Journal of Managed Care*, September 2012; 18(9): 534–544

[386] Lola Butcher, "Specialty Medical Homes Taking Root," *Physician Executive Journal*, May-June 2013. http://www.acpe.org/publications/pej

treated, we can show with pretty good certainty that claims costs for those individuals were less than claims costs for matched controls in that period."

However, that is offset by the additional monies paid out to medical practices to reorganize themselves into medical homes and to deliver better care to healthy people as well. While preventive care got better—and access improved for healthy people and the worried well—there were no claims-cost savings because those people didn't cost very much before.

"Between 2011 and 2012, we were unable to show claims-cost savings across the board," Liss said. Nevertheless, Independence Blue Cross remains committed to the PCMH model and has considerably expanded its efforts. About 37 percent of the payer's primary care providers in its network have now achieved recognition as a PCMH and are paid a financial incentive.

Liss sees a mixed future for the PCMH concept. Right now it is faltering under the weight of unreasonable expectations, he thinks, and is more likely to endure as an interim step toward the accountable care organization (ACO) than as an independent model.

"One of the mistakes of the PCMH movement was trying to take the position that it would lead to lower costs near term," Liss said. It should have positioned itself as offering better coordinated and organized care, which in the long run may reduce costs. He also thinks some experiments will fail because the finances can't be made to work. "We're going to learn from those. What are the values, how do we get better care outcomes, and is there a way to maintain that, and is there a better financing mechanism?"

"What I predict is, the pilot programs that are only for PCMH will wither a bit and you'll see more attention on efforts at bigger ACO-type arrangements." Liss sees evidence of this happening already in the announcements from major national insurance carriers and big integrated delivery systems. "To the extent you can roll in the primary care arrangement (into an ACO), I think that's the flavor we'll see."

Section 8.3: Technical Appendix: The Patient-Centered Medical Home (PCMH)

8.3.1 Introduction:

- Through the provisions of the ACA of 2010, a number of value-based incentive programs have been implemented to encourage the delivery of cost-effective quality patient care for Medicare beneficiaries.

- By using data captured by provider-submitted claims and cost and quality metrics reported through the Inpatient Quality Reporting (IQR) and the Physician Quality Reporting System (PQRS), Medicare has implemented programs such as the Hospital Value-Based Purchasing (VBP) Program, the Hospital Readmissions Reduction Program (HRRP), the Hospital-Acquired Conditions (HAC) program, and the Physician Value-Based Payment Modifier (VBM) program.

- To encourage all providers to more fully utilize the technological potential of electronic health reporting, Medicare established the EHR incentive program.

- To further leverage enhancements made to patient care as a result of these initiatives, the ACA supported the development, testing, and implementation of specific **care coordination** models of care. Such models overlay the value-based initiatives to help reduce fragmentation of health care services and improve both cost efficiency and quality:

  o Identified by the Institute of Medicine (IOM) in 2003 as a national priority area for transforming health care, **care coordination** was one of two "cross-cutting" priorities that impacted all aspects of health care transformation.[387]

---

[387] *Priority Areas for National Action: Transforming Health Care Quality (2003), http://www.nap.edu/catalog.php?record_id=10593*

- ○ The IOM defined care coordination as: "The deliberate organization of patient care activities between two or more participants (including the patient) involved in a patient's care to facilitate the appropriate delivery of health care service. Organizing care involves the marshalling of personnel and other resources needed to carry out all required patient care activities and is often managed care."[388]

- The ACA mandated funding to support the testing and development of two complementary care-coordination models: the **PCMH** and **ACO** (see Chapter 9 on Accountable Care Organizations):

  - ○ Both models support the IOM care-coordination priority and serve as a platform for the delivery of high-quality and efficient care across the health care system.

  - ○ These models were created to be mutually complementary and are structured to work in tandem to more effectively provide comprehensive coordinated patient care:

    - **The PCMH** provides broad-based direct coordination of patient care services. With a central focus of care coordination and primary care services, the PCMH serves as a "building block" for the ACO.

    - ACOs are composed of many elements of the health care system, including primary and specialty care physicians, hospitals, and other providers/suppliers. Incentives are provided to facilitate collaboration across different types of providers and components of the health care system with the goal of high-quality care at lower overall costs.

---

[388] *Care Coordination, Quality Improvement, Agency for Healthcare Research and Quality, http://www.ahrq.gov/clinic/tp/caregaptp.htm*

8.3.2 Overview: PCMH Health Care Model

Background:

Initially introduced by the American Academy of Pediatrics (AAP) in 1967 as a model for centrally archiving a child's medical records, the PCMH has been studied for decades as a patient care model used to describe an expert and evidence-based set of expectations regarding how to organize primary care in a manner to most effectively deliver the core functions of primary health care for all patients and their families.[389]

- The PCMH is a patient care delivery model that enhances the physician-patient relationship by moving from traditional (reactive) episodic care, which results in greater fragmentation of services and less coordinated care, to a more progressive form of coordinated (proactive) care that includes a more robust and ongoing relationship with a physician-led "care team."

- In a PCMH, the patient is the central member of the care team composed of physicians, nurses, and office staff, who all work together to provide quality care for the individual. The care team is responsible for providing all the patient's health care needs, including appropriate referral to other qualified physicians and coordinating additional health care services *for* the patient as needed. Emphasis is placed on open scheduling, expanded hours, and strong communication among patients, physicians, and staff.

Significant Events in PCMH Model Adoption[390]

- **2006:** Over time, various professional societies representing physicians published a number of guidelines for establishment of an effective PCMH. The result was the implementation of different types of the PCMH with varying degrees of success:

---

[389] *Patient-Centered Medical Home: The Call to Action, SuccessEHS,* http://www.successehs.com/item/what-is-a-medical-home.htm

[390] *Joint Principles of the Patient-Centered Medical Home, Patient-Centered Primary Care Collaborative,* http://www.aafp.org/dam/AAFP/documents/practice_management/pcmh/initiatives/PCMHJoint.pdf

- ○ The American Academy of Family Physicians (AAFP) and the ACP developed their own models for improving patient care called the "medical home" (AAFP, 2004) or "advanced medical home" (ACP, 2006).

- **2007:** Recognizing the disparity in PCMH standards, in 2007 the AAFP, the AAP, the American College of Physicians (ACP), and the American Osteopathic Association (AOA) developed joint principles of the patient-centered medical home to provide consistent guidance to primary care practices seeking to adopt the PCMH model. The resulting set of seven principles established the foundational criteria upon which today's PCMH model was built.

Joint Principles of the PCMH:[391]

1. **Personal physician:** Each patient has an ongoing relationship with a personal physician trained to provide first contact, continuous, and comprehensive care.

2. **Physician-directed medical practice:** The personal physician leads a team of individuals at the practice level that collectively takes responsibility for the ongoing care of patients.

3. **Whole-person orientation:** The personal physician is responsible for providing for all the patient's health care needs or taking responsibility for appropriately arranging care with other qualified professionals. This includes care for all stages of life, acute care, chronic care, preventive services, and end-of-life care.

4. **Care is coordinated and/or integrated across all elements of the complex health care system** (e.g., subspecialty care, hospitals, home health agencies, nursing homes) and the patient's community (e.g., family, public, and private community-based services). Care is facilitated by registries, information technology, health information exchange, and other means to ensure that patients get the indicated

---

[391] *Joint Principles of the Patient-Centered Medical Home, Patient-Centered Primary Care Collaborative,*
http://www.aafp.org/dam/AAFP/documents/practice_management/pcmh/initiatives/PCMHJoint.pdf

care when and where they need and want it in a culturally and linguistically appropriate manner.

5. **Quality and safety are hallmarks of the medical home**:

   a. Practices advocate for their patients to support the attainment of optimal, patient-centered outcomes that are defined by a care planning process driven by a compassionate, robust partnership among physicians, patients, and the patient's family.

   b. Evidence-based medicine and clinical decision-support tools guide decision making.

   c. Physicians in the practice accept accountability for continuous quality improvement through voluntary engagement in performance measurement and improvement.

   d. Patients actively participate in decision making and feedback is sought to ensure that patients' expectations are being met.

   e. Information technology is used appropriately to support optimal patient care, performance measurement, patient education, and enhanced communication.

   f. Practices go through a voluntary recognition process by an appropriate nongovernmental entity to demonstrate that they have the capabilities to provide patient-centered services consistent with the medical home model.

   g. Patients and families participate in quality improvement activities at the practice level.

6. **Enhanced access to care is available** through systems such as open scheduling, expanded hours, and new options for communication among patients, their personal physician, and practice staff.

7. **The payment appropriately recognizes the added value** provided to patients who have a PCMH. The payment structure should be based on the following framework:

a. It should reflect the value of the patient-centered care management work done by physician and nonphysician staff that falls outside the face-to-face visit.

b. It should pay for services associated with coordination of care both within a given practice and among consultants, ancillary providers, and community resources.

c. It should support adoption and use of health information technology for quality improvement.

d. It should support the provision of enhanced communication access such as secure email and telephone consultation.

e. It should recognize the value of physician work associated with remote monitoring of clinical data using technology.

f. It should allow for separate FFS payments for face-to-face visits. (Payments for care management services that fall outside the face-to-face visit, as described above, should not result in a reduction in the payments for face-to-face visits).

g. It should recognize case-mix differences in the patient population being treated within the practice.

h. It should allow physicians to share in savings from reduced hospitalizations associated with physician-guided care management in the office setting.

i. It should allow for additional payments for achieving measurable and continuous quality improvements.

2008: In 2008, the NCQA began a PCMH certification and recognition program based on the 2007 joint principles. Between 2008 and early 2011, more than 8,300 clinicians at more than 1,500 practice sites across the country earned PCMH recognition through the NCQA.[392]

---

[392] *Patient-Centered Medical Home (PCMH) 2011 Recognition Program, NCQA, http://www.ncqa.org/portals/0/Public%20Policy/PCMH_2011_fact_sheet.pdf*

2009: On September 18, 2009, the assistant secretary of defense issued Policy Memorandum: (HA POLICY 09-015) **Implementation of the "Patient-Centered Medical Home" Model of Primary Care in Military Treatment Facilities (MTFs)**. This policy mandated the establishment of the PCMH model in primary care settings at all military treatment facilities, across all services.[393]

8.3.3 The PCMH and the Affordable Care Act (ACA)

Section 3021: Establishment of the CMS Innovation Center (CMI):[394]

- Recognizing the potential value of the PCMH model as a means to reduce costs and improve care quality, Section 3021 of the ACA identified the PCMH as a model of patient care to be developed and evaluated by the newly established CMI:

  - Section 3021 directed the creation of the CMI and tasked it with the responsibility for testing innovative payment models that could result in more cost-efficient care, without compromising quality.

  - The PCMH was identified as a model of patient care to be evaluated by the CMI for its potential to provide cost-efficient, quality care with a central focus on patient care coordination. The definition of a medical home provided in the legislation mirrors the components identified in the PCMH joint principles.

  - Implementation of the PCMH model testing was to be accomplished in a budget-neutral manner and was to begin by January 1, 2011.

---

[393] *Policy Memorandum Implementation of the 'Patient-Centered Medical Home' Model of Primary Care in MTFs, http://www.health.mil/libraries/HA_Policies_and_Guidelines/09-015.pdf*

[394] *Section 3021: Patient Protection and Affordable Care Act, http://www.gpo.gov/fdsys/pkg/BILLS-111hr3590enr/pdf/BILLS-111hr3590enr.pdf*

Section 3502: Establishing Community Health Teams:[395]

- Endorsing a definition of the PCMH that mirrors the 2007 joint principles, Section 3502 of the ACA contained specific directives to encourage the development of the infrastructure needed to support the PCMH.

- Section 3502 establishes a federal grant program to assist "eligible entities" in creating community-based interdisciplinary **health teams** to support primary care providers in the creation of PCMHs:

  - eligible entities include:

    - a state or state-designated entity

    - an Indian tribe or tribal organization

  - Community health teams work with primary care practices as part of a PCMH, helping to coordinate care and provide access to a range of health services:

    - Payment for services of contracted practices participating as a PCMH is provided by the health team.

  - Community health teams might provide support and establish contractual relationships with a number of physicians and/or networks of providers, or could be established by a provider group to support their clinicians.

- Such state-supported health teams eligible for grant funding are required to:

  - submit plans for achieving long-term financial sustainability within three years

  - submit plans for integrating prevention initiatives, patient education, and care-management resources with care delivery

  - create an interdisciplinary health team (primary care teams eligible for capitated payments to include medical specialists, nurses, pharmacists, nutritionists, dieticians, social workers, behavioral and mental health providers, doctors of chiropractic

---

[395] Section 3502: Patient Protection and Affordable Care Act, http://www.gpo.gov/fdsys/pkg/BILLS-111hr3590enr/pdf/BILLS-111hr3590enr.pdf

medicine, licensed complementary and alternative medicine practitioners, and physician assistants)

- o provide services to eligible patients with chronic conditions

- Health teams are required to meet basic responsibilities, including:
  - o establishing contractual agreements with primary care providers for support services

  - o supporting patient-centered medical homes

  - o collaborating with local primary care providers and existing state and community-based resources to coordinate disease prevention and chronic disease management

  - o developing and implementing interdisciplinary and inter-professional care plans with local health care providers

  - o incorporating health care providers, patients, caregivers, and authorized representatives into the design and oversight of the program

  - o providing coordination and support to local primary care providers so that they can provide access to high-quality health care services, preventive services, specialty care and inpatient services, culturally appropriate patient and family-centered health care, and pharmacy services

- A provider who contracts with a health team is accountable for providing comprehensive personal health care needs while practicing in the context of family and community. The PCMH provider does not serve in a "gatekeeper" capacity and the model is not designed or incentivized to prevent appropriate referrals to a specialist; instead, the PCMH provider is expected to make referrals based on his or her clinical judgment and current evidence-based practice. As such, support of the health team is needed to effectively coordinate complementary and alternative services such as:
  - o promoting strategies for treatment planning, as well as monitoring health outcomes and resource use, sharing information, and organizing care to avoid duplication of services

  - o providing local access to individuals implementing patient care

- o collecting and reporting relevant data that allows for evaluation of the success of the collaborative efforts on the patients' health

- o establishing a coordinated system of identification for children at risk of developmental or behavioral problems

- o providing 24/7 care management and support during transitions in care settings (e.g., discharge planning and counseling support, and referrals for mental health and behavioral health services)

- o serving as a liaison to community prevention and treatment programs

- In order for the health team to fully meet its responsibilities, individual contracted providers/groups are required to:

  - o provide a care plan to the care team for each patient participant

  - o provide access to participant health records

  - o meet regularly with the care team to ensure integration of care

AHRQ Attributes and Functions of the PCMH

In developing a framework for CMI evaluation, the AHRQ identified the following five essential functions and attributes for effective PCMHs:[396]

- **comprehensive care:** The primary care medical home is accountable for meeting the large majority of each patient's physical and mental health care needs, including prevention and wellness, acute care, and chronic care.

- **patient-centered:** The primary care medical home provides primary health care that is relationship-based with an orientation toward the whole person. Partnering with patients and their families requires understanding and respecting each patient's unique needs, culture, values, and preferences.

- **coordinated care:** The primary care medical home coordinates care across all elements of the broader health care system, including

---

[396] http://pcmh.ahrq.gov/page/implementing-pcmh

specialty care, hospitals, home health care, and community services and supports.

- **accessible services:** The primary care medical home delivers accessible services with shorter waiting times for urgent needs, enhanced in-person hours, around-the-clock telephone or electronic access to a member of the care team, and alternative methods of communication such as email and telephone care.

- **quality and safety:** The primary care medical home demonstrates a commitment to quality and quality improvement by ongoing engagement in such activities as:

  - using evidence-based medicine and clinical decision-support tools to guide shared decision making with patients and families

  - engaging in performance measurement and improvement

  - measuring and responding to patient experiences and patient satisfaction

  - practicing population health management

  - Sharing robust quality and safety data and improvement activities publicly is also an important marker of a system-level commitment to quality.

8.3.4 Payment and Incentive Models for the PCMH

Patient-Centered Primary Care Collaborative (PCPCC) Three-Part Model

- The **Patient-Centered Primary Care Collaborative (PCPCC)** is a leading proponent of the PCMH and advocates a three-part payment model for it:[397]

---

[397] *Patient-Centered Primary Care Collaborative, http://www.pcpcc.org/*

- ○ Founded in 2006, the PCPCC is "dedicated to advancing an effective and efficient health system built on a strong foundation of primary care and the patient-centered medical home (PCMH)."

- ○ The PCPCC represents more than 1,000 medical home stakeholders and supporters throughout the United States that aim to:

  - **disseminate results and outcomes** from medical home initiatives and clearly communicate their impact on patient experience, quality of care, population health, and health care costs

  - **advocate for public policy** that advances and builds support for primary care and the medical home, including payment reform, patient engagement, and employer benefit initiatives

  - **convene health care experts, thought leaders, and consumers** to promote knowledge and awareness of the medical home model as well as innovative thinking about this model

- The three-part payment model supported by the PCPCC combines the traditional FFS for office visits with:[398]

  - ○ a monthly care coordination payment for the physician and nonphysician work that falls outside a face-to-face visit and for the system infrastructure (e.g., heath information technologies) needed to achieve better outcomes

  - ○ a visit-based FFS component that recognizes visit-based services that are currently paid under the present FFS payment system and maintains an incentive for the physician to see the patient in an office-visit when appropriate

  - ○ a performance-based component that recognizes achievement of quality and efficiency goals

---

[398] *Military Health System Patient Centered Medical Home Guide,*
http://www.tricare.mil/tma/ocmo/download/MHSPCMHGuide.pdf

- Current PCMH reimbursement models incorporate some, or all, aspects of the PCPCC three-part reimbursement model:

  o As of December 2013, fifty-one PCMH initiatives had been implemented in thirty-two states. In addition, two national initiatives (one in Veterans Administration Hospitals and one in active military treatment facilities for the Air Force, Army, and Navy) have been implemented since 2009 and are currently in place.[399]

  o An example of a multi-component PCMH reimbursement model that combines payment methodologies with a shared savings component is provided by the **Maryland Multi-Payer PCMH (MMPP) Program.**

The Maryland Multi-Payer PCMH (MMPP) Payment Model:[400]

- This three-year program (beginning in 2011) involved the selection of sixty primary care practices in the Maryland, out of an applicant pool of 179.

- The goals of the MMPP program were to test the following value propositions:

  o Enhanced primary care will improve health status and outcomes for patients (especially for the chronically ill).

  o The result of these improved outcomes will be fewer complications, ER visits, and hospitalizations.

  o Savings from these improved outcomes can be used to fund increased payment to primary care practices.

- To incentivize participants to meet these goals, a per-member per-month (PMPM) payment was established for each carrier (commercial insurers, Medicaid, and Medicare) based on the level of accreditation

[399] *The Medical Home's Impact on Cost & Quality, PCPCC,*
http://www.pcpcc.org/resource/medical-homes-impact-cost-quality

[400] *Maryland Health Quality and Cost Council, Appendix B: Healthiest Maryland Businesses,*
http://dhmh.maryland.gov/mhqcc/Documents/MD%20Health%20Quality%20and%20Cost%20Co
uncil%20%202011%20Annual%20Report%201-12-2012.pdf

attained through the NCQA and the number of assigned beneficiaries. The various levels of PMPM for the MMPP are shown below:

Table 1: Reimbursement Rates for the Maryland Multi-Payer PCMH Program

Commercial Population

PHYSICIAN PRACTICE SIZE	LEVEL OF PCMH RECOGNITION / ACCREDITATION BY NCQA		
# OF PATIENTS	LEVEL 1+ NCQA	LEVEL 2 +NCQA	LEVEL 3+ NCQA
< 10,000	$4.68	$5.34	$6.01
10,000–20,000	$3.90	$4.45	$5.01
>20,000	$3.51	$4.01	$4.51

Note: Level 1+ only applies to the first year of the program. In years two and after, the PCMH must achieve Level 2 or better to receive the applicable payment.

Medicaid Population

PHYSICIAN PRACTICE SIZE	LEVEL OF PCMH RECOGNITION / ACCREDITATION BY NCQA		
# OF PATIENTS	LEVEL 1+ NCQA	LEVEL 2 +NCQA	LEVEL 3+ NCQA
all practices regardless of size	$4.54	$5.19	$5.84

Note: Level 1+ only applies to the first year of the program. In years two and after, the PCMH must achieve Level 2 or better to receive the applicable payment. Fixed payments will not be available for federally qualified health centers (FQHCs).

Medicare Advantage Population

PHYSICIAN PRACTICE SIZE	LEVEL OF PCMH RECOGNITION / ACCREDITATION BY NCQA		
# OF PATIENTS	LEVEL 1+ NCQA	LEVEL 2 +NCQA	LEVEL 3+ NCQA
all practices	$8.66	$9.62	$11.54

Other PCMH reimbursement models incorporate aspects contained in the MMPP with accreditation requirements as a base component.

8.3.5 Accreditation of Physician Practices as a PCMH

Background:

- Through the establishment of a recognition and accreditation program for PCMH participation, based on the 2007 joint principles and guidelines, a physician practice is recognized as meeting the criteria as a successful PCMH. As a "yardstick" for determining the qualifications and capabilities of a practice to function as a PCMH, accreditation plays a significant role in determining the levels of reimbursement received from various payers.

- In March 2011, four organizations representing more than 350,000 primary care physicians developed joint guidelines for patient-centered medical homes recognition and accreditation programs:[401]

- These guidelines were created by the:
    - AAFP
    - AAP
    - ACP
    - AOA

- The 2011 guidelines build on the joint principles of the PCMH created by these four groups in 2007 and have been incorporated into current PCMH recognition and certification programs. The guidelines state that all PCMH recognition or accreditation programs should:
    - incorporate the joint principles of the PCMH
    - address the complete scope of primary care services
    - ensure the incorporation of patient- and family-centered care, emphasizing engagement of patients, their families, and their caregivers

---

[401] http://www.medicalhomeinfo.org/national/recognition_programs.aspx

- o engage multiple stakeholders in the development and implementation of the program

- o identify essential standards, elements, and characteristics

- o align standards, elements, characteristics, and/or measures with meaningful use requirements

- o address the core concept of continuous improvement that is central to the PCMH model

- o allow for innovative ideas

- o care coordination within the medical neighborhood

- o clearly identify PCMH recognition or accreditation requirements for training programs

- o ensure transparency in program structure and scoring

- o apply reasonable documentation/data collection requirements

- o conduct evaluations of the program's effectiveness and implement improvements over time

Accreditation Programs:

- Several national programs offer PCMH recognition, including:[402]

  - o the Accreditation Association for Ambulatory Health Care (AAAHC)

  - o The Joint Commission (TJC)

  - o URAC, formerly known as the Utilization and Review Accreditation Commission

  - o the NCQA

---

[402] *Primary Care Medical Home Certified Organizations, Joint Commission,* http://www.jointcommission.org/pcmh_certified_providers/

8.3.6 NCQA Recognition and Accreditation Program for the PCMH

Background:

- Beginning in 2008, the NCQA provided one of the first PCMH recognition and accreditation programs. The NCQA PCMH accreditation model is now the most widely accepted PCMH accrediting model in the country.

- Starting from 214 clinicians at 28 practices in 2008, when the NCQA program began, the program now has now 29,505 NCQA-recognized clinicians in 49 states, representing more than 6,000 physician practices (September 2013). (In comparison, through 2013, there are 1,028 practice sites involving 2,400 clinicians that are Joint Commission PCMH accredited). The NCQA receives approximately 150 new applications per week for PCMH accreditation.[403]

- Practices that achieve NCQA's PCMH recognition are positioned to take advantage of financial incentives offered by health plans and employers, as well as those that may be offered by federal- and state-sponsored pilot programs. As of January 1, 2014, PCMH adoption includes:[404]

  o more than ninety commercial and not-for-profit plans

  o Twenty-five state Medicaid programs

  o federal agencies, including:

    ▪ **Medicare**

    ▪ **the Federal Employee Health Benefits Program (FEHB)**

    ▪ **the US military**: On September 18, 2009, the assistant secretary of defense issued Policy Memorandum: (HA POLICY 09-015) **Implementation of the Patient-Centered Medical Home Model of Primary Care in**

---

[403] *NCQA News Release: September 24, 2013,*
http://www.ncqa.org/Newsroom/2013NewsArchives/NewsReleaseSeptember242013.aspx

[404] *Patient-Centered Medical Home: The Call to Action, SuccessEHS,*
http://info.successehs.com/Portals/157799/docs/wp-pcmh-v5.pdf

MTFs. This policy mandated the establishment of the PCMH model in primary care settings at **all** military treatment facilities, across all services.[405]

- **the US Department of Veterans Affairs (VA)**: In a concept paper published January 15, 2014, the VA announced its intention to adopt the PCMH model for all patients receiving primary care services through the VA system. Such patients represent 80–90 percent of all VA beneficiaries and the VA estimates some 5 million patients will benefit from the PCMH initiative.[406]

- **Federally Qualified health Centers (FQHCs)**: As part of its FY2013 Congressional Budget Justification, the Department of Health and Human Services Health Resources and Services Administration (DHHS HRSA) established **a "priority" goal of having 25 percent of FQHC grantees recognized as PCMHs by the end of 2013.**[407]

  o and several of the nation's largest employers, including:[408]

   - Boeing

   - Safeway

   - Intel

   - Lockheed Martin

- Practices earning NCQA recognition may qualify for additional bonuses or payments based on the level of accreditation achieved during the accreditation period. Higher incentive payments may be offered by health plans and employers for achievement of higher levels.

---

[405] *Policy Memorandum Implementation of the 'Patient-Centered Medical Home' Model of Primary Care in MTFs,http://www.health.mil/libraries/HA_Policies_and_Guidelines/09-015.pdf*

[406] *Patient-Centered Medical Home Concept Paper,* http://www.va.gov/health/services/PrimaryCare/docs/pcmh_ConceptPaper.doc

[407] *FY2013 HRSA Congressional Budget Justification,* http://www.hrsa.gov/about/budget/budgetjustification2013.pdf

[408] *The Patient-Centered Medical Home's Impact on Cost & Quality, PCPCC,* http://www.pcpcc.org/resource/medical-homes-impact-cost-quality

NCQA Accreditation Requirements[409]

Overview:

- NCQA accreditation is based on a set of standards that is revised every three years, beginning with 2008.

- NCQA accreditation is accomplished through the use of standardized survey tools that are completed by practices applying for accreditation to record performance against standards:

  - Transforming a practice to meet the standards of a successful PCMH takes time. Depending on a practice's current capabilities, this may require as long as three to twelve months to complete the process and produce the documentation required under PMCH 2011 standards.

- NCQA accreditation is valid for a period of three years, after which practices must be reaccredited according to standards in place at that time. During the period of accreditation, practices may raise their recognition level by completing additional relevant survey tool items:

  - NCQA offers three levels of PCMH accreditation (Level 1-lowest to Level 3-highest). Practices that achieve Level 2 or Level 3 NCQA recognition will be provided a streamlined renewal process.

- The current NCQA accreditation standards are based on requirements established in 2011. Revised standards will be introduced by March 31, 2014:[410]

  - Practices currently recognized under the 2011 version will continue to be allowed to upgrade recognition to higher levels (Level 1 to Level 2 or 3) following those standards through the expiration of their current recognition period.

  - The current PCMH 2011 standards will remain active for a period of time after the updated PCMH standards are released in 2014

---

[409] *NCQA's Patient-Centered Medical Home (PCMH) 2011 Standards,*
http://www.lafp.org/connect2014/images/content/Recognition_Programs/NCQA/2._NCQA_PCMH
_2011_Standards_11.21.2011.pdf

[410] *http://www.ncqa.org/PublicationsProducts/RecognitionProducts/PCMHPublications.aspx*

to enable practices that previously purchased the 2011 version and initiated the process to complete and submit their application for recognition.

- ○ June 30, 2014, is the last date to enroll in the NCQA under the 2011 standards and completed survey tools must be submitted by March 31, 2015. Accreditation approved through such submissions will be valid for three years following approval.

- ○ March 31, 2014, is the first day that the 2014 accreditation survey tools may be ordered.

- ○ Participants will be able to submit either 2011 or 2014 PCMH survey tools between March 31, 2014, and March 31, 2015.

Current NCQA Accreditation Standards (2011 Version)[411]

A practice site applying for NCQA PCMH accreditation is scored based on its level of performance against established **standards and elements** (see Table 2 below). Each standard and element has an associated description of the type of documentation and the level of health IT required:

- **standards**: The 2011 version NCQA PCMH accreditation program contains six standards, aligned with the core components of primary care. Each of the standards has a total possible point score determined by performance against specific standard "must-pass" **elements** and elements that are not must-pass.

- **elements:** Each standard contains a number of individual elements that are standard-related measures of evaluated performance. Six elements (one for each standard) are designated as "must-pass" elements. Requirements for must-pass elements have to be met to achieve accreditation, regardless of the total point score attained. Each element has a total possible point score determined by attainment of an assigned number of **factors:**

---

[411] *NCQA's Patient-Centered Medical Home (PCMH) 2011 Standards,* http://www.lafp.org/connect2014/images/content/Recognition_Programs/NCQA/2._NCQA_PCMH_2011 _Standards_11.21.2011.pdf

- o **factors:** Factors are specific actions taken to achieve the element description:
  - Each factor is worth a percentage of the total point values for each element. By combining factor attainments, an element point total is calculated.

- Under the 2011 version of the NCQA PCMH, there are 6 standards, 27 elements, and 149 factors used to determine an accreditation level, based on overall scoring.

- Table 1 lists the standards and elements with the associated attainment points used to determine the total score for an individual practice site:

Table 2: 2011 PCMH Content and Scoring

POINTS	2011 NCQA PCMH STANDARD AND ELEMENT	# OF FACTORS	MUST PASS?
20	PCMH Standard 1: Enhance Access and Continuity	34	
4	Element A: Access During Office Hours	4	**Yes**
4	Element B: Access After Hours	5	No
2	Element C: Electronic Access	6	No
2	Element D: Continuity	3	No
2	Element E: Medical Home Responsibility	4	No
2	Element F: Culturally and Linguistically Appropriate Services	4	No
4	Element G: Practice Organization	8	No

POINTS	2011 NCQA PCMH STANDARD AND ELEMENT	# OF FACTORS	MUST PASS?
17	PCMH Standard 2: Identify and Manage Patient Populations	35	
3	Element A: Patient Information	12	No
4	Element B: Clinical Data	9	No
4	Element C: Comprehensive Health Assessment	10	No
5	Element D: Using Data for Population Management	4	**Yes**

POINTS	2011 NCQA PCMH STANDARD AND ELEMENT	# OF FACTORS	MUST PASS?
17	PCMH Standard 3: Plan and Manage Care	23	
4	Element A: Implement Evidence-Based Guidelines	3	No
3	Element B: Identify High-Risk patients	2	No
4	Element C: Manage Care	7	Yes
3	Element D: Management of Medications	5	No
3	Element E: Electronic Prescribing	6	No

POINTS	2011 NCQA PCMH STANDARD AND ELEMENT	# OF FACTORS	MUST PASS?
9	PCMH Standard 4: Provide Self-Care and Community Support	10	
6	Element A: Self-Care Process	6	Yes
3	Element B: Referrals to Community Resources	4	No

POINTS	2011 NCQA PCMH STANDARD AND ELEMENT	# OF FACTORS	MUST PASS?
18	PCMH Standard 5: Track and Coordinate Care	25	
6	Element A: Test Tracking and Follow-Up	10	No
6	Element B: Referral Tracking and Follow-Up	7	Yes
6	Element C: Coordinate with Facilities/Care Transitions	8	No

POINTS	2011 NCQA PCMH STANDARD AND ELEMENT	# OF FACTORS	MUST PASS?
20	PCMH Standard 6: Measure and Improve Performance	22	
4	Element A: Measures of Performance	4	No
4	Element B: Patient/Family Feedback	4	No
4	Element C: Implements Continuous Quality Improvement	4	Yes
3	Element D: Demonstrates Continuous Quality Improvement	4	No
3	Element E: Performance Reporting	3	No
2	Element F: Report Data Externally	3	No

POINTS	2011 NCQA PCMH STANDARD AND ELEMENT	# OF FACTORS	MUST PASS?
0	Element G: Use of Certified EHR*	2	No

POINTS	2011 NCQA PCMH STANDARD AND ELEMENT	# OF FACTORS	MUST PASS?
100	Six Standards and 27 Scored Elements	149	6

*Element G: **Use of Certified EHR** is a non-scored element containing two non-scored factors. This measure is used only for the practice site's EHR Meaningful Use Report and will not be used in accreditation determination.

Scoring:

- The NCQA survey tool is used for the practice site to self-assess attainment of standards and to calculate a total score.

- Each element is individually scored through an assessment of factor completion as shown below:

Figure A: Survey Tool Element Scoring Example

PCMH 1: Enhance Access and Continuity   20 points

The practice provides access to culturally and linguistically appropriate routine care and urgent team-based care that meets the needs of patients/families.

Element A: Access During Office Hours Must-Pass   4 points

The practice has a written process and defined standards and demonstrates that it monitors performance against the standards for:

	YES	NO	NA
1. providing same-day appointments	☐	☐	☐
2. providing timely clinical advice by telephone during office hours	☐	☐	☐
3. providing timely clinical advice by secure electronic messages during office hours	☐	☐	☐
4. documenting clinical advice in the medical record	☐	☐	☐

Scoring

100%	75%	50%	25%	0%
The practice meets all four factors.	The practice meets three factors, including factor 1.	The practice meets two factors, including factor 1.	The practice meets factor 1.	The practice meets no factors or does not meet factor 1.

- Each element of the standard is similarly scored to determine the total number of points earned for each standard.

- Based upon the total element review points and "must-pass" elements obtained, a practice can be recognized as a Level 1 (lowest) to Level 3 (highest) for PCMH 2011, as follows:

no recognition	34 points or fewer and/or fewer than six must-pass elements;
Level 1	35–59 points and all six must-pass elements;
Level 2	60–84 points and all six must-pass elements;
Level 3	85–100 points and all six must-pass elements.

8.3.7 Effectiveness of the PCMH in Reducing Costs and Improving Quality:[412]

- The PCPCC released a report in January 2014 that summarized findings from thirteen peer-reviewed articles and seven industry reports on PCMH demonstrations during 2012 and 2013. The group concluded that this body of work clearly demonstrates success in increasing the quality of care and in reducing cost of care on some measures.

[412] *The Patient-Centered Medical Home's Impact on Cost & Quality, PCPCC,* http://www.pcpcc.org/resource/medical-homes-impact-cost-quality

Table 3: PCMH Studies from August 2012 to December 2013 Reporting Outcomes

	Total Studies	Cost Reductions	Fewer ED Visits	Fewer Inpatient Admissions	Fewer Readmissions	Improvement in Population Health	Improved Access	Increase in Preventive Services	Improvement in Satisfaction
Peer Review Reported Outcomes	(n=13)	61% (n=8)	61% (n=8)	31% (n=4)	13% (n=1)	31% (n=4)	31% (n=4)	31% (n=4)	23% (n=3)
Industry Reports Reported Outcomes	(n=7)	57% (n=4)	57% (n=4)	57% (n=4)	29% (n=2)	29% (n=2)	14% (n=1)	29% (n=2)	14% (n=1)

Note: The percentages reflect the number of studies reporting the indicated outcome. They do not reflect a percentage increase or decrease in the listed outcome. However, the full report contains data associated with each study for determination of amounts or percentage of outcomes performance.

Selected Study Results Included in the PCPCC January 2014 Report:

- **Veterans Health Administration Patient Aligned Care Team (PACT):**
  - national PCMH program
  - 5 million patients
  - published July 2013
  - **results:**
    - 8 percent fewer urgent care visits
    - 4 percent fewer inpatient admissions
    - decrease in face-to-face visits
    - increase in phone encounters, personal health record use, and electronic messaging to providers

- **Blue Cross/Blue Shield of Michigan Physician Group Incentive Program:**
  - statewide (Michigan)
  - 3 million patients
  - published July 2013
  - **results:**
    - 13.5 percent fewer pediatric Emergency Department (ED) visits
    - 10 percent fewer adult ED visits
    - 17 percent fewer inpatient admissions
    - 6 percent fewer hospital readmissions
    - savings of $26.37 per member per month (PMPM)
    - $155 million in total cost savings

- **UPMC Health Plan:**
  - Pennsylvania
  - 23,390 patients
  - published in July 2013
  - **results:**
    - 2.8 percent fewer inpatient admissions
    - 18.3 percent fewer hospital readmissions
    - 2.6 percent reduction in total costs
    - 160 percent return on investment (ROI)
    - 6.6 percent increase in patients with controlled HbA1c
    - 23.2 percent increase in eye exams
    - 9.7 percent increase in LDL screenings

- **CareFirst Blue Cross Blue Shield:**
  - Maryland
  - 1 million patients
  - published June 2013
  - **results:**
    - $98 million in total cost savings
    - 4.7 percent lower costs for physicians who received an incentive award

- **Oregon Health Authority Coordinated Care Organization:**
  - Oregon statewide Medicaid program
  - 600,000 patients
  - published November 2013
  - **results:**
    - 9 percent reduction in ED visits
    - 14–29 percent fewer ED visits for chronic disease patients
    - 12 percent fewer hospital readmissions
    - 18 percent reduction in ED visit spending
    - reduced per capita health spending growth by more than 1.0 percent

Section 8.4: Appendix

Acronym Guide

AAFP........................American Academy of Family Physicians

AAP..........................American Academy of Pediatrics

ACP..........................American College of Physicians

AHRQ.......................Agency for Healthcare Research and Quality

AOA ....American Osteopathic Association

CAHs........................Critical Access Hospitals

CMI ....Center for Medicare & Medicaid Innovation within CMS

CMS ....Centers for Medicare & Medicaid Services

CSW..........................Clinical Social Worker

DHHS........................Department of Health and Human Services

DOB ....Date of Birth

DOJ............................Department of Justice

DRA ....Deficit Reduction Act of 2005 (Public Law 109–171)

DSH ....Disproportionate Share Hospital

EHR ....Electronic Health Record

ESRD..........................End-Stage Renal Disease

eRx..............................Electronic Prescribing Incentive Program

FFS ....Fee-for-Service

FQHCs.........................Federally Qualified Health Centers

HAC ....Hospital-Acquired Conditions

HHAs ....Home Health Agencies

HHS ....Department of Health and Human Services

HIT ....Health Information Technology

HITECH ....Health Information Technology for Economic and Clinical Health

HMO.............................Health Maintenance Organization

HRRP............................Hospital Readmissions Reduction Program

HRSA............................Health Resources and Services Administration

HVBP ....Hospital Value-Based Purchasing

IOM .... Institute of Medicine

IQR............................. Inpatient Quality Reporting

LTCHs........................ Long-Term Care Hospitals

MA.............................. Medicare Advantage

MAPCP .... Multi-Payer Advanced Primary Care Practice

MedPAC .... Medicare Payment Advisory Commission

MHCQ........................ Medicare Health Care Quality

MMA .... Medicare Prescription Drug, Improvement, and Modernization Act

MMPP .... Maryland Multi-Payer Program

MSSP........................ Medicare Shared Savings Program

MTF........................... Military Treatment Facilities

NCQA........................ National Committee for Quality Assurance

NP .... Nurse Practitioner

NPI .... National Provider Identifier

NQF .... National Quality Forum

PACFs....................... Post-Acute Care Facilities

PCMH .... Patient-Centered Medical Home

PCPCC .... Patient-Centered Primary Care Collaborative

PFS .... Physician Fee Schedule

PGP .... Physician Group Practice

PMPM .... Per Member Per Month

PPS........................... Prospective Payment System

PQRS........................ Physician Quality Reporting System

QPS .... Quality Performance Standard

RBRVS .... Resource-Based Relative Value Scale

RIA .... Regulatory Impact Analysis

SNFs........................ Skilled Nursing Facilities

SSA........................... Social Security Administration

SSN........................... Social Security Number

TIN .... Taxpayer Identification Number

VBM .... Value-Based Modifier

VBP........................... Value-Based Purchasing

CHAPTER 9

The Accountable Care Organization (ACO)

Section 9.1: Flash Read!

The Affordable Care Act (ACA) has established an agenda for accelerating and testing adoption of Accountable Care Organizations (ACOs) through the Medicare program. ACOs have been in existence since Medicare first piloted the Physician Group Practice Demonstration in 2003, and this model for grouping doctors, hospitals, and other health care providers together to provide coordinated care to patients has shown some promise in reducing costs and improving health outcomes. The aim of ACOs is to ensure that patients get the right care at the right time in the right setting, thereby reducing redundancy and inefficiency in the health care system and improving outcomes. There are currently more than 500 recognized ACOs in the United States, including approximately 200 commercial model ACOs:

- The scope of an ACO is much broader than that of the Patient-Centered Medical Home (PCMH) and it involves groups of physicians, hospitals, and other health providers who come together voluntarily to deliver coordinated care to patients. Incentives are provided to facilitate collaboration across these different types of providers and components of the health care system with the goal of delivering high-quality care at lower overall costs.

- Currently there are 366 Medicare ACOs:
  - 343 Medicare Shared Savings Program (MSSP) ACOs, including 123 new ACOs that began participating on January 1, 2014
  - 23 Pioneer ACOs under the CMS Innovation Center (CMI) (in late 2013, nine of the original thirty-two Pioneer ACOs dropped out of the program)
- Medicare beneficiaries are not required to enroll in an ACO and retain their rights to seek care from any provider (hospital or physician) authorized to treat Medicare beneficiaries.
- ACO providers are not subject to a capitated model of payment. They continue to bill and receive fee-for-service payments from Medicare.
- In order for an ACO to share in any savings (as part of the MSSP), specific quality standards must be met.
- The purpose of the ACO is not to avoid at-risk patients, but rather to achieve savings through coordination and quality of care.

MSSP Model:

- ACOs are identified as a collection of Tax Identification Numbers (TINs) (hospitals, physician groups or networks, and other providers/suppliers) working together under the MSSP.
- Participating ACOs must agree to a three-year period of participation called an **agreement period.**
- As established under the ACA, MSSP ACOs may elect to participate during the agreement period as a Track 1 or Track 2 ACO:
  - **Track 1**: shared savings only (one-sided model; low risk):
    - Meeting quality reporting standards in each year of the agreement period qualifies Track 1 ACOs to share in up to 50 percent of annual savings.
    - ACOs that elect Track 1 must transition to Track 2 beginning with their second agreement period.

- **Track 2**: shared savings and shared losses (two-sided model; higher risk):

  - Track 2 ACOs meeting quality reporting standards are qualified to share in up to 60 percent of savings and will be liable for repaying a share of any losses, based on their quality scores.

- Regardless of track:

  - Year 1 of the agreement period requires only reporting of quality measures. For Track 2 ACOs, evaluations against quality performance benchmarks are made for years two and three of the agreement period.

  - Each ACO must have a minimum adjusted number of 5,000 attributed Medicare FFS beneficiaries during each year of the agreement period.

- **MSSP ACO Quality Standards and Reporting:**

  - For 2014 and 2015, there are thirty-three individual quality measures assigned to four equally weighted domains:

Table 1: Summary of 2014–2015 Quality Measures by Domain and Total Points[413]

DOMAIN	# OF INDIVIDUAL MEASURES	TOTAL MEASURES FOR SCORING PURPOSES	TOTAL POSSIBLE POINTS	DOMAIN WEIGHT
Patient/ Caregiver Experience	7	seven measures of the individual survey module*	14	25%
Care Coordination/Patient Safety	6	six measures (the EHR measure is double weighted to equal four points)	14	25%
Preventive Health	8	eight measures	16	25%

---

[413] http://www.cms.gov/Medicare/Medicare-Fee-for-Service-Payment/sharedsavingsprogram/Downloads/MSSP-QM-Benchmarks.pdf

		seven measures, including the five-component Diabetes Composite Measure and the two-component Coronary Artery Disease Composite		
At-Risk Population	12		14	25%
Total in All Domains	33	28	58	100%

*Clinicians and Group Consumer Assessment of Healthcare Providers and Systems (CG-CAHPS) patient experience survey:

- ACOs must successfully meet quality requirements to earn at least 70 percent of the total points available for a given domain to qualify for shared savings.

  Note: Failure to meet the EHR measure will result in a score of less than 70 percent of total domain points for the Care Coordination/Patient Safety domain.

Determining Shared Savings:

- ACOs that meet quality standards with average per beneficiary costs below a CMS-established benchmark are eligible to share in savings as determined by their final quality score and the maximum rate of shared savings for their selected track of participation.

- CMS has established a maximum level of shared savings **(sharing cap)** equal to a percentage of the benchmark according to the track of participation selected:

  - for Track 1, shared savings cannot exceed **10 percent** of the ACO's adjusted benchmark

  - for Track 2, shared savings cannot exceed **15 percent** of the ACO's adjusted benchmark

Determining Shared Losses:

- For Track 2 participants, any annual losses (average per beneficiary spending in excess of the benchmark) will be shared between the ACO and Medicare.

- CMS establishes a **minimum loss rate (MLR)** at 2.0 percent **above** the benchmark as a "buffer" against normal variations in spending.

- ACOs with expenditures above the benchmark, but below the MLR, will not be liable for repaying any losses.

- ACOs with expenditures at or above the MLR will be responsible for repaying a share of losses to Medicare.

- The payable share of losses is determined by applying the inverse of the final sharing rate (1.00 minus the final sharing rate) to losses meeting or exceeding the MLR.

- CMS has established a maximum loss rate (sharing loss rate), above which an ACO is not liable for additional losses. The sharing loss rate is a percentage of the adjusted benchmark according to the year of the agreement period:
  - **Year 1:** 5 percent
  - **Year 2**: 7.5 percent
  - **Year 3**: 10 percent

- CMS requires losses to be repaid within ninety days of notification.

Section 9.2: Provider Perspectives

If US health care costs too much and the quality of care varies across providers, one salient reason is the fragmentation of care into silos controlled by various provider entities that are not financially responsible for the entirety of the patient's diagnosis and treatment. Hospitals don't always talk to nursing homes, nursing homes don't always talk to doctors, and doctors don't always talk to each other. The toll in duplication and failed hand-offs is enormous, both clinically and financially.

The accountable care organization (ACO) concept is intended to redress this endemic failing by unifying the piecework nature of care delivery under a single overarching umbrella organization. It is supposed to make different service streams within the continuum of care conceive of themselves and behave as one.

9.2.1 Rationale

Fundamentally, the purpose of ACOs is to change the way people in health care think. Consider the University of Michigan Health System (UMHS). UMHS and its 1,700 physicians have been active, engaged participants in the ACO concept from the beginning, in 2005. They have made a lot of progress and have gained many insights.

What they're working on now is the role of subacute nursing facilities. When the health system's leaders took a hard look at the data for orthopedics, they discovered that every patient who has a knee replacement who goes to subacute care stays nineteen to twenty days. The ACO wants to get it down to seven days.

"Our people told us we couldn't get discharged before nineteen days," said David Spahlinger, MD, senior associate dean for clinical affairs at the University of Michigan Medical School and executive director of the faculty group practice. "Well, the length of benefit is twenty-one days. That's their business model. Medicare pays them per diem.

"If you're not in an ACO model, you don't think this way," Spahlinger continued. "You don't think upstream or downstream about what you do." Before, it wouldn't have made any difference to the hospital or its doctors how long the knee patients stayed in the subacute facility or how much it cost; it wasn't their problem.

"The point is to think more globally about how you deliver care," Spahlinger said. "It's a culture change. You're working your way to a new way of thinking."[414]

The ACO concept may be useful for either the post-65 cohort or the commercially insured non-Medicare population. Indeed, some of the most advanced ACOs in operation, such as Advocate Health Care in northeastern Illinois, were built before the ACA was passed or Medicare formalized its shared savings program. Yet as a payment model, the ACO may be particularly appropriate for an older population. A young person who breaks her leg is happy when she gets her cast removed; she goes through rehab, and then goes dancing and resumes her life. An elderly person, by contrast, has far fewer resources—physical, psychological, social or financial, to get back on her feet.

"It reminds me of the last scene in *Gone With the Wind*," commented Stuart Guterman, a vice president with The Commonwealth Fund. "'But doctor, where will I go, what will I do?' The health care system is telling them, 'I don't give a damn.' The hospital says, 'Congratulations, Mrs. Jones, you're ready to leave the hospital now.' But you're not always ready. For elderly people with chronic conditions, you're not cured."[415]

The episode in the hospital is "a spike. You're still at some level of below-level functioning, you leave the hospital, and you're panic stricken. 'Where do I go next?' They recommend you get post-acute care or home health or rehab, and you say, 'OK, where do I get that?' You go into the hospital—you don't know anything about the health care system—it's very difficult. They tell you, 'Here's a list of places in the area, tell us where to ship your mother.' That's scary. There's very little continuity; the doctors in this facility have never talked to the doctors who treated you in the hospital. Nobody talks to anybody else. Nobody coordinates your care, especially if you have multiple problems. Nobody is overseeing the whole package of treatment to ensure you're at the maximum

---

[414] David Spahlinger, MD, telephone interview, August 26, 2013.
[415] Stuart Guterman, telephone interview, September 3, 2013.

level of health. Instead you get duplicate tests, people bouncing around, back and forth."

These pieces could be woven together in a coherent way, Guterman proposed. The ACO is a structural concept that allows for the gathering of groups of providers that are willing to take responsibility for "the whole bundle" of care for their patients. The providers will be rewarded if they manage down the costs of that care while maintaining quality; one can't go without the other. "Paying less for a quality outcome that's not worth anything is not higher value. ACO says providers have to stop thinking about the patient in front of them and think more about the whole set of care the patient needs—and where can they get it."

Thus the ACO concept marries two objectives: payment reform and delivery-system reform, with the first driving the second.

9.2.2 Summary

An ACO takes responsibility for the full continuum of care for a defined population of patients or Medicare beneficiaries. Typically it is a fully integrated delivery system that includes primary care physicians, specialty physicians, and inpatient facilities. These providers arrange among themselves to provide coordinated evidence-based care. They have to figure out: how to organize this care among their constituent parts; how to keep track of data on care, quality, and costs, and report them to CMS; and how to distribute savings or expenses among their members. At Advocate, for example, the savings are distributed 48 percent to specialists, 36 percent to primary care physicians, and 16 percent to hospitals.[416]

Because an emphasis on costs alone would lead to providers potentially stinting on care, CMS has proscribed specific quality metrics that ACOs must meet. In 2013, those metrics focused on diabetes, hypertension, ischemic vascular disease, heart disease, and coronary heart disease. CMS is evaluating performance in four areas: Patient/Caregiver Experience; Care Coordination and Patient Safety; Preventive Health; and At-Risk Populations. ACOs are being judged on thirty-three quality measures: seven are derived from patient surveys, three from claims, one from the electronic health record, and twenty-two through

---

[416] http://www.advocatehealth.com/mssp

the Group Practice Reporting Option (GPRO) in the Physician Quality Reporting System (PQRS).

Medicare has offered three types of ACOs: first came the Physician Group Practice Demonstration (PGPD), which ran from 2005 to 2010. The ACA introduced the shared savings model, which includes the vast majority of Medicare ACOs. In addition, CMS created the Pioneer Model ACO for experienced, high-performing health systems that were prepared to take on a higher level of risk.

- **PGPD**: Ten respected multispecialty groups were chosen as pilot sites for this early demonstration of what would evolve into the ACO. During the five years of the project, they attained strong quality results but had less success hitting their cost-savings goals. Only five of the ten sites achieved the required two percent savings after three years, and one, the Marshfield Clinic, drew in half the total bonuses.[417]

- **Shared Savings Model**: The ACO and its providers agree to be held accountable for the "quality, cost, and overall care of the Medicare fee-for-service beneficiaries assigned to the ACO," according to the language of the CMS ACO contract.[418] If the shared savings ACOs save money and improve quality, they will get back a portion of those savings from Medicare, but not until about two years after the start of the program year. All the upfront investments in population health management infrastructure, chronic disease management programs, IT capabilities, PCMHs, care coordinators, etc., are incurred prospectively by the ACO out of its own resources. If it doesn't achieve savings, it doesn't get any rebate from Medicare.

- **Pioneer Model**: This three-year experiment started on January 1, 2012. In the first two years of the model, participants test a shared savings and shared losses arrangement with higher levels of risk than the shared savings model. That means, if they don't generate savings or perhaps even generate losses, they may have to repay Medicare part of their reimbursements. This is what is referred to as "downside risk." In the third

---

[417] Gail R. Wilensky, "Lessons from the Physician Group Practice Demonstration—A Sobering Reflection," New England Journal of Medicine 2011; 365:1659–1661, November 3, 2011. http://www.nejm.org/doi/full/10.1056/NEJMp1110185

[418] http://www.cms.gov/Medicare/Medicare-Fee-for-Service-Payment/sharedsavingsprogram/Shared-Savings-Program-ACO-Agreement.html

year, ACOs that have demonstrated savings can move to a population-based payment episode, in which case FFS payments would be replaced by a prospective per-member-per-month (PMPM) amount, otherwise known as capitation. CMS would let providers know at the beginning of the performance period which patients' cost and quality they will be held accountable for, based on where the beneficiaries have been receiving the plurality of their primary care. However, patients retain the right to receive services from any provider accepting Medicare beneficiaries—an issue that is causing much consternation among ACO leaders. The minimum size for a Pioneer ACO is 15,000 aligned beneficiaries, unless located in a rural zone, in which case they must have 5,000 beneficiaries.

9.2.3 Current State

Starting from a few dozen at the end of 2010, the ranks of ACOs of all kinds swelled to almost 500 by September 2013, covering about 20.1 million lives, according to *Health Affairs*.[419] About 343 of those were MSSP ACOs and 23 were Pioneer ACOs.

By December 2011, thirty-two organizations signed up to become Pioneer ACOs. Since that time, nine of them dropped out. Seven of them recategorized themselves as Medicare Shared Savings Program (MSSP) ACOs, and two—Plus, in northern Texas, and Presbyterian Healthcare Services, in Albuquerque, New Mexico—withdrew as Medicare ACOs entirely. The University of Michigan, which achieved 0.3 percent savings, notably shifted into the less-risky MSSP program.

In July 2013, CMS announced the first-year results for the Pioneer cohort. Costs for the 669,000 enrolled beneficiaries rose by 0.3 percent in 2012, while costs for traditional Medicare beneficiaries rose 0.8 percent in the same period—thus, a 0.5 percent savings. Thirteen of the thirty-two ACOs produced favorable financial results, accumulating gross savings of $87.6 million, of which $33 million accrued to the Medicare Trust Funds. Just two of the Pioneers had

---

[419] David Muhlestein, "Why Has ACO Growth Slowed?" *Health Affairs* blog, October 31, 2013. http://healthaffairs.org/blog/2013/10/31/why-has-aco-growth-slowed/#!

shared losses, totaling $4.0 million. Savings were driven in part by reductions in hospital admissions and readmissions, CMS said.[420]

CMS characterized the results as "positive and promising," but didn't offer much granular detail. The agency chose to highlight the quality outcomes:

- **readmissions**: Twenty-five of thirty-two Pioneer ACOs had lower hospital readmission rates than average FFS beneficiaries.

- **hypertension**: Pioneers achieved 68 percent blood pressure control among people with diabetes versus 55 percent for the average in managed-care plans.

- **cholesterol**: Diabetes patients in Pioneer ACOs had markedly better LDO control than typical managed-care populations.

- **patient experience**: Pioneers won higher scores than FFS providers on all four patient experience indicators.

Despite all that, the financial picture is still indeterminate. Some observers see reasons for optimism, yet many are skeptical that the concept can ever live up to the ambitions placed upon it. The Medicare Payment Advisory Commission (MedPAC) noted that even though the savings from Pioneer in the first year were 0.5 percent, the costs to providers of hiring care coordinators and administering these programs ran 1 to 2 percent in 2012.[421]

Health care quality expert Michael L. Millenson acknowledges that "ACOs have gotten a lot of publicity," but he worries that "how much it's affecting individual institutions is yet to be seen."[422]

"We've now got six full years of field testing of the Medicare shared savings idea," wrote analyst Jeff Goldsmith after CMS released preliminary results for the Pioneer Model ACOs in July 2013, "and the prognosis for Medicare ACOs is not encouraging. If the most sophisticated provider-based managed-care enterprises cannot master this program, neither will most of the nation's

---

[420] http://www.cms.gov/Newsroom/MediaReleaseDatabase/Press-Releases/2013-Press-Releases-Items/2013-07-16.html

[421] Rebecca Adams, "MedPAC Plans Closer Look at Medicare ACOs," Commonwealth Fund blog, September 12, 2013. http://www.commonwealthfund.org/Newsletters/Washington-Health-Policy-in-Review/2013/Sep/September-16-2013/MedPAC-Plans-Closer-Look-at-Medicare-ACOs.aspx

[422] Michael L. Millenson, telephone interview, August 15, 2013.

community hospitals, even with the help of an avid corps of consultants and policy cheerleaders."[423]

Lack of Patient "Skin in the Game"

More than a handful of prominent, forward-looking health systems have scrutinized the government's ACO and demurred. Geisinger Health System in Pennsylvania is widely regarded as an innovator in care delivery and financing, but it's not doing an MSSP ACO. Similarly, Baptist Health South Florida, an eight-hospital system in Miami with 14,000 employees, has embraced the evolution of medicine toward managing population health. The system recognizes that inpatient hospitalizations are bound to decline and it is preparing to assume more risk in partnership with payers, so that it receives a share of the savings.

Baptist was interested, on a conceptual level, in creating an MSSP ACO. But when Ralph E. Lawson, Baptist's executive vice president and chief financial officer, read the 700 pages of "enormously complex" implementing regulations, his enthusiasm declined. The major stumbling block was that "a Medicare beneficiary could go out of network anytime they wanted to, just like traditional Medicare," he said. "I didn't think it was going to be very easy to be successful with the concept. So I decided to work with our commercial payers. It will be simpler and easier. You can call them up and say, 'This thing isn't working, what can we do to fix it?' You can't do that with the federal government."[424]

There is a fair amount of dispute about what an ACO really is. "I find ACO to be a confusing and imprecise term," said Martin Love, CEO of the Humboldt-Del Norte Independent Practice Association in Eureka, California. The Medicare ACO is a well-defined set of requirements and activities, he notes, yet many things referred to as ACOs "are not that similar to what Medicare ACOs are. So I think it's sometimes not a useful term."

---

[423] Jeff Goldsmith, "Pioneer ACOs Disappointing First Year," Health Affairs blog, August 15, 2013. http://healthaffairs.org/blog/2013/08/15/pioneer-acos-disappointing-first-year/

[424] Ralph E. Lawson, telephone interview, November 7, 2013.

Here is what a real ACO means to Love:

- a defined population

- accountability around total cost

- utilization management

- contractual arrangements with providers

- some sort of shared savings arrangement around total costs

Those shared savings arrangements may take a variety of forms. "What differs a lot is, outside the Medicare world, whether the population can opt in and opt out," Love said. In the commercial market, part of the goal, realistically speaking, is to postpone expenses and reduce the disease burden until the patient goes on Medicare. A commercial plan, with a preponderance of younger, healthier people, may have different operational goals and strengths, whereas "nobody lives to pass out of the Medicare market, everybody dies." For Medicare ACOs, therefore, end-of-life strategies are critical.

The other significant differentiator among ACOs is whether: they are organized around a physician and ambulatory perspective; or that of an aggregation of hospitals that contracts with physicians practices; or centered around a payer. These three models may have markedly different orientations.

For Mount Sinai Health System, which went live with its MSSP ACO on July 1, 2012, the really big problem—the one facing all participants in the ACO experiment—is that by design, it's not permitted to incentivize patients who are counted in the Mount Sinai ACO to stay at Mount Sinai for all their care. If they drift off to another hospital, "We're responsible for that cost of care," said Mark Callahan, MD, CEO of the Mount Sinai Care ACO.

This is the dreaded "attribution issue," source of much muttering in the halls of well-intentioned ACOs across the land. Patients can wander wherever they want and have no obligation to stick with the ACO to which they have been attributed by CMS. They may not even know they've been assigned to one hospital or physicians group instead of another.

From a patient-care perspective or a financial perspective, it makes no sense to set it up this way, but in the end it's a matter of "patient choice" and thus a political issue. Congress is unwilling to put restrictions on the Medicare population, afraid of pushback from beneficiaries, Callahan said. "In addition to going to the doctor, they vote a lot," he remarked.

The only way the hospital and its affiliated physicians can make it work is to "create green pastures to attract them to come to us." The downside is, some populations like to doctor shop. And New York City is home to thousands of snowbirds who go to South Florida in the wintertime, a very high-cost Medicare region with plenty of patient churning and overutilization. "We have zero control of what happens down there," he said. "It does make us concentrate on the patient experience."

In Goldsmith's view, the attribution problem will weigh especially heavily against physician-centric Pioneer organizations, because they will have trouble diverting these free-floating patients from hospitalization or reducing the use of expensive out-of-network services. "It's really tough to practice managed care without the patient's knowledge or consent or sharing some of savings with them—the fundamental flaw in ACO program design," he said.

While Robert A. Berenson, MD, a former vice chair of MedPAC, believes that ACOs really do make sense, he also believes it's worthwhile to alter incentives so that providers take on more risk for the health of populations they serve. "It's going to be easier to measure the performance of an organization than of individual doctors," he said.

The problem is that CMS's payment model, retrospective attribution, doesn't serve the purpose. It asks nothing of the patient, who may not even understand she is in an ACO, and puts all the responsibility on the providers. "The thinking was, they didn't want the ACO to treat the patients in the ACO differently from the patients who were seeing them but not in the ACO," Berenson said of the drafters of the regulations at CMS. "They thought the ACO would have to treat everybody well. It's a nice theory, but the negatives outweigh it. I don't see how it can work."

Instead, Berenson said, CMS should adopt a prospective attribution based on a previous pattern of care. CMS should tell the beneficiary, "It looks like you get your care from Dr. Jones. He's part of ACO XYZ. Here's how an ACO works. Your choices won't be limited but you are now part of an ACO." The patient can decide to opt out, but most will probably stay if they like their doctor.

Other Challenges

While patient attribution is the biggest challenge facing the ACO experiment, many organizations say, other issues are also front and center. For example,

CMS gave Mount Sinai Health System its historical data for spending on patients for the three years previous to launch. The ACO is responsible for reducing costs against its own baseline. CMS sends Mount Sinai quarterly reports on how it's faring on quality and utilization.

"Right now our data looks like we are saving money, spending less than if we were not in the ACO," Callahan said. "Knock on wood, we're moving in the right direction." He wasn't in a position to share financial numbers yet, but proudly shared that Mount Sinai got 100 percent on its quality reporting.

The investment required to make the transformation from FFS to population payment has been enormous, he said. It required managing the doctors, human resources, and IT. They started with IT, building a series of population management reports and tools in the electronic health record (EHR) and then "crosswalked that with all the claims data we get from Medicare."

"We identify prospectively patients who are not getting the right care or are doing poorly," Callahan said. "For example, with diabetes, we want to screen for retinal disease, kidney disease, peripheral neuropathy." To do that, the patient needs to come in. The problem is, the patient who doesn't come to see you is the one who's getting in trouble.

"So we added people resources, to find the patients who are falling through the cracks," Callahan explained. "They've got transport issues, they have a broken elevator in their building, they have a problem with benefits, can't get medications. We work to close the social problems that lead to poor patient outcomes. That is not paid for in fee-for-service. Who's going to pay for extra staff for home visits, outreach? Who's going to pay for the EHR to generate these data? We don't get an extra payment per member per month. This is all from the Bank of Mount Sinai right now, with the hope that we will save enough to get a shared savings payment from Medicare to cover those costs."

The savings target is 2.5 percent off baseline costs, but Callahan has no assurance that he will reach it. For Mount Sinai, the potential optimum payday would be on the order of "multiple millions of dollars." Once Medicare takes its split, "we would get roughly half of that." They've been dancing the ACO tango for about sixteen months and won't see the payout for a good long time yet. The first savings cycle is eighteen months and then CMS waits ninety days for the laggard claims to come in. CMS calculates the claims after that, taking another three months. "So it's two years between when we start and when we get some money," Callahan said. In the meantime, the hospital and physicians are fronting an extra $2 million per year on operating costs, not including IT investments. "You have to be committed to it—and have deep pockets," he said.

To gain buy-in from doctors, Callahan arranged for primary care physicians—the backbone of the ACO—to receive "a significant bonus payment for their efforts. The behavioral economists say bonuses have to be within a range of 10 to 20 percent of their salary in order for people to pay attention to something," Callahan said. "With the quality performance programs from the managed-care companies, it's a 1 percent or 2 percent upside. It's not enough to influence behavior."

There are other complications as well. At first, the data from CMS were mangled and it took awhile to clean that up. Second, the doctors need a lot of support. "You can't just mail them a report; you have to continuously be out there talking and working with them." Each of the eighteen affiliated medical practices gets its own data report, which has to be problem-solved in person.

If an ACO can be thought of as composed of components—primary care physician, specialty physician, imaging, laboratory, physical therapy, management, etc.—the critical point is that "every one of those components has to demonstrate efficiency and effectiveness to the overall enterprise," said Bruce Bagley, MD, a quality leader at the American Academy of Family Physicians (AAFP) and CEO of its TransforMED consulting subsidiary. It's no longer possible for each individual component to act as an autonomous profit maximizer.

This affects all parties in the ACO, but it is particularly consequential for hospitals, Bagley believes. "No longer is the hospital a place where we put heads in beds. It's now the place we use only if we really need it because we can't get it done as an outpatient."

A more robust primary care framework and more integration of care will inevitably result in less need for inpatient hospital stays. "That's where most people think we're going to save the money," Bagley said. "It's not one more glucose test. It's unnecessary procedures and hospitalizations, and excessive workups, fruitless care at the end of their life." Enlightened hospital executives understand they will have to be transformative, he said. "They know they have to add value and not be a cost center. There are others who are hanging on desperately and trying to crank it until the future comes."[425]

---

[425] Bruce Bagley, MD, telephone interview, September 14, 2013.

Keith M. Starke, MD, is one of the forward-looking physician hospital executives. Chief quality officer and chairman of the department of medicine at Mercy Hospital St. Louis, he is trying to get an MSSP ACO up and running by January 2015. The date was pushed back to 2015 because there were so many things that needed to be accomplished first. "It's a huge challenge. You have to have an ambulatory EHR—for the inpatient side as well—as well as a database analysis and ability to extract data for the physicians."

Second, Starke noted, you have to have a large enough primary care base plus specialty physicians to which you can refer patients. "You've got to be able to demonstrate that patients who stay within the ACO group have better outcomes," he said. That raises a problematic issue: How do you change behavior in cities where there's a lot of competition and patients do not feel bound to any one hospital or physicians group or coherent delivery continuum? Patients move at will among a variety of physicians—"a renal specialist down at Missouri Baptist, a cardiologist at Barnes. How do you manage them and provide better value, and have the data to make sure you're able to do that?"

Starke doesn't have a good answer and neither do many other physicians and hospital leaders trying in good faith to realize this concept on the ground. Callahan took a conservative approach by signing Mount Sinai up for the MSSP model and not the Pioneer model, mainly because of the risk of the downside penalty if the ACO spent more than its baseline. "We didn't want to be writing checks to Medicare," he said.[426]

The quality metrics and how they determine the amount of financial sharing with the government is stacked against providers in the Pioneer model, Callahan said. There are thirty-three quality metrics. In the first year, ACOs merely report them. In subsequent years, the performance determines the financial result, whether you receive or pay back money to the government. "They give percentile ranking against the other ACOs around the country. If you're at the 90th percentile or above, you get two points for that metric," he said. "If you're at the 30th percentile or below, you get zero points. You sum all those points for the quality metrics and you get your shared savings, with how close you are to 100 percent on all your metrics." It's extremely hard to land above the 90th percentile. There's also no correction for urban versus rural disadvantages.

---

[426] *Mark Callahan, MD, telephone interview, October 17, 2013.*

Even if everybody improves quality and reduces expenses, somebody has to lose. "The University of Michigan is a great system; they have great quality," he said. "They didn't see how they could make it," so they withdrew from the Pioneer program. "It's not whether you do a good job, it's how you stack up against all the other ACOs in the country. By the definition, people will lose money," Callahan said.

Although some have complained that CMS has been inflexible in its rule making and interpretation, Callahan sees the problem embedded in the legislation itself. There's only so much CMS can do to ease the strictures in the law as written, he said.

You can be completely on board with the overall intention of refocusing US providers on patient safety, value for money, clinical excellence, and yet still bristle at "the inherent unfairness" of how Medicare has structured these risk-and-reward models, Starke agreed. "I do think good places will figure out how to make it work and how to survive. There will be lots of stresses and pressures on those organizations." But if the government is going to put those kinds of penalties in place for not meeting the targets, the metrics should be rock solid and indisputable, he added.

Part of the problem is the CMS Innovation Center (CMI) doesn't understand how people make decisions on risk, suggested William L. Rich III, MD, an ophthalmologist in northern Virginia. "If you look at the main two goals, increasing access and constraining costs, in simple summary they are all going to fail—their entire construct from ACOs to global payments. Does that mean they are doomed to fail? No. The way they were constructed by CMI, there is no evidence they will succeed."

The cost basis is not the region in which you are practicing. "It's your own efficient system that you developed," Rich said. If you're a relatively efficient provider in a metropolitan area like Minneapolis or Albuquerque, "Where's the fat? Where's the savings?" Among the ACOs that signed up for the Pioneer model, the savings were only 0.5 percent. "The cost to the institutions to run these things was 2 percent. That means they lost money," Rich said. "These guys were the most sophisticated of the lot. This was perfectly predictable, the way these things were constructed."

The University of Michigan's story is worth a longer look. The health system started down the road of accountable care with the Physician Group Practice Demonstration in 2005 and made money on it. "We were relatively successful," Spahlinger said. "We didn't go in with the idea that we would have success.

566

We went in with the idea that we would learn how to make medical care more coordinated." The health system invested $4 million—$800,000 a year for five years. Medicare sent Michigan back $17 million, "a lot more than our investment." There were also other benefits: Michigan got full credit for its PQRS, which it could apply to other parts of the Medicare pay-for-value reimbursement revolution.

Michigan's withdrawal from the Pioneer program was taken by many observers as an omen of the program's inherent failings. But Spahlinger said UM withdrew largely because it was operating two ACOs in parallel: the Pioneer, with 24,000 beneficiaries in southeastern Michigan, and an MSSP (known as the POM ACO) covering the whole state, with 82,000 beneficiaries. From an administrative perspective, it had become too complicated to manage them both.

Running an ACO is "not without its difficulties," Spahlinger said. The main problem is you are working against your own previous outcomes. In addition, if they were good, and you improved quality and saved money, "You get rebased. Every time you make savings and you get rebased, you have to come up with new ways to improve."

That makes it hard to keep going. "If you're going to be rebased every three years, it's not really shared savings," Spahlinger said. "It's a transition to a global budget at some point."

Glenn Hackbarth, MedPAC chairman, said at a meeting in September 2013, "If people are losing money because they're being punished for being efficient in the past, there's going to be a lot of unhappiness."[427]

Or, as Goldsmith put it, "Orchards full of low-hanging fruit (e.g., very high levels of previously unexamined Medicare spending) appear to be an essential precondition of ACO success."

---

[427] *Adams, Commonwealth Fund blog, September 12, 2013.*

9.2.4 The Road Ahead

The health care providers and organizational leaders quoted in this chapter each have substantial experience with ACOs and have labored in good faith to reform their health systems in accordance with the goals of policy makers in Congress and CMS. Many of them, however, aren't optimistic that the ACO model is going to be successful in the long run. When pressed, many of them express skepticism on a wide range of issues.

The MSSP ACO "is probably a transitional model," said Callahan, likely to be succeeded by something else in two or three years.

Love doesn't think either the Pioneer or the MSSP ACOs will be successful. The big savings will have to be extracted first from hospitals and second from specialists. But to gain any savings at all, there must first be cooperation among providers and facilities. It defies common sense to expect these interest groups to work together toward their own diminishment. "Health care communities are like coral reefs," Love said. "Every fish is trying to eat every other fish."

ACOs as presently structured will lead to the financial suicide of their parent organizations, said John Toussaint, MD, chief executive officer of the ThedaCare Center for Healthcare Value in Appleton, Wisconsin. As providers become more efficient working with Medicare beneficiaries, these gains bleed over into the commercial payer population. As hospital admissions and readmissions decline—a consequence of more proactive primary care and smoother care transitions—reimbursements and utilization for the 80 percent of the population that is still FFS must also decline. This quickly puts the hospital affiliated with the ACO into financial peril. Indeed, hospitals are already reporting lower net income and have started laying off personnel.

Those provider systems that have reduced their total cost of care are being penalized with corresponding declines in revenue. They're still competing with other organizations that are not participating in the ACO program and that are still able to charge full rates. "We can't have the 'haves' and 'have nots' here," Toussaint added.

The MSSP ACO concept will fail, Toussaint said, because retrospective FFS payments are not aggressive enough. Providers should be paid up front to care for a defined population. "If it costs $100 to take care of them last year, let's set a price for what it will cost next year. A population capitation—that's the experiment we need to run next, the sooner the better." This would shift the financial risk to the providers, but that's what Medicare is doing anyway. This interim stage, as Toussaint calls it, "is like a foot in two graves. We can't win in either scenario." The only solution, as he sees it, is "to run payment experiments that are much more radical than what we're doing now."

Goldsmith thinks policy makers are ignoring the obvious solution staring them in the face: the growing enrollment in the "politically incorrect" Medicare Advantage (MA) Program, which offers beneficiaries "a much better deal financially and logistically than regular Medicare." The MA program allows plans to use more effective tools to manage care, discipline beneficiaries, and squeeze payment concessions from providers, compared to the relatively lever-less ACOs.

Spahlinger, at the University of Michigan, likes MA plans but thinks an Advantage PPO is just "fee-for-service all over again," he said. "I think Advantage plans are important, I think ACOs are important. I wish the government would say Advantage plans have to be HMOs and not PPOs. The problem is, nobody has had the political will to move everybody into Advantage plans."

The value in the ACO is that it is one mechanism to try to reduce fragmentation in care, Spahlinger said. "I don't think anybody believes this is a panacea, the secret sauce, for our health care problems." Mainly it provides "an incentive for physicians to work together for better care. It moves us toward an integrated health system a few years down the road."

Perhaps we should still give ACOs, which are very much in their infancy, the benefit of the doubt. The process of becoming an ACO—converting from volume to value—requires significant investments in technology, in process improvement, in care coordination, in data management, and in clinical team redesign. In other words, it takes time.

Craig Samitt, MD, formerly CEO of the Dean Clinic in Wisconsin, an MSSP ACO, suggested that it's still too early to assess the ACOs' performance. "Many ACOs are developing skills and muscle they didn't have before," he said. "From my vantage point, this will only continue to help the beneficiary, will only improve access, improve service, and reduce cost. It's culture change. It takes several years to facilitate."

Zirui Song wrote on the *Harvard Business Review* blog that the ACO concept is essential "because it enables delivery-system reform to make economic sense and it provides physicians the opportunity to lead in this reform. With

10,000 Americans turning 65 every day over the next two decades, for Medicare, at least, this opportunity will look increasingly like an imperative."[428]

Millenson concurs that the ACO concept is valid. Yet, he wonders, "at the payment levels, the specific payment regulations put together by Medicare, is the prize worth it?"[429]

To many organizations, the answer will be no. "I don't know if all this stuff is going to work," said Arthur Palamara, MD, a cardiovascular surgeon who's on the ACO steering committee at Memorial Health System in Hollywood, Florida. "If we save 5 percent of our expenses in 2011, we all get a bonus. Then we divide it by 1,000 people. I'm not sure it's enough money to change the practice patterns of many doctors."[430]

Mitchell Goldman, a health care lawyer in Philadelphia who works closely with doctors and hospitals on risk and malpractice issues, argued that ACOs are not going to be the models of the future. "The whole notion of shared savings is ridiculous," he said. "We've tried it numerous times and it always fails." They started off well because they trimmed the fat—easily done. But as the system became more efficient and benchmarks were lowered, fewer hospitals and physicians could find the windfalls that buoyed them in the beginning and failed to benefit from any shared savings surplus. The current Medicare programs may deliver a short-term impact, but they won't be sustainable in the long term, he said.

"What we're going to learn from ACOs, we're going to get everybody focused on population health and we will improve care coordination," Goldman said. "I believe in my heart, my care will be better. We'll have the electronic health record and incentives to coordinate care. Those things in and of themselves for me are enough to do the ACO experiment," he said, but they are not going to work for providers. The Pioneer dropouts are just the first indication of what is in store, he added.

In fact, the growth rate of ACOs slowed in 2013. After "significant growth" through January of 2013, the formation of ACOs slowed to just thirty-five in the rest of the year, according to David Muhlestein, who, as director of research at

---

[428] Zirui Song, "Pioneer Accountable Care Organizations: Lessons from Year 1," *Harvard Business Review* blog, October 8, 2013. http://blogs.hbr.org/2013/10/pioneer-accountable-care-organizations-lessons-from-year-1/

[429] Michael L. Millenson, telephone interview, August 15, 2013.

[430] Arthur Palamara, MD, telephone interview, August 25, 2013.

Leavitt Partners, is actively tracking ACO contracts. He hypothesized that the "trailblazers" are already engaged and working on issues of managing population health, even if the endgame is uncertain, but the "followers," who are less willing or able to bear risk, are waiting for a proven model to follow.[431] After this slowdown in ACO growth in 2013, growth resumed in 2014 as 126 new ACOs began participating in the MSSP.

The most useful bellwether we have for the future of Medicare ACOs will be the renewal rate of existing contracts. The initial high rate of renewal gives reason for optimism, but CY2014 will be critical, Muhlestein said. ACOs that have been in operation for a year or two will have the opportunity to renew or cancel their contracts. If more than 95 percent of them renew, "expect the growth of ACOs to begin again in earnest as the follower organizations begin to choose successful models to emulate." If a large number of ACOs decline to renew, then "future growth will be weak, if it continues at all."[432]

Goldsmith has observed that in health policy, silver-bullet solutions have had "a transient high-concept appeal only to be revealed later not to work. Solving Medicare's problems is most likely going to require doing a dozen smaller things right, rather than one big thing."[433]

---

[431] Muhlestein, Health Affairs blog. http://healthaffairs.org/blog/2013/10/31/why-has-aco-growth-slowed/#!

[432] Muhlestein, Health Affairs blog. http://healthaffairs.org/blog/2013/10/31/why-has-aco-growth-slowed/#!

[433] Goldsmith, Health Affairs blog, August 15, 2013.

Section 9.3: Technical Appendix: The Accountable Care Organization (ACO)

9.3.1 The Accountable Care Organization (ACO)

Overview:

- As defined by the CMS, ACOs (under the MSSP) are "groups of doctors, hospitals, and other health care providers who come together voluntarily to deliver coordinated high-quality care to their Medicare patients. The goal of such coordinated care is to ensure that patients, especially the chronically ill, get the right care at the right time, while avoiding unnecessary duplication of services and preventing medical errors."[434]

- From the regulatory perspective, CMS further defines the ACO as:

  - a legal entity that is: recognized and authorized under applicable state law, as identified by a TIN; composed of an eligible group of ACO participants that works together to manage and coordinate care for Medicare FFS beneficiaries; and has established a mechanism for shared governance that provides all ACO participants with an appropriate proportionate control over the ACO's decision-making process:[435]

    - **ACO participant**: Medicare-enrolled provider of services and/or a supplier, as identified by a TIN.

    - **ACO provider/supplier:** a provider of services and/or a supplier that bills for items and services it furnishes to

---

[434] http://www.cms.gov/Medicare/Medicare-Fee-for-Service-Payment/ACO/index.html?redirect=/ACO/

[435] Page 67974: Federal Register/Vol. 76, No. 212/Wednesday, November 2, 2011, http://www.ncua.gov/Legal/Documents/Regulations/FIR20111027CommDevRev.pdf

Medicare beneficiaries under a Medicare billing number assigned to the TIN of an ACO participant in accordance with applicable Medicare rules and regulations.

- As of January 1, 2014, there are some 600 ACOs in the United States:

  - more than 200 commercial ACOs (as estimated by Leavitt Partners, a consultancy working in this area):[436]

    - Cigna has committed to expanding its ACO models (called collaborative accountable care (CAC)) to 100 by the end of 2014, citing reductions in annual cost growth of 50 percent for patients who are CAC members as compared to those covered by traditional FFS. Currently, Cigna has eighty-six CACs in thirty-one states serving 880,000 patients.[437]

  - 366 Medicare Model ACOs:[438]

    - 343 ACOs participating under the MSSP

    - 23 Pioneer Model ACOs under the CMI

- An estimated 5.3 million Medicare beneficiaries are now in an ACO, and, combined with the private sector, more than 428 hospitals have already signed up. Overall, some 14 percent of the US population is now being served by an ACO.

Legislative Background on the Medicare Shared Savings Program (MSSP):

- Under provisions contained in the Medicare Prescription Drug, Improvement, and Modernization Act of 2003 (MMA), Medicare implemented the Medicare Physician Group Practice (PGP) Demonstration and the Medicare Health Care Quality Demonstration as initial steps toward improving patient care through provider coordination and increased responsibility. Outcomes of these two

---

[436] http://leavittpartners.com/aco-publications/

[437] Cigna Newsroom, Accountable Care Organizations (ACOs), http://newsroom.cigna.com/KnowledgeCenter/ACO/

[438] http://www.cms.gov/Newsroom/MediaReleaseDatabase/Press-Releases/2013-Press-Releases-Items/2013-12-23.html

demonstration projects formed the building blocks for development of the ACO:

- o **The PGP saved** $137 million over five years **across ten participating physician groups, an average of $114 per year per beneficiary.**[439]

- The "father" of the ACO concept is Elliott Fisher, director of the Center for Health Policy Research at Dartmouth Medical School, who first introduced the term "accountable care organization" during a discussion at a public MedPAC meeting in 2006.[440]

- In December 2006, Fisher introduced his views on the basic concepts of the ACO in an article titled, "Creating Accountable Care Organizations: The Extended Hospital Staff." This seminal article introduced the ACO concept to the health care community as a more robust model of improving patient care through care coordination and shared accountability:[441]

  - o In January 2009, Fisher proposed a new approach to "help achieve more integrated and efficient care by fostering local organizational accountability for quality and costs through performance measurement and 'shared savings' payment reform." This proposal, in an article titled, "Fostering Accountable Care: Moving Forward in Medicare," outlined the fundamental structure of what would be adopted in the ACA as the MSSP.[442]

  - o During the development of the ACA, Fisher's ACO concept was so widely supported for inclusion by congressional Democrats that it was included in all three draft health care "reform" bills prepared in early 2009.

---

439 *Physician Group Practice Demonstration-Centers for Medicare,*
http://www.cms.gov/Medicare/Demonstration-
Projects/DemoProjectsEvalRpts/downloads/PGP_Fact_Sheet.pdf

440 *The History and Definition of the "Accountable Care Organization," PNHP,*
http://pnhpcalifornia.org/2010/10/the-history-and-definition-of-the-%E2%80%9Caccountable-care-
organization%E2%80%9D/

441 *E. S. Fisher, et al., Creating Accountable Care Organizations: The Extended Hospital*
Medical Staff, Health Affairs, December 11, 2007,
http://www.ncbi.nlm.nih.gov/pmc/articles/PMC2131738/

442 *E. S. Fisher, et al., Fostering Accountable Health Care: Moving Forward in Medicare, Health*
Affairs, March 16, 2009, http://www.ncbi.nlm.nih.gov/pubmed/19174383

The 2010 Affordable Care Act (ACA):

- Section 3022 of the ACA amended Title XVIII of the Social Security Act (SSA) (42 U.S.C. 1395 et seq.) by adding new Section 1899 to the SSA to establish a **shared savings program** (known as the **MSSP)** that:[443]
  - promotes accountability for a patient population
  - coordinates items and services under Medicare Parts A and B
  - encourages investment in infrastructure and redesigned care processes for high-quality and efficient service delivery
  - provides incentives for higher-value care

- Section 3022 identified the **ACO** as the primary mechanism through which the goals of the MSSP were to be achieved. Participation in the MSSP as an ACO is purely voluntary and the MSSP is structured to assist Medicare FFS to become an ACO.

  →KEY TERM: **ACO professional**: An ACO professional is defined as a physician (Doctor of Medicine or Osteopathy) or a Practitioner (Physician Assistants, Nurse Practitioners, and Clinical Nurse Specialists):

  - ACOs of various compositions are allowed under the MSSP, including:

    - ACO professionals (as defined above) in group practice arrangements:

    - networks of individual practices of ACO professionals

    - partnerships or joint venture arrangements between hospitals and ACO professionals

    - hospitals employing ACO professionals

    - critical access hospitals (CAHs) that bill under Method II*

    - rural health clinics (RHCs)*

---

[443] *Section 3022: Patient Protection and Affordable Care Act,*
http://www.gpo.gov/fdsys/pkg/BILLS-111hr3590enr/pdf/BILLS-111hr3590enr.pdf

- federally qualified health centers (FQHCs)*

- such other groups of providers of services and suppliers as the HHS secretary determines appropriate

*In the November 2, 2011 Final Rule, the HHS secretary added certain CAHs, FQHCs, and RHCs as eligible to participate in the MSSP, without participating as an ACO.

Note: To participate as an ACO, each of these groups must have a "shared governance mechanism" in place that provides ACO participants with at least 75 percent control of the governing body and includes beneficiary representation.

- For ACOs to qualify for participation in the MSSP and receive incentives in the form of a percentage of shared savings, the following requirements must be met:

  - The ACO must be willing to become accountable for the quality, cost, and overall care of the Medicare beneficiaries assigned to it.

  - The ACO must enter into an agreement with the HHS secretary to participate for no fewer than three years (agreement period).

  - The ACO must have a formal legal structure that allows it to receive and distribute payments for shared savings.

  - The ACO must have a minimum of 5,000 attributed Medicare beneficiaries.

  - The ACO must include primary care providers who are sufficient for the number of assigned Medicare beneficiaries.

  - ACOs must provide information necessary for beneficiary attribution and assessment of quality of care.

  - ACOs must have a leadership and management structure that includes clinical and administrative systems.

  - ACOs must define internal processes to:

    - promote evidence-based medicine and patient engagement

    - report quality and cost measures

- coordinate care, to include use of "enabling technology" such as telehealth and remote patient monitoring

  - ACOs must demonstrate "patient-centeredness" through use of patient and caregiver assessments or individualized care plans.

42 CFR Part 425

To provide specific guidelines for ACO participation, CMS finalized new rules under the ACA on October 20, 2011. These Final Rules were published in the Federal Register on November 2, 2011, as **42 CFR Part 425: Medicare Program; Medicare Shared Savings Program: Accountable Care Organizations; Final Rule:**[444]

- The goals of the MSSP, as described in Section 3022 of the ACA, were further defined to:

  - support attainment of the Institute of Healthcare Improvement's (IHI) "triple aim" for improving health care quality, which includes:

    - better care for individuals

    - better health for populations

    - lower per-capita cost of health care

  - and develop quality performance standards (QPS) for ACOs to determine their eligibility to receive payments for shared savings.

- The MSSP ACO model is different from HMOs and other managed-care models in several aspects:

  - participating Medicare FFS beneficiaries:

    - retain their right to see any physician of their choosing

    - are not required to enroll in an ACO, and are assigned where, and by whom, they have chosen to receive care during the course of a performance period

---

[444] *Federal Register/Vol. 76, No. 212/Wednesday, November 2, 2011, http://www.ncua.gov/Legal/Documents/Regulations/FIR20111027CommDevRev.pdf*

- o ACO provider participants are not subject to a capitated model of payment. They continue to bill and receive FFS payments for services provided.

- o In order for an ACO to share in any savings, specific quality standards must be met.

- o The purpose of the ACO is not to avoid at-risk patients, but rather to achieve savings through coordination and quality of care.

9.3.2 Three Medicare ACO Models:[445]

MSSP ACO:

- MSSP ACOs facilitate coordination and cooperation among providers to improve the quality of care for Medicare FFS beneficiaries and reduce unnecessary costs. Participants who meet quality measure standards and are successful in reducing costs may share in overall savings.

The Advance Payment ACO Model:[446]

- This model is a CMI initiative to provide additional support to physician-owned and rural providers participating in the MSSP who would benefit from additional start-up resources to build the necessary infrastructure, such as new staff or IT systems.

- Currently, a subset of thirty-five Advance Payment Model ACOs participates under the MSSP.

---

[445] *http://www.cms.gov/Medicare/Medicare-Fee-for-Service-Payment/sharedsavingsprogram/News.html*

[446] *Center for Medicare and Medicaid Innovations (Innovation Center), http://innovations.cms.gov/*

The Pioneer ACO Model:[447]

- The Pioneer ACO Model is a CMI initiative designed to support organizations with experience operating as ACOs or in similar arrangements designed to provide more coordinated care to beneficiaries at a lower cost to Medicare.

- The Pioneer ACO Model is designed to test the impact of different payment arrangements in helping these organizations achieve the goals of providing better care to patients and reducing Medicare costs.

- Thirty-two Pioneer ACOs were selected through an open and competitive process from a large applicant pool for operations, beginning January 1, 2012.

- In 2012 and 2013, the Pioneer Model tested a shared savings and shared losses payment arrangement with higher levels of reward and risk than in the MSSP. These shared savings were to be determined through comparisons against an ACO's benchmark, which is based on previous CMS expenditures for the group of patients aligned to the Pioneer ACO.

- Participants generally must have a minimum of 15,000 aligned beneficiaries, unless located in a rural area, in which case they are to have a minimum of 5,000 beneficiaries.

- In late 2013, nine organizations dropped from enrollment in the Pioneer ACO program. Five of these indicated that they would reapply for participation under the MSSP ACO model.[448] From the remaining twenty-three Pioneer ACOs (in 2014), those that have shown savings over the first two years will be eligible to move to a population-based payment model:

  o Population-based payment is a per-beneficiary per-month payment amount intended to replace some or all of the ACO's FFS payments with a prospective monthly payment.

[447] Pioneer ACO Fact Sheet (PDF), http://innovation.cms.gov/Files/fact-sheet/Pioneer-ACO-General-Fact-Sheet.pdf

[448] Pioneer ACO Model, http://innovation.cms.gov/initiatives/Pioneer-ACO-Model/

9.3.3 CMS Identification of MSSP ACO Participants[449]

Eligible Participants:

CMS identifies an ACO operationally as a "collection of Medicare-enrolled Tax Identification Numbers (TINs), defined as ACO participants." Additionally, ACOs that participate in the MSSP must meet state law requirements to operate in that state:

- The set of TINs participating in a given ACO would identify a network of independent practices that forms an ACO.

- Organizations applying to be an ACO must provide not only their TINs but **also** a list of associated National Provider Identifiers (NPIs) for all ACO professionals, including a list that separately identifies physicians who provide primary care:

    o ACOs must maintain, update, and annually report to CMS the TINs of its ACO participants and the NPIs associated with the ACO providers/suppliers.

- ACO participant TINs on which beneficiary assignment is based (TINs providing primary care services) will be exclusive to one ACO agreement in the MSSP.

- ACO participants (TINs) upon which beneficiary assignment is not dependent (TINS not providing primary services) are not required to be exclusive to a single MSSP ACO.

- Individual providers may participate in more than one ACO **as long as they bill under another TIN,** not associated with the ACO selected for participation.

---

[449] *Page 67808: Medicare Shared Savings Program, http://www.gpo.gov/fdsys/pkg/FR-2011-11-02/pdf/2011-27461.pdf*

Exclusions to MSSP ACO Participation[450]

- Section 1899(b)(4) of the SSA states that participants in other shared savings programs are excluded from participating in the MSSP ACO. These include:

  - a model tested or expanded under Section 1115A (CMI) that involves shared savings or any other program or demonstration project that involves such shared savings

  - the Independence At Home Medical Practice Pilot Program

- In the November 2, 2011 Final Rule, participation in the following programs would also exclude MSSP ACO participation:

  - the Independence at Home Medical Practice Demonstration Program

  - Medicare Health Care Quality (MHCQ) Demonstration Programs

  - the Multi-Payer Advanced Primary Care Practice (MAPCP) Demonstration

  - the PGP Transition Demonstration

- State initiatives to integrate care for dually eligible (Medicare/ Medicaid) individuals in partnership with the CMI **will not** preclude participation in the MSSP ACO.

- Applications to the MSSP that include TINs that are already participating in another program or demonstration involving shared savings will be rejected.

Participation Agreement:[451]

ACOs participating in the MSSP must enter into an agreement with the HHS secretary to participate in the program for not less than a three-year period (the

---

[450] Page 67830: Medicare Shared Savings Program, http://www.gpo.gov/fdsys/pkg/FR-2011-11-02/pdf/2011-27461.pdf

[451] Page 67807: Medicare Shared Savings Program, http://www.gpo.gov/fdsys/pkg/FR-2011-11-02/pdf/2011-27461.pdf

agreement period), although some agreements may be longer than three years:

- The participation agreement is signed by an executive of the ACO who also must certify that all entities providing services for the ACO would be compliant with ACO requirements.

- All ACO participants are to be provided with a copy of the participation agreement.

MSSP Participation Tracks 1 and 2:

Based on an ACO's willingness and readiness to accept risk, CMS provides for two tracks of participation during the agreement period:[452]

- **Track 1:** ACOs wanting to participate in the MSSP under the one-sided model of shared savings only, to earn up to 50 percent of shared savings. Track 1 is available as an option for the duration of the first agreement period **only,** for those ACOs needing more experience before taking on risk.

- **Track 2:** ACOs willing and able to take on performance-based risk in exchange for higher reward (up to 60 percent of shared savings) and willing and able to share in any losses. Track 2 participation is available for ACOs during **all a**greement periods and is **mandatory** beginning with an ACO's second agreement period.

*Note: Regardless of the track selected, the first year of the agreement period requires only successful **reporting** of quality measures.*

Required Number of Beneficiaries:

- The minimum number of assigned beneficiaries for ACO participation in the MSSP is 5,000:

    o Determination of the number of beneficiaries is based on historical assignment of beneficiaries to ACO participants in each of the

---

[452] *Page 67976: Medicare Shared Savings Program, http://www.gpo.gov/fdsys/pkg/FR-2011-11-02/pdf/2011-27461.pdf*

three years before the start of the agreement period, using the beneficiary attribution methodology described in Section 9.3.11 below.

- CMS established this number of assigned beneficiaries based on maintaining "statistical stability" for purposes of calculating per capita expenditures and assessing quality performance.

- If an ACO's assigned population falls below 5,000 during the course of the three-year agreement period, CMS will take the following actions:

  - CMS will issue a warning and place the ACO on a corrective action plan (CAP). During the year in which a warning was issued, the ACO would remain eligible for shared savings.

  - CMS will terminate an ACO's participation agreement if the ACO fails to meet the eligibility criteria of having more than 5,000 beneficiaries by the completion of the **next** performance year. The ACO would not be eligible to share in savings for that year.

  - CMS also reserves the right to review the status of the ACO while on the corrective action plan and terminate the agreement on the basis that the ACO no longer meets eligibility requirements.

- ACOs are required to have a number of primary care physicians who are "sufficient to the number of assigned beneficiaries:"

  - CMS determines sufficiency of primary care providers by examining historically assigned beneficiaries over a three-year benchmarking period using the ACO participant TINs. If the number of beneficiaries exceeds the 5,000 threshold for each year, Medicare considers the level of primary care to be sufficient.

9.3.4 Beneficiary Attribution to MSSP ACOs[453]

Overview:

- **Medicare FFS beneficiary**: an individual who is enrolled in the original Medicare FFS program under both Parts A and B and not enrolled in any of the following:

  - an MA plan under Part

  - HMOs or other entities with risk-sharing contracts with Medicare, as described under Section 1876 of the SSA

  - the Program of All-inclusive Care for the Elderly (PACE)

- Beneficiary assignment to an ACO is only for purposes of determining the population of Medicare FFS beneficiaries for whose care the ACO is accountable and determining whether an ACO has achieved savings.

- ➔IMPORTANT! **assignment to a particular ACO in no way restricts the rights of beneficiaries to exercise free choice in determining where to receive health services:**

  - Beneficiaries are notified that they have been assigned to a physician participating in an ACO and that the physician may receive compensation for providing cost-effective quality care.

  - Beneficiaries may "opt out" of ACO assignment.

  - Unlike managed-care restrictions, beneficiaries are not "locked in" to receiving care from only their assigned physician.

  - Whether or not the beneficiary chooses to receive care from an assigned ACO physician, the ACO remains accountable for total costs and quality of care for assigned beneficiaries.

- Medicare assigns beneficiaries in a preliminary manner at the beginning of a performance year based on most recent data available:

---

[453] *ACO Quality Measures and Performance Standards, CMS, http://www.cms.gov/Medicare/Medicare-Fee-for-Service-Payment/sharedsavingsprogram/Quality_Measures_Standards.html*

- ○ The assignment will be updated quarterly based on the most recent twelve months of data.

- ○ The final assignment is determined after the end of each performance year, based on data from the performance year.

Two-Step Beneficiary Attribution Process:

CMS employs a two-step attribution process for assignment of Medicare FFS beneficiaries who have had **at least one** primary care service with a physician who is a participant in an MSSP ACO:

Step 1: Identify **all primary care services** provided by **primary care physicians** during one of the following:

- the most recent twelve months (for purposes of preliminary prospective assignment and quarterly updates to the preliminary prospective assignment)

- or the performance year (for purposes of final assignment).

- **primary care physician:** a physician who has a primary specialty designation of internal medicine, general practice, family practice or geriatric medicine.

- **primary care services:** the set of services identified by the following Healthcare Common Procedure Coding System (HCPCS) codes:

  - ○ 99201 through 99215

  - ○ 99304 through 99340

  - ○ 99341 through 99350

  - ○ G0402 (the code for the Welcome to Medicare visit)

  - ○ and G0438 and G0439 (codes for the annual wellness visits)

The beneficiary is assigned to an ACO if the total allowed charges for primary care services furnished to the beneficiary by all the primary care physicians who are in the ACO are greater than the total allowed charges for primary care services furnished by primary care physicians who are:

- ACO providers/suppliers in any other ACO

- not affiliated with any ACO

- identified by a Medicare-enrolled TIN.

Step 2: This step considers the remainder of the beneficiaries who have received **at least one** primary care service from an ACO physician. The beneficiary will be assigned to an ACO if the allowed charges for primary care services furnished to the beneficiary **by all ACO professionals** who are ACO providers/suppliers in the ACO are greater than the allowed charges for primary care services furnished by:

- all ACO professionals who are ACO providers/suppliers in any other ACO

  - **ACO professional:** a physician (Doctor of Medicine or Osteopathy) or a practitioner (Physician Assistants, Nurse Practitioners, and Clinical Nurse Specialists) providing services to Medicare FFS beneficiaries.

- other physicians, Nurse Practitioners, Physician Assistants, or Clinical Nurse Specialists who are unaffiliated with an ACO and are identified by a Medicare-enrolled TIN

Note: Although this method does not necessarily assign the beneficiary to the entity that saw the patient most frequently, the beneficiary will be assigned to the entity that provided the highest complexity and intensity of primary care services. This method also results in the assignment of the responsibility for containing costs to the provider who generates the most costs.

9.3.5 Quality Measures and Reporting

Overview:

- To qualify to receive amounts of shared savings under the MSSP, participant ACOs must meet quality standards for measures of success in providing high-quality health care at the individual and population levels.

- Evaluation of ACO quality of care is made through the comparison of ACO performance on thirty-three quality measures against CMS-established benchmarks:

- o Measures are divided among four equally weighted domains:
    - Patient/Caregiver Experience
    - Care Coordination/Patient Safety
    - Preventive Health
    - At-Risk Populations
- Adopted measures include patient experience, outcomes, and evidence-based care processes.
- CMS selected measures to align with the "triple aim" of health care to provide:
    - o better care for individuals
    - o better health for populations
    - o lower growth in expenditures
- Reporting on quality measures associated with a given performance calendar year of the ACO agreement period will generally be done in the spring of the following calendar year. For example, an ACO will submit quality measures for the 2014 reporting period in early 2015.

2014 Quality Measures:[454]

For 2014, there are thirty-three individual quality measures, assigned for reporting under domains:

Table 2: MSSP ACO Quality Measures for 2014

DOMAIN	MEASURE	DESCRIPTION OF MEASURE
Patient/Caregiver Experience	ACO #1	Getting Timely Care, Appointments, and Information
Patient/Caregiver Experience	ACO #2	How Well Your Doctors Communicate

---

[454] Page 1156: CMS-1600-FC, http://www.gpo.gov/fdsys/pkg/FR-2013-12-10/pdf/2013-28696.pdf

DOMAIN	MEASURE	DESCRIPTION OF MEASURE
Patient/Caregiver Experience	ACO #3	Patient's Rating of Doctor
Patient/Caregiver Experience	ACO #4	Access to Specialists
Patient/Caregiver Experience	ACO #5	Health Promotion and Education
Patient/Caregiver Experience	ACO #6	Shared Decision-Making
Patient/Caregiver Experience	ACO #7	Health Status/Functional Status
Care Coordination/ Patient Safety	ACO #8	Risk-Standardized, All Conditions Readmissions
Care Coordination/ Patient Safety	ACO #9	Ambulatory Sensitive Condition (ASC) Admission: COPD or Asthma in Older Adults
Care Coordination/ Patient Safety	ACO #10	ASC Admission: Heart Failure
Care Coordination/ Patient Safety	ACO #11	Percent of PCPs Who Qualified for EHR Incentive Payment
Care Coordination/ Patient Safety	ACO #12	Medication Reconciliation
Care Coordination/ Patient Safety	ACO #13	Falls: Screening for Fall Risk
Preventive Health	ACO #14	Influenza Immunization
Preventive Health	ACO #15	Pneumococcal Vaccination
Preventive Health	ACO #16	Adult Weight-Screening and Follow-up
Preventive Health	ACO #17	Tobacco Use Assessment and Cessation Intervention
Preventive Health	ACO #18	Depression Screening
Preventive Health	ACO #19	Colorectal Screening
Preventive Health	ACO #20	Mammography Screening
Preventive Health	ACO #21	Proportion of Adults Who Had Blood Pressure Screened in Past Two Years
At-Risk Population: Diabetes	ACO #22– ACO #26	ACO #22: Hemoglobin A1c Control (HbA1c) (<8%) ACO #23: Low Density Lipoprotein (LDL) (<100mg/dl) ACO #24: Blood Pressure (BP) <140/90 ACO #25: Tobacco Non Use ACO #26: Aspirin Use
At-Risk Population: Diabetes	ACO #27	Percent of Beneficiaries With Diabetes Whose HbA1c is in Poor Control (>9%)

DOMAIN	MEASURE	DESCRIPTION OF MEASURE
At-Risk Population: Hypertension	ACO #28	Percent of Beneficiaries with Hypertension Whose BP< 140/90
At-Risk Population: Ischemic Vascular Disease (IVD)	ACO #29	Percent of Beneficiaries With IVD with Complete Lipid Profile and LDL Control < 100mg/dl
At-Risk Population: Ischemic Vascular Disease (IVD)	ACO #30	Percent of Beneficiaries With IVD Who Use Aspirin or Other Antithrombotic
At-Risk Population: Heart Failure (HF)	ACO #31	Beta-Blocker Therapy for LVSD
At-Risk Population: Coronary Artery Disease (CAD)	CAD Composite ACO #32–33	ACO #32. Drug Therapy for Lowering LDL Cholesterol ACO #33. ACE Inhibitor or ARB Therapy for Patients with CAD and Diabetes and/or LVSD

Note: Specifications for administration of the CG-CAHPS are contained in the 2014 Quality Performance Standards Narrative Measure Specifications document at: http://www.cms.gov/Medicare/Medicare-Fee-for-Service-Payment/sharedsavingsprogram/Quality_Measures_Standards.html

Quality Measures Data Sources:

- ACO performance on quality measures includes data reported/ collected from:

    o Medicare claims

    o clinical quality data reported by the GPRO web-based interface

    o **CG-CAHPS** patient experience surveys

    o the EHR incentive program

Quality Measures Data CMS-Extracted From Claims:

- For 2014, there are three quality measures contained in the Care Coordination/Patient Safety Domain, which rely on data that is extracted by CMS from Medicare Part A claims:

    o Risk-Standardized All Conditions Readmission

- o Ambulatory Sensitive Conditions (ASCs) Admissions: Chronic Obstructive Pulmonary Disease (COPD or Asthma in Older Adults
- o ASCs Admissions: Heart Failure (HF)

Quality Measures Reported by the CG-CAHPS:

- The CG-CAHPS survey is a global measure of patient assessment of the Patient/Caregiver Experience.

- For 2012 and 2013, CMS funded the collection of information for the CG-CAHPS for ACOs participating in MSSP. Beginning in 2014, ACOs will be responsible for selecting and paying for a CMS-certified vendor to administer the CG-CAHPS survey.

- The following seven components of the CG-CAHPS are included in the Patient/Caregiver Domain and are reportable for 2014–2015:

  - o Getting Timely Care, Appointments and Information
  - o How Well Your Provider Communicates
  - o Patient's Rating of Provider
  - o Access to Specialists
  - o Health Promotion and Education
  - o Shared Decision-Making
  - o Health Status/Functional Status

- **New for 2014–2015:** The seven Patient Experience of Care measures within the Patient Experience of Care Quality domain are now equally weighted (with a possible two points per measure) and the value of the patient experience of care domain is raised from four points to fourteen points.[455]

Note: Beginning in 2014, CMS will publicly report results of the CG-CAHPS survey on the Physician Compare website at the ACO level only. The initial reports will be based on 2013 reporting of CG-CAHPS surveys that will be conducted in early 2014.

---

[455] *Medicare Shared Savings Program Quality Measure Benchmarks, http://www.cms.gov/Medicare/Medicare-Fee-for-Service-Payment/sharedsavingsprogram/Downloads/MSSP-QM-Benchmarks.pdf*

Quality Measures Reported by the (GPRO) Web-based Interface:[456]

- Twenty-two of the thirty-three 2014 quality measures must be reported through the CMS GPRO web-based interface.

- In 2014, the ACO, on behalf of its ACO providers/suppliers (eligible professionals), must submit all of the ACO GPRO measures for purposes of the PQRS program to avoid a penalty payment adjustment of -2.0 percent under the MSSP for 2016.

- Individual eligible professionals (EPs) within the ACO may only participate under their ACO participant TIN as a group practice under the PQRS.

- If an ACO, on behalf of its individual ACO EPs, does not satisfactorily report required measures through the GPRO web-based interface in 2014, each ACO provider/supplier who is an EP will receive a payment adjustment of -2.0 percent in 2016 for all Medicare Part B covered professional services.

- Successful GPRO reporting in 2014 also qualifies the ACO participant TIN for the +.5 percent incentive payment adjustment under the PQRS program.

- Individual ACO participants who bill under another non-ACO TIN during a performance year must participate in PQRS reporting outside the ACO GPRO.

Note: For detailed information on the GPRO web-based interface, see Chapter 5: The Physician Quality Reporting System (PQRS, Process-Payments-Penalties).

Quality Measure Reported by EHR:

- One EHR-reportable quality measure is contained in the Care Coordination/Patient Safety Domain for 2014:

    - Percent of Primary Care Physicians Who Successfully Qualify for an EHR Incentive Payment.

---

[456] *Pages 67904–67909: Medicare Shared Savings Program, http://www.gpo.gov/fdsys/pkg/FR-2011-11-02/pdf/2011-27461.pdf*

9.3.6 Quality Measures Scoring for the 2014 MSSP ACO Program

Key Terms:

- **agreement period:** a three-year time frame is required by CMS for ACO participation in the MSSP. All ACOs must agree to participate for this period and may renew their application for another agreement period at the end of the three-year period.

- **benchmark:** a CMS-established measure performance rate an ACO must achieve to earn a corresponding number of quality points.

- **composite measure:** a clinical measure consisting of supporting individual component measures. One benchmark is established by CMS to apply to all individual component measures in determining the Total Composite Score.

- **domain:** a collection of related quality measures used to determine a total weighted domain score.

- **performance year:** the calendar year aligned with each year of the three-year ACO agreement period. Data is collected during the performance year to determine qualification for shared savings.

- **quality performance standard (QPS):** annual pay-for-reporting (P4R) or pay-for-performance (P4P) requirements for each quality measure. The QPS is aligned with each year of the ACO agreement period.

Scoring Overview:

- ACOs are required to completely and accurately report quality data on the thirty-three quality measures used to calculate and assess quality performance to qualify for shared savings under the MSSP program.

- The thirty-three quality measures of the 2014 MSSP ACO program are divided into four weighted domains composed of related measures:

  - Each domain is assigned a total possible point score, determined by individual measure scoring against a CMS-established benchmark.

- o For scoring purposes, there are twenty-six individual quality measures and two composite measures (which include five and two individual component measures, respectively).

- o CMS establishes a benchmark for each quality measure, against which individual ACO performance is evaluated:

  - ▪ For the two composite measures, CMS will establish a **single benchmark** that applies to **all** individual measures of the composite measure.

- Domain weighting and total points possible are shown below:

Table 3: Summary of 2014–2015 Quality Measures by Domain and Total Points[457]

DOMAIN	# OF INDIVIDUAL MEASURES	TOTAL MEASURES FOR SCORING PURPOSES	TOTAL POSSIBLE POINTS	DOMAIN WEIGHT
Patient/Caregiver Experience	7	seven measures of the individual survey module*	14	25%
Care Coordination/ Patient Safety	6	six measures (the EHR measure is double weighted to equal four points)	14	25%
Preventive Health	8	eight measures	16	25%
At-Risk Population	12	seven measures, including the five-component Diabetes Composite Measure and the two-component Coronary Artery Disease Composite	14	25%
Total in All Domains	33	28	58	100%

* CG-CAHPS patient experience survey

---

[457] *Medicare Shared Savings Program Quality Measure Benchmarks,* http://www.cms.gov/Medicare/Medicare-Fee-for-Service-Payment/sharedsavingsprogram/Downloads/MSSP-QM-Benchmarks.pdf

9.3.7 Annual Quality Performance Standards (QPS)[458]

Overview:

- ACOs are required to completely and accurately report quality data used to calculate and assess their quality performance according to an annual **QPS** for each year (performance year) of the three-year agreement period:

  - **The QPS** specifies measures considered under P4R or P4P for a given year of the three-year agreement period.

  - In the first performance year of the agreement period, ACOs are required to **only accurately report** (P4R) all measures performance to meet the annual QPS. CMS will not score any measures for ACOs reporting quality measures in their first year of the agreement period:

    - This first-year requirement allows ACOs to ramp up, invest in their infrastructure, engage ACO providers/suppliers, redesign care processes to capture and provide data back to their ACO providers/suppliers, and begin to transform care at the point of care.

  - During the second year of the agreement period, CMS will phase in performance scoring (P4P) against benchmarks for eight of thirty-three quality measures.

  - In the third year, performance scoring against benchmarks will be phased in for thirty-two of thirty-three quality measures.

  - The table below summarizes QPS requirements for 2014:

---

[458] *2013 Quality Performance Standards Narrative Measure Specifications, http://www.cms.gov/Medicare/Medicare-Fee-for-Service-Payment/sharedsavingsprogram/Downloads/ACO-NarrativeMeasures-Specs.pdf*

Table 4: Annual QPS Summary[459]

PERFORMANCE YEAR OF THE AGREEMENT PERIOD	PAY-FOR-REPORTING QUALITY MEASURES: REPORTED ONLY	PAY-FOR-PERFORMANCE QUALITY MEASURES: PERFORMANCE-SCORED	TOTAL QUALITY MEASURES
1	33	0	33
2	8	25	33
3	1	32	33

Note: *One measure (health status/functional status) remains as P4P for all years.*

- The table below summarizes 2014 quality measures to include domain assignment, method of reporting required, and annual QPS P4R and P4P requirements:

---

[459] *2013 Quality Performance Standards Narrative Measure Specifications,* http://www.cms.gov/Medicare/Medicare-Fee-for-Service-Payment/sharedsavingsprogram/Downloads/ACO-NarrativeMeasures-Specs.pdf

Table 5: <u>2014 Quality Measures Reporting Summary</u>[460]

Domain	ACO#	Measure Title	Method of Data Submission	P4P Phase-In PY1	P4P Phase-In PY2	P4P Phase-In PY3
Patient/Caregiver Experience	ACO #1	Getting Timely Care, Appointments, and Information	CAHPS Survey	R	P	P
Patient/Caregiver Experience	ACO #2	How Well Your Doctors Communicate	CAHPS Survey	R	P	P
Patient/Caregiver Experience	ACO #3	Patient's Rating of Doctor	CAHPS Survey	R	P	P
Patient/Caregiver Experience	ACO #4	Access to Specialists	CAHPS Survey	R	P	P
Patient/Caregiver Experience	ACO #5	Health Promotion and Education	CAHPS Survey	R	P	P
Patient/Caregiver Experience	ACO #6	Shared Decision-Making	CAHPS Survey	R	P	P
Patient/Caregiver Experience	ACO #7	Health Status/Functional Status	CAHPS Survey	R	R	R
Care Coordination/Patient Safety	ACO #8	Risk-Standardized, All Conditions Readmissions	Claims	R	R	P
Care Coordination/Patient Safety	ACO #9	Ambulatory Sensitive Condition (ASC) Admission: COPD or Asthma in Older Adults	Claims	R	P	P
Care Coordination/Patient Safety	ACO #10	ASC Admission: Heart Failure	Claims	R	P	P
Care Coordination/Patient Safety	ACO #11	Percent of PCPs who Qualified for EHR Incentive Payment	EHR Incentive Program Reporting	R	P	P
Care Coordination/Patient Safety	ACO #12	Medication Reconciliation	GPRO Web Interface	R	P	P
Care Coordination/Patient Safety	ACO #13	Falls: Screening for Fall Risk	GPRO Web Interface	R	P	P
Preventive Health	ACO #14	Influenza Immunization	GPRO Web Interface	R	P	P
Preventive Health	ACO #15	Pneumococcal Vaccination	GPRO Web Interface	R	P	P
Preventive Health	ACO #16	Adult Weight-Screening and Follow-up	GPRO Web Interface	R	P	P
Preventive Health	ACO #17	Tobacco Use Assessment and Cessation Intervention	GPRO Web Interface	R	P	P
Preventive Health	ACO #18	Depression Screening	GPRO Web Interface	R	P	P
Preventive Health	ACO #19	Colorectal Screening	GPRO Web Interface	R	R	P
Preventive Health	ACO #20	Mammography Screening	GPRO Web Interface	R	R	P
Preventive Health	ACO #21	Proportion of Adults who had Blood Pressure screened in past 2 years	GPRO Web Interface	R	R	P
At-Risk Population - Diabetes	ACO #22- ACO #26	ACO #22: Hemoglobin A1c Control (HbA1c) (<8%) ACO #23: Low Density Lipoprotein (LDL) (<100mg/dl) ACO #24: Blood Pressure (BP) <140/90 ACO #25: Tobacco Non Use ACO #26: Aspirin Use	GPRO Web Interface	R	P	P
At-Risk Population- Diabetes	ACO #27	Percent of beneficiaries with diabetes whose HbA1c is in poor control (>9%)	GPRO Web Interface	R	P	P
At-Risk Population- Hypertension	ACO #28	Percent of beneficiaries with hypertension whose BP< 140/90	GPRO Web Interface	R	P	P
At-Risk Population – Ischemic Vascular Disease (IVD)	ACO #29	Percent of beneficiaries with IVD with complete lipid profile and LDL control < 100mg/dl	GPRO Web Interface	R	P	P
At-Risk Population - – Ischemic Vascular Disease (IVD)	ACO #30	Percent of beneficiaries with IVD who use Aspirin or other antithrombotic	GPRO Web Interface	R	P	P
At-Risk Population – Heart Failure (HF)	ACO #31	Beta-Blocker Therapy for LVSD	GPRO Web Interface	R	P	P
At-Risk Population – Coronary Artery Disease (CAD)	CAD Composite ACO #32 -33	ACO #32. Drug Therapy for Lowering LDL Cholesterol ACO #33. ACE Inhibitor or ARB Therapy for Patients with CAD and Diabetes and/or LVSD	GPRO Web Interface	R	R	P

*P4P – Pay for performance   R- Reporting Only   P-Measures Reported and Performance Scored

---

[460] *2013 Quality Performance Standards Narrative Measure Specifications, http://www.cms.gov/Medicare/Medicare-Fee-for-Service-Payment/sharedsavingsprogram/Downloads/ACO-NarrativeMeasures-Specs.pdf*

596

9.3.8 2014–2015 Quality Measures Benchmarks[461]

Overview:

- In the 2014 IPPS Final Rule, CMS finalized a proposal that requires:

    - Benchmarks for the 2014 reporting year to be determined in advance, using data submitted in 2013 for the 2012 reporting year.

- The benchmarks established for 2014 would be used for two reporting years (specifically, the 2014 and 2015 reporting years).

- Benchmarks discussed below apply to MSSP ACOs whose second or third performance years of their three-year agreement period occur in 2014 or 2015:

    - The QPS for the first performance year requires only **reporting** of quality measures and benchmark comparison does not apply.

    - The quality measure data collected from surveys is administered to the larger Medicare FFS population, including beneficiaries participating in P4P demonstrations.

Data Sources for Individual Measures Benchmarks:

- Benchmarks for most measures in the Care Coordination/Patient Safety, Preventive Health and At-Risk Population domains were established using all available FFS data from CY2012 collected under the PQRS and reported in 2013. Data sources include:

    - data collected from ACOs participating in the MSSP and the Pioneer ACO Model, and other groups that satisfactorily reported data through the PQRS GPRO web-based interface

---

[461] *Medicare Shared Savings Program Quality Measure Benchmarks, http://www.cms.gov/Medicare/Medicare-Fee-for-Service-Payment/sharedsavingsprogram/Downloads/MSSP-QM-Benchmarks.pdf*

- o data collected from EPs and group practices eligible for the PQRS incentive payment reporting through all available submission mechanisms for the PQRS, including, for example, claims, registry, EHR, and measures group

- Benchmarks for measures of the Care Coordination/Patient Safety domain were determined as follows:

  - o benchmarks calculated using 2012 Medicare FFS claims data using TIN-level data for physicians and groups who had at least twenty cases:

    - ACO #8 All-Condition Readmission Measure

    - ACO #9 Ambulatory Sensitive Condition Admissions Measure for Chronic Obstructive Pulmonary Disease (COPD) or Asthma in Older Adults

    - ACO #10 Ambulatory Sensitive Condition Admissions Measure for Heart Failure

  - o For the EHR measure (ACO #11), results from MSSP and Pioneer ACO Model are used.

- Benchmarks for measures in the Patient/Caregiver Experience domain were developed as follows:

  - o Benchmarks were developed based on survey data collected from beneficiaries with FFS Medicare in **2013** regarding their care experiences during CY2012. These data include:

    - initiatives by beneficiaries assigned to ACOs participating in the MSSP or the Pioneer ACO Model

    - responses to CMS's Medicare FFS CAHPS survey by beneficiaries with FFS Medicare, including beneficiaries receiving services under FFS demonstrations

    Note: CMS has not defined a benchmark for the ACO #7 Health Status/Functional Status measure of the Patient/Caregiver Experience domain because the measure remains P4P in all performance years of an ACO's agreement period.

Scoring for Individual Quality Measures Points:

In the November 2, 2011 Final Rule, CMS established a minimum attainment level of ACO measure performance against benchmarks (lower threshold) required to earn quality points. The minimum threshold was set at a national flat percentage rate of 30 percent **or** the national 30th percentile level of performance for the national FFS rates.[462]

Benchmarks Established Using the National Flat Percentage Rate:

In the November 2, 2011 Final Rule, CMS specified that for any measure benchmark for which the performance at the 60th percentile was **equal to or greater** than 80 percent for individual measures, benchmarks would be set using a flat national percentage rate:

- This scoring method allows ACOs with high scores to earn maximum or near-maximum quality points while allowing room for improvement and rewarding that improvement in subsequent years.

- Quality points are earned based on a sliding scale of performance (see Table 8).

- Attainment percentiles for scoring begin at the 30th percentile threshold and increase by 10 percentile increments up to the 90th+ percentile.

- For 2014, there are nine measures with benchmarks established under the national flat rate (see Table 7).

- An example of the application of the national flat rate follows in Table 6:

---

[462] *Page 67984: Federal Register/Vol. 76, No. 212/Wednesday, November 2, 2011, http://www.ncua.gov/Legal/Documents/Regulations/FIR20111027CommDevRev.pdf*

Table 6: Methodology for Setting Benchmarks using National Flat Percentages[463]

PERCENTILE	30TH	40TH	50TH	60TH	70TH	80TH	90TH
performance rates using all available FFS data	85.83	86.21	86.76	87.15	87.65	88.21	89.23
revised benchmark using flat percentages when the 60th percentile is 80 percent or more	30.00	40.00	50.00	60.00	70.00	80.00	90.00
quality points earned by the ACO*	1.10	1.25	1.40	1.55	1.70	1.85	2.00

*Point assigned would be double for the EHR measure

Note: *CMS will also use the national flat percentages when data are unavailable, inadequate or unreliable to set quality performance benchmarks.*

Benchmarks Established Using the National Fee-for-Service (FFS) Rate:

- In the 2014 Final IPPS Rule, CMS finalized establishment of national FFS benchmarks for quality measures during 2014–2015 using a national sample of all available and applicable Medicare FFS claims data for 2012 (reported in 2013) to include:

  - quality data reported through the PQRS by physicians and groups of physicians (through both the GPRO tool and other quality reporting mechanisms)

  - quality measure data calculated from Medicare claims data submitted by physicians and groups of physicians

  - **new for 2014–2015:** quality data reported by MSSP ACOs, including ACOs participating in the Pioneer ACO Model for 2014–2015 and subsequent years[464]

---

[463] *Page 1147: CMS-1600-FC, http://www.gpo.gov/fdsys/pkg/FR-2013-12-10/pdf/2013-28696.pdf*
[464] *Page 1145: CMS-1600-FC, http://www.gpo.gov/fdsys/pkg/FR-2013-12-10/pdf/2013-28696.pdf*

- In the 2014 Final IPPS Rule, CMS also did not finalize a proposal to use MA data alone or in combination with FFS data in the short term. CMS intends to revisit the policy of using MA data in future rule making.

- ACO performance against National FFS benchmarks will be measured in a graduated fashion (sliding scale), with points assigned to attainment of each graduation.

- National FFS benchmarks are established on a percentile basis, beginning with 30 percent attainment of the full benchmark, up to 90+ percent attainment.

- The 2014 and 2015 quality measure benchmarks used for determination of MSSP ACO quality performance are shown in Table 7 below:

Table 7: 2014–2015 MSSP ACO Quality Measures Benchmarks[465]

ACO# and Domain	ACO #	Measure Title	30th Perc.	40th Perc.	50th Perc.	60th Perc.	70th Perc.	80th Perc.	90th Perc.
Patient/Caregiver Experience	ACO #1	Getting Timely Care, Appointments, and Information	30.00	40.00	50.00	60.00	70.00	80.00	90.00
Patient/Caregiver Experience	ACO #2	How Well Your Doctors Communicate	30.00	40.00	50.00	60.00	70.00	80.00	90.00
Patient/Caregiver Experience	ACO #3	Patient's Rating of Doctor	30.00	40.00	50.00	60.00	70.00	80.00	90.00
Patient/Caregiver Experience	ACO #4	Access to Specialists	30.00	40.00	50.00	60.00	70.00	80.00	90.00
Patient/Caregiver Experience	ACO #5	Health Promotion and Education	54.71	55.59	56.45	57.63	58.22	59.09	60.71
Patient/Caregiver Experience	ACO #6	Shared Decision-Making	72.87	73.37	73.91	74.51	75.25	75.82	76.71
Patient/Caregiver Experience	ACO #7	Health Status/Functional Status	N/A	N/A	N/A	N/A	N/A	N/A	N/A
Care Coordination/Patient Safety	ACO #8	Risk-Standardized, All Conditions Readmissions	16.62	16.41	16.24	16.08	15.91	15.72	15.45
Care Coordination/Patient Safety	ACO #9	Ambulatory Sensitive Condition (ASC) Admission: COPD or Asthma in Older Adults	1.24	1.02	0.84	0.66	0.52	0.36	0.00
Care Coordination/Patient Safety	ACO #10	ASC Admission: Heart Failure	1.22	1.03	0.88	0.72	0.55	0.40	0.18
Care Coordination/Patient Safety	ACO #11	Percent of PCPs who Qualified for EHR Incentive Payment	51.35	59.70	65.38	70.20	76.15	84.85	90.91
Care Coordination/Patient Safety	ACO #12	Medication Reconciliation	30.00	40.00	50.00	60.00	70.00	80.00	90.00
Care Coordination/Patient Safety	ACO #13	Falls: Screening for Fall Risk	17.12	22.35	27.86	35.55	42.32	51.87	73.38
Preventive Health	ACO #14	Influenza Immunization	29.41	39.04	48.29	58.60	75.93	97.30	100.00
Preventive Health	ACO #15	Pneumococcal Vaccination	23.78	39.94	54.62	70.66	84.55	96.64	100.00
Preventive Health	ACO #16	Adult Weight-Screening and Follow-up	40.79	44.73	49.93	66.35	91.34	99.09	100.00
Preventive Health	ACO #17	Tobacco Use Assessment and Cessation Intervention	30.00	40.00	50.00	60.00	70.00	80.00	90.00
Preventive Health	ACO #18	Depression Screening	5.31	10.26	16.84	23.08	31.43	39.97	51.81
Preventive Health	ACO #19	Colorectal Screening	19.81	33.93	48.49	63.29	78.13	94.73	100.00
Preventive Health	ACO #20	Mammography Screening	28.59	42.86	54.64	65.66	76.43	88.31	99.56
Preventive Health	ACO #21	Proportion of Adults who had Blood Pressure screened in past 2 years	30.00	40.00	50.00	60.00	70.00	80.00	90.00
Diabetes Composite: At-Risk Population - Diabetes	Diabetes Composite: ACO #22- ACO # 26	ACO #22: Hemoglobin A1c Control (HbA1c) (<8%) ACO #23: Low Density Lipoprotein (LDL) (<100mg/dl) ACO #24: Blood Pressure (BP) <140/90 ACO #25: Tobacco Non Use ACO #26: Aspirin Use	17.39	21.20	23.48	25.78	28.17	31.37	36.50
At-Risk Population- Diabetes	ACO #27	Percent of beneficiaries with diabetes whose HbA1c is in poor control (>9%)	70.00	60.00	50.00	40.00	30.00	20.00	10.00
At-Risk Population- Hypertension	ACO #28	Percent of beneficiaries with hypertension whose BP< 140/90	60.00	63.16	65.69	68.03	70.89	74.07	79.65
At-Risk Population – Ischemic Vascular Disease (IVD)	ACO #29	Percent of beneficiaries with IVD with complete lipid profile and LDL control < 100mg/dl	35.00	42.86	51.41	57.14	61.60	67.29	78.81
At-Risk Population - – Ischemic Vascular Disease (IVD)	ACO #30	Percent of beneficiaries with IVD who use Aspirin or other antithrombotic	45.44	56.88	68.25	78.77	85.00	91.48	97.91
At-Risk Population – Heart Failure (HF)	ACO #31	Beta-Blocker Therapy for LVSD	30.00	40.00	50.00	60.00	70.00	80.00	90.00
At-Risk Population – Coronary Artery Disease (CAD) Composite	CAD Composite ACO #32 ACO #33	ACO #32. Drug Therapy for Lowering LDL Cholesterol ACO #33. ACE Inhibitor or ARB Therapy for Patients with CAD and Diabetes and/or LVSD	54.08	61.44	66.11	69.96	72.32	76.40	79.84

Note: *Shaded areas indicate measures with benchmarks determined by the national flat percentage rate as described above.*

Note: *The diabetes and CAD composites are considered to be "all-or-nothing" measures and all sub-measures would need to be reported in order to earn any credit for these measures.*

---

[465] *Medicare Shared Savings Program Quality Measure Benchmarks, http://www.cms.gov/Medicare/Medicare-Fee-for-Service-Payment/sharedsavingsprogram/Downloads/MSSP-QM-Benchmarks.pdf*

9.3.9 Total Quality Scoring Methodology[466]

Individual Quality Measures Scoring:

- Scoring will be accomplished for years two and three of the ACO agreement period. The first year of the agreement period only requires informational reporting of all measures to qualify for shared savings:

  - One hundred percent reporting of quality measures during the first year of the agreement period qualifies ACOs to receive 100 percent of the shared-savings percentage assigned to their chosen model (Track 1: one-sided: 50 percent or Track 2: two-sided: 60 percent).

  - For years two and three of the agreement period, the percent of potential shareable savings will vary based on the ACO's performance on the measures as compared with the measure benchmarks under P4P scoring.

- Quality points are earned by ACOs for each of the quality measures by achieving a certain level of performance as measured against the benchmark standard for that measure:

  - A maximum of two points may be earned for each measure **except for** the EHR measure, which is worth up to four points. This "double-weighting" of the EHR measure is to provide additional incentive for greater levels of EHR adoption and use by physicians and groups.

  - Quality points are earned on a "sliding scale" that establishes an upper and lower threshold for each benchmark (see Table 8, below).

- Performance below the minimum attainment level for a measure will receive zero points for that measure.

---

[466] *Pages 67896–67900: Medicare Shared Savings Program, http://www.gpo.gov/fdsys/pkg/FR-2011-11-02/pdf/2011-27461.pdf*

- Performance equal to or greater than the minimum attainment level for a measure will earn points on a sliding scale based on the level of performance.

- Those measures designated as all-or-nothing measures (CAD and Diabetes Composite measures) will receive the maximum available points if all criteria are met and zero points if one or more of the criteria are not met.

- Performance at or above 90 percent or the 90th percentile of the performance benchmark earns the maximum points available for the measure.

Sliding Scale Measures Scoring:

Scoring for individual measures will be accomplished through the use of a sliding scale, as illustrated in Table 8.

Table 8: Sliding Scale Measure Scoring Approach[467]

ACO PERFORMANCE LEVEL	QUALITY POINTS (ALL MEASURES EXCEPT EHR)	EHR MEASURE QUALITY POINTS
90+ percentile FFS Rate **or** 90+ percent national flat rate	**2.00 points**	**4.0 points**
80+ percentile FFS Rate **or** 90+ percent national flat rate	**1.85 points**	**3.7 points**
70+ percentile FFS Rate **or** 90+ percent national flat rate	**1.70 points**	**3.4 points**
60+ percentile FFS Rate **or** 90+ percent national flat rate	**1.55 points**	**3.1 points**
50+ percentile FFS Rate **or** 90+ percent national flat rate	**1.40 points**	**2.8 points**
40+ percentile FFS Rate **or** 90+ percent national flat rate	**1.25 points**	**2.5 points**
30+ percentile FFS Rate **or** 90+ percent national flat rate	**1.10 points**	**2.2 points**
<30 percentile FFS Rate **or** <30+ percent national flat rate	**no points**	**no points**

[467] Pages 67896–67900: Medicare Shared Savings Program, http://www.gpo.gov/fdsys/pkg/FR-2011-11-02/pdf/2011-27461.pdf

Quality Domain Scoring:[468]

- **Step 1:** Scoring for individual quality measures will be made according to the sliding scale in Table 8 for all measures within a domain.

- **Step 2:** Individual measure scores are then summed and divided by the total points available for the domain to produce an overall domain score of the percentage of points earned versus points available.

- **Step 3**: The percentage score for each domain will be summed and divided by four (reflecting the equal weighting of the domains) to determine the Aggregated Domain Score (ADS) (also known as the final sharing rate).

- The ADS will then be applied to the Maximum Sharing rate (MSR) or the Maximum Loss Rate (MLR) under either the one-sided or two-sided options for purposes of determining its shared savings payment or share of losses penalty:

  - **application of the ADS for shared savings**: If CMS determines that savings are available for sharing under the MSSP, the ADS percentage is applied to the maximum rate of shared savings to determine the percent of shared savings available to the ACO (Track 1 (one-sided model) maximum shared savings 50 percent; Track 2 (two-sided model) 60 percent).

  - **application of the ADS for shared losses**: The ADS percentage, minus 1.00, is multiplied by the amount of excess expenditure (loss) above a fixed minimum loss rate benchmark percentage. The results represent the ACO's portion of loss to be repaid to CMS.

---

468 Pages 67896–67900: Medicare Shared Savings Program, http://www.gpo.gov/fdsys/pkg/FR-2011-11-02/pdf/2011-27461.pdf

Table 9 provides an example of the calculation of an ADS:

Table 9: Example of Aggregated Domain Score Calculation

DOMAIN	NUMBER OF INDIVIDUAL MEASURES	TOTAL POSSIBLE QUALITY POINTS	TOTAL EARNED QUALITY POINTS	UNWEIGHTED DOMAIN SCORE (TOTAL POINTS EARNED/TOTAL POSSIBLE POINTS)	AGGREGATE WEIGHTED DOMAIN SCORE (25% EACH DOMAIN)
Patient/Caregiver Experience	7	14	14	1.0000	.25
Care Coordination/ Patient Safety	6	14	11.25	.8035	.2008
Preventive Health	8	16	12.74	.7963	.1990
At-Risk Population	12	14	13.45	.9607	.2401
Total in All Domains	33	58	51.44	3.5605	.89 or 89%

Note: The ADS is used to calculate shared savings/losses as follows:

- **shared savings**: The ADS of .89 indicates that the ACO would receive 89 percent of up to 50 percent of the total savings generated by the ACO under the Track 1 one-sided model or 89 percent of 60 percent of the total savings generated by the ACO under the Track 2 two-sided risk model.

- **shared losses:** Using the ADS of .89 minus 1.00 (-.11 percent) equals the percentage of shared losses that the ACO must repay to CMS.

Minimum Attainment Levels:[469]

- ACOs must achieve the minimum attainment threshold on at least 70 percent of the measures in each domain in order to continue in the program.

---

[469] *Pages 67896–67900: Medicare Shared Savings Program, http://www.gpo.gov/fdsys/pkg/FR-2011-11-02/pdf/2011-27461.pdf*

- If an ACO **fails to achieve** the minimum attainment level on at least 70 percent of the measures in each domain:
  - ○ CMS will give the ACO a warning with an opportunity to resubmit and reevaluate the following year.
  - ○ If the ACO continues to underperform in the following year, the agreement would be terminated.
  - ○ In any year that an ACO scores a zero for an entire measure domain, it would not be eligible to share in any savings generated.
  - ○ If an ACO fails to report one or more measures:
    - ▪ CMS will send the ACO a written request to submit the required data by a specified date and to provide a reasonable explanation for its delay in reporting the required information.
    - ▪ If the ACO fails to report by the requested deadline or does not provide a reasonable explanation for delayed reporting, CMS would immediately terminate the ACO for failing to report quality measures and it would be disqualified from sharing in any savings.

→IMPORTANT! *If an ACO fails to completely and accurately report the EHR measure, the ACO would miss the 70 percent cut-off for the Care Coordination domain, since this measure is double weighted for both scoring purposes and for purposes of determining poor performance.*

9.3.10 Determination of Shared Savings:[470]

Five-Step Process:

CMS evaluates ACO performance through a comparison of annual average per capita Medicare expenditures against a benchmark established for the ACO at the beginning of the three-year agreement period. If the ACO's average

---

[470] *Pages 67927–67936: Medicare Shared Savings Program, http://www.gpo.gov/fdsys/pkg/FR-2011-11-02/pdf/2011-27461.pdf*

per capita expenditure level is below the benchmark by a predetermined amount, based on the number of assigned beneficiaries, the ACO will be qualified to share in the resulting savings, as long as the ACO successfully met the quality standards for that year. To determine shared savings amounts, CMS takes the following actions:

- **Step 1:** Determine the ACO-specific per capita benchmark for Medicare Parts A and B expenditures for assigned beneficiaries.

- **Step 2:** Compare the benchmark to the ACO's assigned beneficiary average per capita expenditure rate in the performance year to determine savings.

- **Step 3:** Compare percent of savings to the appropriate minimum savings rate (MSR) to determine ACO eligibility to share in savings.

- **Step 4:** Determine the appropriate sharing rate for ACOs that have realized savings against the benchmark, met or exceeded the MSR, and met QRS.

- **Step 5:** Test the final savings amount against the sharing cap (payment limit) established for the appropriate ACO participation track.

Step 1: Determine the ACO-Specific Per Capita Benchmark for Medicare Parts A and B

Expenditures for Assigned Beneficiaries:

- The shared savings benchmark is an ACO-specific projection by CMS of average per capita Medicare Parts A and B expenditures incurred during the three-year agreement period of an ACO participating in the MSSP. It is annually adjusted and updated for national Medicare growth trends, patient case mix, severity, and number of assigned beneficiaries.

- To determine the benchmark, CMS takes the following actions:
    - Compute the per capita Medicare Parts A and B FFS benchmark expenditures for an individual ACO participating in the MSSP:
        - CMS will calculate a fixed "historical" benchmark that is annually adjusted for historical growth and beneficiary characteristics in each year of the three-year ACO agreement period.

608

- ○ CMS determines the per capita Part A and B FFS expenditures for beneficiaries that would have been assigned to the ACO in **any** of the three most recent years prior to the agreement period using the ACO participants' TINs identified at the start of the agreement period.

- ○ CMS calculates payment amounts included in Part A and B FFS claims using three-month claims run-out (claims to be processed ninety days after the completion of a reporting calendar year). Payment calculations also consider individual beneficiary identifiable payments made under CMS demonstration, pilot or time-limited programs:

  - Calculations **exclude** indirect medical education (IME) and disproportionate share hospital (DSH) payments in setting the shared-savings benchmark.

  - In determining the average per capita expenditure benchmark, CMS performs a separate expenditure calculation for each of the following populations of beneficiaries: end-stage renal disease (ESRD); disabled; aged/dual eligible Medicare and Medicaid beneficiaries; and aged/non-dual eligible Medicare and Medicaid beneficiaries.

  - CMS will adjust expenditures for changes in severity and case mix using prospective hierarchical condition code (HCC) risk scores.

  - To minimize variations in calculations created by exceptionally large claims, CMS truncates the total amount considered of an assigned beneficiary's total annual Part A and B FFS per capita expenditures at the 99th percentile of national Medicare FFS expenditures as determined for each benchmark year. In the November 2, 2011 Final Rule, CMS estimated this amount to be approximately $100,000.

- Using CMS Office of the Actuary national Medicare expenditure data for each of the years making up the historical benchmark, CMS determines national growth rates and trends expenditures (for each benchmark year (BY1 and BY2) to the third benchmark year (BY3) dollars) forward to current dollars. Per capita costs are then averaged using the weights described below to obtain the benchmark for the first agreement period:

- To account for different beneficiary characteristics in trending expenditures forward, CMS makes separate calculations for expenditure categories for each of the following populations of beneficiaries: ESRD; disabled, aged/dual eligible Medicare and Medicaid beneficiaries; and aged/non-dual eligible Medicare and Medicaid beneficiaries.

- CMS uses this method of utilizing category-specific data in creating the benchmark to increase the accuracy and relevance of the benchmark to the assigned beneficiary population.

- CMS will apply weights to each year of the benchmark using the following percentages:
  - BY3 (most recent year) at 60 percent
  - BY2 at 30 percent
  - BY1 at 10 percent

- Based on the weighted benchmark calculations, CMS determines the agreement period benchmark used (with annual adjustments) to determine annual shared savings/ losses.

Updating and Adjusting the Initial Agreement Period Benchmark:

To reflect annual changes in care-related expenditures and assigned beneficiary composition, CMS will update and adjust the agreement period benchmark annually:

- **assigned beneficiary adjustment**: CMS estimates that an ACO may have as many as 25 percent of beneficiaries change during a given year. As such, the ACO's benchmark may be adjusted annually to account for the addition and removal of ACO participants or ACO providers/suppliers during the term of the agreement period.

- **growth in national expenditures adjustment:** To account for annual increases or decreases in care-related expenditures, CMS will update the benchmark by the projected absolute amount of growth in national per capita expenditures for Parts A and B services under the original Medicare FFS program using data from the CMS Office of the Actuary:

- To develop an appropriately updated benchmark that reflects the different expected growth rates for separate types of beneficiaries, CMS makes expenditure calculations for separate categories for each of the following populations: ESRD; disabled; aged/dual eligible Medicare and Medicaid beneficiaries; and aged/non-dual eligible Medicare and Medicaid beneficiaries.

- **resetting the benchmark**: An ACO's benchmark will be recalculated using the methodology described above and reset at the start of each agreement period.

Step 2: Compare the benchmark to the ACO's assigned beneficiary average per capita expenditure rate in the performance year to determine savings:

- During each year of an agreement period, CMS will determine the average per capita expenditure rate for Medicare Parts A and B FFS beneficiaries assigned to an ACO.

- This average ACO per capita expenditure rate will be compared to the benchmark average per capita rate to determine participation in savings or losses.

Step 3: Compare percent of savings to the appropriate MSR to determine ACO eligibility to share in savings:

- The **minimum savings rate (MSR)** is a specified percentage level of savings established **below** the benchmark that an ACO must meet or exceed to qualify for shared savings. The MSR is set below the benchmark to account for normal variation in expenditures and is specified by a sliding scale based on the number of assigned beneficiaries for Track 1 ACOs and by a flat rate for Track 2 ACOs:

  - **Track 1**: one-sided model: savings only, no risk

  - **Track 2**: two-sided model: participates in shared savings and accepts risk for losses

- In order to qualify for a shared savings payment, the ACO's average per capita Medicare expenditures for the performance year must be below the applicable updated benchmark by at least the **MSR** established for the ACO.

- ACOs that generate savings that are below the benchmark, but do not meet the MSR, will not qualify for shared savings.

- CMS will establish the applicable MSRs based on the adjusted number of assigned beneficiaries for a given year:

    o The MSR for Track 2 (two-sided model) ACO participants has been established in the November 2, 2011 Final Rule as **2.0 percent**, regardless of the number of assigned beneficiaries. That is, the average per capita expenditure level for Track 2 ACOs in a given year must be at least 2.0 percent **less** than the benchmark in order to qualify for shared savings.

    o The MSR for Track 1 (one-sided model) ACO participants is based upon the number of Medicare FFS beneficiaries assigned to an ACO according to the following sliding scale:

Table 10: Minimum Savings Rate by Number of Assigned Beneficiaries (One-Sided Model)[471]

| Number of Assigned Beneficiaries | RANGE OF MINIMUM SAVINGS RATES (MSRS)* | |
	MSRs for the Minimum Number of Assigned Beneficiaries	MSRs for the Maximum Number of Assigned Beneficiaries
5,000–5,999	3.9	3.6
6,000–6,999	3.6	3.4
7,000–7,999	3.4	3.2
8,000–8,999	3.2	3.1
9,000–9,999	3.1	3.0
10,000–14,999	3.0	2.7
15,000–19,999	2.7	2.5

---

[471] Page 67928: Medicare Shared Savings Program, http://www.gpo.gov/fdsys/pkg/FR-2011-11-02/pdf/2011-27461.pdf

20,000–49,999	2.5	2.2
50,000–59,999	2.2	2.0
60,000+	2.0	2.0

CMS will establish MSRs between the minimum and maximum rates based on the actual adjusted number of assigned beneficiaries for a given year.

- The MSR, in combination with the savings rate, will determine the amount of shared savings that an ACO can receive. For example, fewer savings would be shared if the MSR were set closer to the benchmark (i.e., a 2 percent MSR). Conversely, shared savings would be higher if the MSR were set further below the benchmark (i.e., a 3.9 percent MSR).

Step 4: Determine the appropriate sharing rate for ACOs that have realized savings against the benchmark, met or exceeded the MSR, and met quality reporting standards (QRS):

Sharing Rate:

The sharing rate is a percentage of the difference between the annually adjusted agreement period benchmark and the estimated ACO average per capita Medicare expenditures for a given year of the agreement period, which may be paid to the ACO as shared savings. The sharing rate represents the total "potential" for shared savings and the remainder of the shared amount is to be retained by CMS:

- To participate in shared savings, an ACO must have met the annual quality standards.

- The sharing rate has been established by CMS and the applicable percentage is determined by the election of the ACO to participate the MSSP through:

  - **Track 1** (one-sided model, savings only): up to 50 percent of total annual ACO savings, as compared to the benchmark:

    - ACO must meet or exceed the annual MSR as established by the number of assigned beneficiaries in the sliding scale.

- ACOs must meet annual quality reporting requirements.

- A **final sharing rate** is determined by applying the ADS to the percent of Track 1 potential savings (50 percent):

  - for example: an ACO with an ADS of 89 percent would receive (.89 x.50) = 44.5 percent of available total savings.

- **Track 2** (two-sided model, savings and loss risk): up to 60 percent of total annual ACO savings, as compared to the benchmark:

  - ACOs must meet or exceed the 2.0 percent MSR established for Track 2 participants.

  - ACOs must meet annual quality reporting requirements.

  - A **final sharing rate** is determined by applying the ADS to the percent of Track 2 potential savings (60 percent).

    - for example: an ACO with an ADS of 89 percent would receive (.89 x.60) = 53.4 percent of available total savings.

Step 5: Test the final savings amount against the sharing cap (payment limit) established for the appropriate ACO participation track:

- Section 1899(d) (2) of the SSA requires the HHS secretary to "establish limits on the total amount of shared savings that may be paid to an ACO." Therefore, CMS established a "sharing cap" for determining the maximum allowed performance payment an ACO may receive in any given performance year.

- The sharing cap applies only to the savings paid to the ACO, not to the total amount of savings subject to sharing between the ACO and CMS.

- The sharing cap is established as a percentage of an ACO's updated benchmark for a given performance year, based on ACO election to participate under Track 1 or Track 2:

  - **Track One** (one-sided model): **sharing cap = 10 percent** (shared savings payments made cannot exceed a limit equal to 10 percent of the ACO's adjusted benchmark).

- ○ **Track Two** (two-sided model): **sharing cap = 15 percent** (shared savings payments made cannot exceed a limit equal to 15 percent of the ACO's adjusted benchmark).

Calculating the Total Dollar Amount of Shared Savings to be Paid to the ACO:

If the ACO has achieved savings at a rate at least equaling the MSR requirement and successfully reported required quality measures, the total dollar amount due to the ACO under the MSSP can be estimated as follows:

- Subtract the annual adjusted ACO performance rate for average per capita Medicare expenditures from the annually adjusted benchmark average per capita rate to determine **average beneficiary savings.**

- Multiply the average beneficiary savings by the total annual adjusted number of assigned beneficiaries to determine the **total amount of shared savings**.

- Apply the ADS to the level of total possible sharing percentage for the associated track (Track 1, 50 percent or Track 2, 60 percent) to determine the **final sharing rate.**

- Multiply the final sharing rate by the total amount of shared savings to determine the **final dollar amount due to the ACO.**

- Test the final dollar amount due to the ACO against the sharing cap percentage aligned with the appropriate track (Track 1, 10 percent or Track 2, 15 percent) as follows:
  - ○ Multiply the adjusted benchmark average per capita rate by the appropriate sharing cap to determine the capped dollar amount:
    - ▪ Compare this result with the total dollar amount due to the ACO:
      - If the capped dollar amount exceeds the total dollar amount due to the ACO, no adjustment is required.
      - If the capped dollar amount is below the total dollar amount due to the ACO, then the ACO may only receive the capped dollar amount.

Example of Shared Savings Calculation:

Background Information for ACO A:

- **ACO A** is a Track 2 participant just completing its second year of its first MSSP agreement period with a total adjusted number of 9,845 assigned beneficiaries. ACO A met all year two quality reporting requirements and earned an ADS Score of 89 percent.

Step 1: Determine the ACO-specific per capita benchmark for Medicare Parts A and B expenditures for assigned beneficiaries:

- CMS determined that ACO A's adjusted average per capita expenditure benchmark for assigned Medicare beneficiaries is **$12,018** in year two.

Step 2: Compare the benchmark to the ACO's assigned beneficiary per capita Medicare expenditures in the performance year to determine the amount of any savings:

- **ACO A's** performance year average for per capita expenditures for assigned Medicare beneficiaries is **$10,000** for year two.
  - ACO A saved $2,108 in per capita expenditures ($12,018-$10,000).

Step 3: Compare percent of savings to the appropriate MSR to determine ACO eligibility to share in savings:

- From the sliding scale (Table 10), ACO A has an MSR of 3.0 percent, based on having 9,845 assigned beneficiaries:
  - ACO A must save an amount equal to or greater than 3 percent ($360.57) of the benchmark per capita average (12018 x .03).
  - ACO A actually saved $2,018 on per capita expenditures (16.7 percent lower than the benchmark) and qualifies for shared savings ((12018–10000)/ (12018)) by exceeding the MSR of 3.0 percent.
  - To determine the dollar amount available for shared savings:

- Based on 9,845 assigned beneficiaries and a savings of $2,018 per capita, a total of (9845 x 2018) = $19,867,210 is available for shared savings.

Step 4: Determine the appropriate sharing rate for ACOs that have realized savings against the benchmark and met or exceeded the MSR.

- Determine the sharing rate:

  - As a Track 2 (two-sided model) participant, ACO A is eligible to receive up to 60 percent of total savings of ($19,867,210 x .60) = **$11,920,326**. (This amount must be adjusted by application of the ACO A's earned ADS to determine the final amount of shared savings due to the ACO.)

- Determine the final shared savings rate:

  - Based on successful reporting of annual quality measures and earning an ADS of 89 percent, ACO A would receive an adjusted amount of savings as follows:

  - ADS x shared rate or

  - (.89 x.60) = .534 or 53.4 percent of total savings

- The adjusted final amount of savings due to ACO A is determined by multiplying the total savings by the final savings rate:

  - ($19,867,210 x .534) = **$10,609,090**

Step 5: Test the final savings amount against the sharing cap (payment limit) established for the appropriate ACO participation track:

- test of shared savings rate against payment limit:

  - The payment limit for Track 2 ACOs is set at 15 percent of the ACO benchmark or ((number of assigned beneficiaries x ACO benchmark) x .15) = ((9845 x $12,018) x .15) = **$17,747,581**

  - The calculated shared savings rate for ACO 1 ($10,609,090) is less than the payment limit ($17,747,581) and **ACO A will receive shared savings in the amount of $10,609,090.**

- o Of total savings ($19,867,210), CMS will retain the remaining ($19,867,210-$10,609,090)=**$9,258,120**.

9.3.11 Determination of Shared Losses:[472]

Overview:

- For ACOs participating in Track 2 (two-sided, risk-sharing model), any calculated annual losses will be shared between the ACO and Medicare. Losses are defined by an ACO's annual per capita expenditures exceeding the benchmark established by CMS for a given year:

  - o ACO participation in Track 2 is optional for the first agreement period of participation in the MSSP.

  - o Beginning with an ACO's second three-year agreement period, participation in Track 2 is mandatory.

- The methodology used to determine shared losses mirrors the shared savings methodology, composed of:

  - o a formula for calculating shared losses based on the final loss sharing rate

  - o use of a minimum loss ratio (MLR) to protect the ACO against losses resulting from random variation

  - o application of a shared loss limit to provide a ceiling on the amount of losses an ACO would be required to repay

Five-Step Process:

- In determining the amount of shared losses requiring ACO repayment, CMS takes the following actions:

  - o **Step 1:** Determine the benchmark used for loss comparison. This is the same benchmark determined for shared savings.

---

[472] *Pages 67936–67941: Medicare Shared Savings Program, http://www.gpo.gov/fdsys/pkg/FR-2011-11-02/pdf/2011-27461.pdf*

618

- o **Step 2:** Compare the ACO's assigned beneficiary per capita Medicare expenditures in the performance year to the benchmark to determine the amount of any losses.

- o **Step 3:** Compare percent of losses to the appropriate MLR to determine ACO responsibility for share losses.

- o **Step 4:** Determine the appropriate loss rate for ACOs that have realized losses against the benchmark and met or exceeded the MLR.

- o **Step 5:** Test the final savings amount against the established sharing loss limit.

Step 1: Determine the benchmark used for loss comparison. This is the same benchmark determined for shared savings:

- See Step 1 under Determination of Shared Savings, above.

Step 2: Compare the ACO's assigned beneficiary per capita Medicare expenditures in the performance year to the benchmark to determine the amount of any losses:

- During each year of an agreement period, CMS will determine the average per capita expenditure rate for Medicare Parts A and B FFS beneficiaries assigned to an ACO.

- This average ACO per capita expenditure rate will be compared to the benchmark average per capita rate to determine participation in savings or losses.

Step 3: Compare percent of losses to the appropriate MLR to determine ACO responsibility for share losses:

- MLR: To help ensure that losses experienced by an ACO during a given year are not the result of random variation, CMS has established the MLR as a percentage "buffer" around the benchmark.

- CMS established the MLR in a similar manner to the minimum savings rate (MSR) under Track 2 for determining shared savings, except the

MLR is established as a flat 2.0 percent **above** the benchmark, regardless of the number of assigned beneficiaries.

- ACOs with expenditures above the benchmark, but below the MLR, will not be responsible for paying a share of the losses.

- ACOs with expenditures equaling or exceeding the MLR would be responsible for paying a share of excess expenditures.

Step 4: Determine the Shared Loss Rate (SLR) for ACOs that have realized losses against the benchmark and met or exceeded the MLR:

- The payable share of losses an ACO is responsible for is determined based on the inverse of its ADS based on quality performance (that is, 1.00 minus the ADS). This amount, the SLR, is multiplied by the total amount of excess per capita expenditures at or above the MLR of +2.0 percent.

- In our example of calculating the ADS, a score of .89 (89 percent) was achieved. To determine the payable share of losses, the SLR is calculated as 1.00-.89) = 0.11. Thus, the ACO would be responsible for 11 percent of losses meeting or exceeding the MLR.

Step 5: Test the final savings amount against the established sharing loss limit:

- In its November 2, 2011 Final Rule, CMS established that the total amount of shared losses for which an eligible ACO is liable may not exceed the following percentages of its updated benchmark (see example below for application of sharing loss limit):

  o 5 percent in the first performance year of participation in a two-sided model under the MSSP

  o 7.5 percent in the second performance year

  o 10 percent in the third performance year

Example of Shared Losses Calculation:

Background Information for ACO B

ACO B is a Track 2 participant in the MSSP in its second year of the agreement period with 9,000 adjusted assigned beneficiaries. ACO B successfully met the QRS for the year and achieved an ADS of .89 (89 percent):

- Step 1: Determine the benchmark used for loss comparison. This is the same benchmark determined for shared savings:

    o CMS established an adjusted year two per capita benchmark of $12,000.

- Step 2: Compare the ACO's assigned beneficiary per capita Medicare expenditures in the performance year to the benchmark to determine the amount of any losses:

    o CMS determined that the ACO's actual per capita expenditure level for year two was $14,000.

Step 3: Compare percent of losses to the appropriate Minimum Loss Rate (MLR) to determine ACO responsibility for shared losses:

- The MLR is established at 2.0 percent above the benchmark or at **$12,240.**

- (($12,000 x .02) + ($12,000)) = $12,240

- ACO B had per capita losses above the MLR of **$1,760** ($14,000 - $12,240).

- **Total losses above the MLR**, based on an adjusted assigned beneficiary population of 9,000, equals **$15,840,000** ($1,760 x 9,000).

Step 4: Determine the SLR for ACOs that have realized losses against the benchmark and met or exceeded the MLR:

- CMS calculated ACO B's SLR as 11 percent (1.00 - ADS) or (1.00 - .89) = .11.

- **The total dollar amount of shared losses that ACO B is responsible for is $1,742,400**

- (SLR x total losses **above** the MLR) or (.11 x $15,840,000) = $1,742,400.

Step 5: Test the final shared loss amount against the established sharing loss limit:

- For an ACO in its second year of MSSP participation under Track 2, CMS has established a limit on repayable losses equal to 7.5 percent of the adjusted benchmark.

- Seven and a half percent of the adjusted benchmark equals $900 ($12,000 x .075).

- The total dollar payment limit, based on 9,000 beneficiaries, is $8,100,000 (900 x 9,000).

- ACO B's total liability of repayable losses of $1,742,000 is below the sharing loss limit for year two.

- **The total amount repayable to CMS by ACO B remains $1,742,000.**

Rules for Repayment of Shared Losses:[473]

- During the application process and annually, ACOs participating in Track 2 (and for all ACOs after the initial three-year participation period) must specify their preferred method for repaying potential losses, and how that process would apply to ACO participants and ACO suppliers/providers (e.g., reinsurance, escrowed funds, surety bond, letter of credit, and the like).

- The selected repayment mechanism must be sufficient to ensure repayment of potential losses equal to at least 1 percent of the total per capita Medicare Parts A and B FFS expenditures for assigned beneficiaries, based either on expenditures for the most recent performance year or expenditures used to establish the benchmark.

- CMS requires that an ACO maintain a capital reserve equaling at least 1 percent of per capita Medicare FFS Parts A and B expenditures for its

---

[473] Pages 67937–67940: Medicare Shared Savings Program, http://www.gpo.gov/fdsys/pkg/FR-2011-11-02/pdf/2011-27461.pdf

assigned beneficiaries. This amount should be based either on expenditures for the most recent available performance year or benchmark year.

- If an ACO incurs shared losses, the ACO must make payment in full to CMS within ninety days of receipt of notification. CMS will not allow losses to be carried forward to other program years or agreement periods.

- ACOs not fully repaying their losses as required may face termination from the program by CMS or have the opportunity to enter into a corrective action plan to address the failure to meet program requirements.

Note: ACOs experiencing a net loss in their initial agreement period may apply to participate in a subsequent agreement period. Such ACOs must identify in their application the cause(s) for the net loss and specify what safeguards are in place to enable the ACO to potentially achieve savings in its next agreement period.

Section 9.4: Appendix

Acronym Guide

ACO .... Accountable Care Organization

ADS .... Aggregated Domain Score

AHRQ .... Agency for Healthcare Research and Quality

ASC .... Ambulatory Sensitive Condition

CAD .... Coronary Artery Disease

CAHPS .... Consumer Assessment of Health Providers and Systems

CAHs .... Critical Access Hospitals

CG-CAHPS .... Clinician Group-Consumer Assessment of Health Providers and Systems

CMI .... Center for Medicare & Medicaid Innovation within CMS

CMS .... Centers for Medicare & Medicaid Services

CMS-HCC .... CMS Hierarchal Condition Category

COPD .... Chronic Obstructive Pulmonary Disease

DHHS .... Department of Health and Human Services

DSH .... Disproportionate Share Hospital

EHR .... Electronic Health Record

ESRD .... End-Stage Renal Disease

FFS .... Fee-for-Service

FQHCs .... Federally Qualified Health Centers

GPRO .... Group Practice Reporting Option

HCC .... Hierarchal Condition Category

HCPCS .... Healthcare Common Procedure Coding System

HHS .... Department of Health and Human Services

HIT .... Health Information Technology

HMO .... Health Maintenance Organization

HRRP .... Hospital Readmissions Reduction Program

HRSA .... Health Resources and Services Administration

HVBP .... Hospital Value-Based Purchasing

IME .... Indirect Medical Education

IOM .... Institute of Medicine

IPPS .... Inpatient Prospective Payment System

IQR........................... Inpatient Quality Reporting

IVD .... Ischemic Vascular Disease

LTCHs....................... Long-Term Care Hospitals

LVSD........................ Left Ventricular Systolic Dysfunction

MA........................... Medicare Advantage

MAPCP .... Multi-Payer Advanced Primary Care Practice

MedPAC .... Medicare Payment Advisory Commission

MHCQ...................... Medicare Health Care Quality

MMA......................... Medicare Prescription Drug, Improvement, and Modernization Act

MLR .... Minimum Loss Rate

MSP .... Minimum Savings Percentage

MSR .... Minimum Savings Rate

MSSP....................... Medicare Shared Savings Program

NCQA...................... National Committee for Quality Assurance

NP .... Nurse Practitioner

NPI .... National Provider Identifier

NQF .... National Quality Forum

PACE .... Program of All-Inclusive Care for the Elderly

PACFs...................... Post-Acute Care Facilities

PFS .... Physician Fee Schedule

PGP .... Physician Group Practice

PMPM .... Per Member Per Month

PPS.......................... Prospective Payment System

PQRS....................... Physician Quality Reporting System

QPS .... Quality Performance Standard

RHCs .... Rural Health Clinics

SNFs .... Skilled Nursing Facilities

SSA.......................... Social Security Administration

SSN.......................... Social Security Number

TIN .... Taxpayer Identification Number

VBM .... Value-Based Modifier

VBP.......................... Value-Based Purchasing

About the Authors

Raymond Paul Tew

CEO and President, Medicus Innovation

As CEO and President, Ray has led the creation of Medicus Innovation and its unique suite of resources on value-based reimbursement and is co-author of the *Provider's Guide to Value-Based Medicare Reimbursement*. Over the last eighteen months, he has worked with a variety of health care organizations to develop their understanding of value-based reimbursement and its financial impact on their business or customers. Prior to the creation of Medicus Innovation, Ray was the president of Summit Leadership Strategies, a consulting company focused on executing strategy during times of organizational change, operational excellence, and leadership effectiveness for Fortune 500 companies and a diverse range of organizations in the United States and abroad. Before starting these two businesses, Ray had a twenty-five-year career with Pfizer, the largest research-based pharmaceutical company in the world. Ray rose through the ranks at Pfizer, building and leading teams and developing performance solutions throughout the United States before ultimately assuming the role of Director of Leadership Development for the US field force. Ray is a graduate of the University of North Carolina at Chapel Hill.

Steven Lee Owen

Chief Operating Officer, Medicus Innovation

Steve's extensive background in a variety of senior leadership roles brings a wealth of real-world experience to Medicus Innovation. Steve is the co-author of the *Provider's Guide to Value-Based Medicare Reimbursement* and has played a critical role in the development of its unique suite of resources on this topic. As the Chief Operating Officer at Medicus Innovation, Steve works with a variety of clients on value-based reimbursement and the development of unique learning programs that build this competency for clients. Prior to Medicus Innovation, Steve was a principal with Summit Leadership Strategies where he led consulting efforts on change management and leadership development.

Prior to working with these two consulting companies, Steve had a career with Pfizer, the largest research-based pharmaceutical company in the world.

As a senior sales leader during multiple corporate acquisitions and subsequent organizational restructuring initiatives, he is exceptionally experienced in achieving peak performance while leading teams through organizational change. Steve has been recognized throughout his career with numerous national leadership awards as a senior leader. Steve is a graduate of Auburn University.

J. Duncan Moore Jr.

Health Care Journalist

Duncan is an accomplished journalist with an extensive background in health care and policy. He is the founder and former president of the Association of Health Care Journalists in the United States and formerly served as communications manager for McKinsey & Company where he helped formulate and articulate health care issues for the company. He has written for the *Washington Post, Los Angeles Times, Kansas City Star, Bloomberg News,* and *KaiserHealthNews.* Duncan is a graduate of Brown University and the Johns Hopkins School of Advanced International Studies.

Alison Szot

Senior Editor and Health Care Communications Consultant

Alison Szot is an experienced health care journalist and communication strategist. She has more than fifteen years of experience working in traditional and corporate journalism and holds a master's degree in health services administration from the University of Michigan School of Public Health.

She recently served as the senior editor and director of external partnerships for The Medicare NewsGroup. She has worked on staff at numerous Chicago-area hospitals and health care organizations, reporting on both clinical and organizational issues, as well as at *Modern Healthcare* and *Modern Physician,* where she served as an online editor.